# Decision Making in
# SKIN ALLERGIES

# Decision Making in
# SKIN ALLERGIES


***Editors***

**Kiran Godse** MD PhD FRCP(Glasgow)
Professor
Department of Dermatology
Dr DY Patil Medical College and Hospital
Navi Mumbai, Maharashtra, India

**Anant Patil** MD
Professor
Department of Pharmacology
Dr DY Patil Medical College and Hospital
Navi Mumbai, Maharashtra, India

***Foreword***

**Ruby Pawankar**



JAYPEE

JAYPEE BROTHERS MEDICAL PUBLISHERS

*The Health Sciences Publisher*

**New Delhi | London**

JAYPEE Jaypee Brothers Medical Publishers (P) Ltd

**Headquarters**
EMCA House
23/23-B, Ansari Road, Daryaganj
New Delhi 110 002, India
Landline: +91-11-23272143, +91-11-23272703
+91-11-23282021, +91-11-23245672
E-mail: jaypee@jaypeebrothers.com

**Corporate Office**
Jaypee Brothers Medical Publishers (P) Ltd.
4838/24, Ansari Road, Daryaganj
New Delhi 110 002, India
Phone: +91-11-43574357
Fax: +91-11-43574314
E-mail: jaypee@jaypeebrothers.com

**Overseas Office**
JP Medical Ltd.
83, Victoria Street, London
SW1H 0HW (UK)
Phone: +44-20 3170 8910
Fax: +44(0)20 3008 6180
E-mail: info@jpmedpub.com

Website: www.jaypeebrothers.com
Website: www.jaypeedigital.com



**Inquiries for bulk sales may be solicited at:** jaypee@jaypeebrothers.com

*Decision Making in Skin Allergies* / ***Kiran Godse, Anant Patil***

*First Edition*: **2025**

ISBN: 978-93-5696-645-1

*Printed in India*

# CONTRIBUTORS

**Abhishek De** MBBS MD
SCE(Dermatology) FAGE IFAAD
FRCP(Edinburgh) PhD(Schl)
Associate Professor
Department of Dermatology
Calcutta National Medical College
and Hospital
Kolkata, West Bengal, India

**Adnan Al Ali** MD
Department of Pediatrics
United Arab Emirates University
Al Ain, United Arab Emirates

**Al Baiyan A Al-Wahshi** MD
Intern, Department of Clinical
Immunology and Allergy
Royal Hospital
Oman

**Aleksandra Wardzyńska** MD
Assistant Professor
Department of Immunology and
Allergy
Medical University of Lodz
Poland, Europe

**Andaç Salman** MD
Associate Professor of Dermatology
Acıbadem Mehmet Ali Aydınlar
University School of Medicine
Department of Dermatology
Acıbadem Healthcare Group
Altunizade Hospital
Istanbul, Turkiye

**Anna Zalewska-Janowska** MD
Professor
Department of Psychodermatology
Medical University of Lodz
Poland, Europe

**Arnab Dutta** MBBS MD
Senior Resident
Department of Dermatology
Calcutta National Medical College
and Hospital
Kolkata, West Bengal, India

**Bushra Al Hinai** RN(Diploma in Nursing)
Specialized Nurse
Department of Clinical Immunology
and Allergy Royal Hospital
Oman

**Busra Kocali** MD
Fellowship Assistant
Department of Pediatric Allergy and
Immunology
Hacettepe University Faculty of
Medicine
Turkiye

**Carly Sillcox** MD Candidate
Faculty of Medicine and Health
Sciences
Trinity College
Dublin, Ireland

**Claudia Arenas** MD MSc MBA
Dermatologist
Dermatologist Service
Universidad Militar Central Nueva
Granada
Colombia

**Deepika Halder** MBBS MD
Senior Resident
Department of Dermatology
Calcutta National Medical College
and Hospital
Kolkata, West Bengal, India

**Delvin Poulose** MBBS MD DVL
Assistant Professor (Former)
Department of Dermatology
Kanachur Institute of Medical Sciences
Mangaluru, Karnataka, India

**Disha Chakraborty** MBBS MD
Postdoctoral Fellow
Department of Dermatology and
Rheumatology, Sacramento VA
Medical Center
California, USA

**Elizabeth Garcia** MD
Allergist
Department of Allergology
Fundacion Santa Fe
Colombia

**Emine Aylin Yılmaz** MD
Department of Pediatric Neurology
Zeynep Kamil Women and Children
Diseases Training and Research
Hospital
Health Science University
Istanbul, Turkiye

**Gatha M Upadya** MBBS MD
Professor
Department of Dermatology
Kasturba Medical College
Mangaluru
Manipal Academy of Higher Education
Manipal, Karnataka, India

**Hristina Breshkovska** PhD
Assistant Professor
Department of Dermatology
University Clinic of
Dermatovenereology
Skopje, North Macedonia

**Hüseyin Bahadır Şenol** MD
Department of Pediatrics
Dokuz Eylül University Faculty of Medicine, Division of Pediatric Neurology
Izmir, Turkiye

**Iman Hamed Nasr** MD FRCP FAAAI
Consultant
Department of Clinical Immunology and Allergy
Royal Hospital
Oman

**Indrashis Podder** MD DNB MNAMS
Assistant Professor
Department of Dermatology
College of Medicine and Sagore Dutta Hospital
Kolkata, West Bengal, India

**Jie Shen (Jason) Fok** MBBS FRACP FRCP(Edinburgh)
Allergist/Immunologist
Associate Professor
Department of Respiratory Medicine
Box Hill Hospital, Eastern Health
Melbourne, Australia
Monash Lung Sleep Allergy Immunology, Monash Health
Melbourne, Australia
Monash University
Melbourne, Australia

**Jorge Sanchez** MD MSc PhD
Professor
Department of Pediatric and Allergy
University of Antioquia
Colombia

**Kiran Godse** MD PhD FRCP(Glasgow)
Professor
Department of Dermatology
Dr DY Patil Medical College and Hospital
Navi Mumbai, Maharashtra, India

**Lisa Jennifer Dsouza** MBBS MD(DVL)
Senior Resident
Department of Dermatology
Kasturba Medical College, Manipal
Manipal Academy of Higher Education
Manipal, Karnataka, India

**Maia Gotua** MD PhD
Professor
Department of Allergy and Immunology
David Tvildiani Medical University
Tbilisi, Georgia

**Maryam Khoshkhui** MD
Associate Professor
Department of Allergy and Clinical Immunology
Mashhad University of Medical Sciences
Mashhad, Iran

**Meghashree G** MBBS MD FRGUHS
Assistant Professor (Former)
Department of Dermatology
Kanachur Institute of Medicine Sciences
Mangaluru, Karnataka, India

**Michael Rudenko** MD PhD FAAAAI
Professor
Consultant in Allergy and Immunology
The London Allergy and Immunology Centre
London, UK

**Mona Al-Ahmad** MD FRCPC FAAAAI
Professor
Department of Microbiology
College of Medicine, Kuwait University
Kuwait

**Moshe Ben-Shoshan** MD MSc
Department of Pediatric Allergy, Immunology and Dermatology
McGill University Health Centre
Montreal, Canada

**Muhammed Burak Yücel** MD
Dermatologist
Department of Dermatology and Venereology
Ergani State Hospital
Diyarbakır, Turkiye

**Nandana C** MBBS
Junior Resident
Department of Dermatology
Kasturba Medical College
Manipal Academy of Higher Education
Manipal, Karnataka, India

**Natasa Teovska Mitrevska** PhD
Assistant Professor
Department of Dermatology
Remedika General Hospital
Skopje, North Macedonia

**Öner Özdemir** MD
Professor
Department of Pediatric Allergy and Immunology
Sakarya Research and Training Hospital, Sakarya University Medical Faculty
Sakarya, Turkiye

**Özlem Su Küçük** MD
Professor
Department of Dermatology and Venereology
Bezmialem Vakif University, School of Medicine
Istanbul, Turkiye

**Prabhakar Mallikarjuna Sangolli** MBBS MD(DVL) DNB DVD
Professor and Head
Department of Dermatology
Sri Siddhartha Institute of Medical Sciences and Research Centre
T-Begur, Karnataka, India

**Priya Bhesaniya** MBBS
Junior Resident
Department of Dermatology
Kasturba Medical College, Manipal
Manipal Academy of Higher Education
Manipal, Karnataka, India

**Raghavendra Rao** MBBS MD DNB
Professor and Unit Head
Department of Dermatology
Kasturba Medical College, Manipal
Manipal Academy of Higher Education
Manipal, Karnataka, India

**Rana Tafrishi**
Fellow
Department of Allergy and Clinical Immunology
Mashhad University of Medical Sciences
Mashhad, Iran

**Regis A Campos** MD PhD
Associate Professor IV
Department of Internal Medicine
Federal University of Bahia
Medical School
Salvador, Brazil

**Rosana Câmara Agondi** MD PhD
Clinical Immunology and Allergy
Division, Hospital das Clínicas,
University of São Paulo, Brazil

**Roy Khalaf** MD
Resident
Faculty of Medicine and Health
Sciences
McGill University Health Centre
Montreal, Canada

**Salma Rashid Al Abri** MD
Specialist, Department of Clinical
Immunology and Allergy
Royal Hospital
Oman

**Sathish Pai B** MBBS MD DVD
Professor
Department of Dermatology
Katurba Medical College, Manipal
Manipal Academy of Higher
Education
Manipal, Karnataka, India

**Shrayan Pal** MBBS MD
Senior Resident
Department of Dermatology
Calcutta National Medical College and
Hospital
Kolkata, West Bengal, India

**Shrutakirthi D Shenoi** MBBS MD DVD
Professor and Head
Department of Dermatology
Kanachur Institute of Medical Sciences
Mangaluru, Karnataka, India

**SK Shahriar Ahmed** MBBS MD
Senior Resident
Department of Dermatology
Calcutta National Medical College and
Hospital
Kolkata, West Bengal, India

**Sofianne Gabrielli** MD
Resident
Faculty of Medicine and Health
Sciences
McGill University Health Centre
Montreal, Canada

**Solange Oliveira Rodrigues Valle**
MD PhD
Internal Medicine, Immunology Service
Clementino Fraga Filho University
Hospital, Brazil

**Subhajit Sadhukhan** MD DNB
Senior Resident
Department of Dermatology
College of Medicine and Sagore Dutta
Hospital
Kolkata, West Bengal, India

**Umit Murat Sahiner** MD
Professor
Department of Pediatric Allergy and
Immunology
Hacettepe University Faculty of
Medicine
Turkiye

**Vesna Trajkova** PhD
Higher Lecturer
Department of Dermatology
General Hospital "8th September"
Skopje, North Macedonia

**Zoya A** MBBS
Junior Resident
Department of Dermatology
Kanachur Institute of Medical
Sciences
Mangaluru, Karnataka, India

# FOREWORD

Skin allergies are quite prevalent across the world. In some patients, these conditions present as acute onset whereas in others and more often these present as chronic conditions with a severe adverse impact on the quality of their lives. While there has been considerable progress in the understanding of these diseases and advances in therapeutic options have evolved over time, we now have a better understanding of the pathomechanisms of these diseases and also have better diagnostic tools for their evaluation as well as protocols for the management of most of these diseases.

Kiran Godse and Anant Patil have excellently compiled the chapters related to skin allergies in this book "*Decision Making in Skin Allergies*". This book comprising 39 chapters is divided into four sections: Urticaria, Atopic dermatitis, Contact dermatitis, and Drug allergy, authored by experts from around the world.

It is my pleasure to write this foreword for the book as I am sure it will help clinicians in better patient care and management of skin allergies.

Wishing all the very best.

**Ruby Pawankar** MD PhD FRCP(UK) FAAAI
Past WAO President
Past APPACI President

# PREFACE

Greetings!

Dear readers,

I am really happy to present this book "*Decision Making in Skin Allergies*" to you. This book is unique in terms of its concept and preparation. This handbook is being published to increase awareness about skin allergy among family physicians, consultant physicians, and postgraduate students of dermatology. Expert authors from India and many other countries have contributed chapters in this book. The book contains a total of 39 chapters divided into four sections: Urticaria, Atopic dermatitis, Contact dermatitis, and Drug allergy.

I am sure readers will appreciate the content of the book. Clinical images, tables, figures, and algorithms have been added to the chapters to make it more reader-friendly. I thank the management of DY Patil Hospital, Nerul, Navi Mumbai, Maharashtra, India, for constant support in academic endeavors. I also thank Dr Anant Patil for his constant support and help in coordinating with authors of all chapters and completing the task.

I wish to thank my family Dr Meenal, Dr Gauri, and Atharva for supporting my academics.

**Kiran Godse**

# PREFACE

Greetings!

Dear readers,

It gives me immense pleasure to write preface of this book "*Decision Making in Skin Allergies*".

This handbook is written with an objective of increasing awareness about skin allergy as well as provide an easy-to-refer resource for family physicians, consultant physicians, and postgraduate students of dermatology while managing skin allergy-related conditions. I personally wish to thank all authors from India and other countries for providing their contributions in the form of chapters to all four sections, i.e., Urticaria, Atopic dermatitis, Contact dermatitis, and Drug allergy. Clinical pictures, images, tables, and flowcharts are the highlights of this book.

I thank the management of DY Patil, deemed to be university, School of Medicine and DY Patil Hospital, Nerul, Navi Mumbai, Maharashtra, India, for constant support and motivation in academic activities. I thank Dr Kiran Godse for his guidance in completing the book.

I also wish to thank my family members Dr Rohini, Anushka, and Aayush for their support.

**Anant Patil**

# CONTENTS

## SECTION 1: URTICARIA

*Section Editors: Kiran Godse and Anant Patil*

## SECTION 2: ATOPIC DERMATITIS

*Section Editors: Abhishek De and Disha Chakraborty*



## SECTION 3: CONTACT DERMATITIS

*Section Editor: Sathish Pai B*

*Assistant Editor: Lisa Jennifer Dsouza*

## SECTION 4: DRUG ALLERGY

*Section Editors: Kiran Godse and Anant Patil*

SECTION

1

# Urticaria

***Section Editors:*** Kiran Godse and Anant Patil

CHAPTER 1.1

# Introduction and Classification of Urticaria

*Natasa Teovska Mitrevska, Vesna Trajkova, Hristina Breshkovska*

## DEFINITION AND CLINICAL PRESENTATION

Urticaria, commonly known as hives, has been recognized since ancient times. However, it is only in the last century that we have gained a clearer understanding of its various forms and complexity. It is an inflammatory condition driven by mast cells.[1]

It significantly affects patients beyond the skin, causing pain, sleep disturbances, fatigue, and substantial psychological impact, including anxiety and depression. Untreated urticaria can lead to significant direct and indirect healthcare costs, as well as a reduced quality of life.[2] The condition often impacts physical function, emotional well-being, sexual relationships, social interactions, and work performance. This highlights the importance of timely diagnosis and effective treatment.

Urticaria is characterized by wheals (hives), angioedema, or both:[1]

- "Wheals" are sharply circumscribed, superficial swellings of varying size and shape, surrounded by erythema. They are usually itchy or sometimes cause a burning sensation and typically resolve within 1–24 hours **(Figs. 1 and 2)**.[1,2]
- "Angioedema" involves deep swelling in the lower dermis, subcutis, or mucous membranes. It is often erythematous or skin-colored and is accompanied by tingling, burning, tightness, and occasionally pain, rather than itching. The skin generally returns to normal within 72 hours **(Fig. 3)**.[1-3]

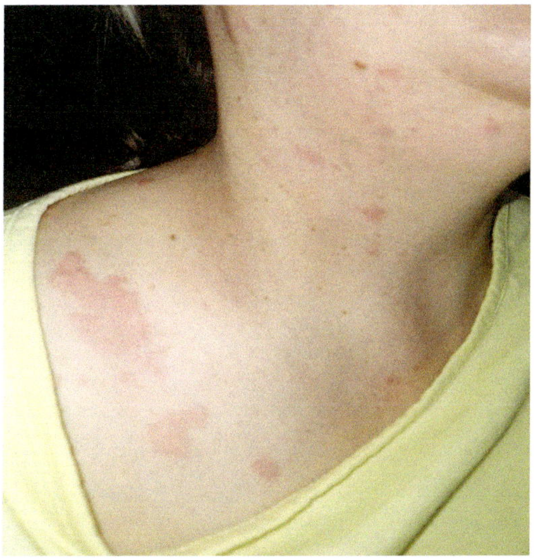

**FIG. 1:** Wheals on the neck.

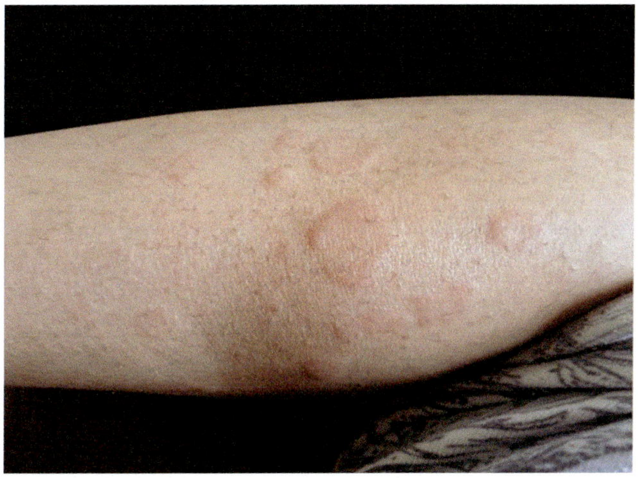

**FIG. 2:** Wheals on lower extremities.

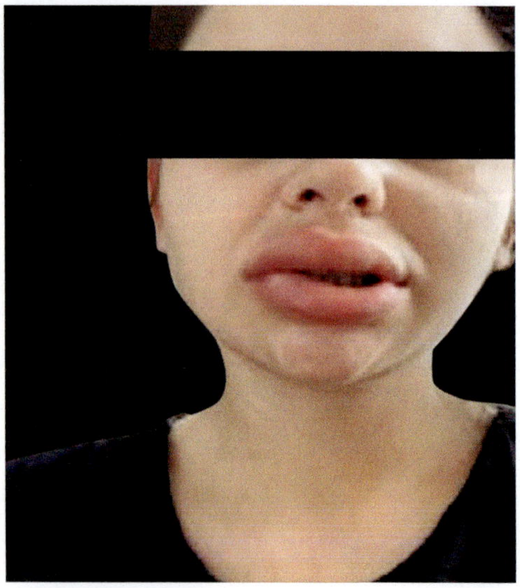

**FIG. 3:** Angioedema on upper lip.

## CLINICAL CLASSIFICATION

Urticaria classification is based on duration and triggers, following the Global Allergy and Asthma European Network ($GA^2LEN$)/the European Academy of Allergology and Clinical Immunology (EAACI)/the World Allergy Organization (WAO)/the European Dermatology Forum (EDF) guidelines (2023) **(Table 1 and Flowchart 1)**.

### Acute Urticaria Overview

Repeated appearance of wheals with or without angioedema lasting up to 6 weeks. Acute urticaria has a lifetime prevalence of approximately 20%.[1,4,5]

Key mediators include histamine, platelet-activating factor, and cytokines. These substances cause blood vessels to dilate and become leaky, leading to fluid accumulation in surrounding tissues and activating sensory nerves. Angioedema, a deeper swelling, can be caused by bradykinin release.[1,6]

**TABLE 1: Classification of urticaria based of duration and triggers and frequency.**[1-3]

| | Duration | Frequency |
|---|---|---|
| *Spontaneous urticaria*: | | |
| • Acute urticaria<br>• *Chronic urticaria*:<br>○ Chronic continuous urticaria<br>○ Chronic recurrent urticaria | • <6 weeks<br>• >6 weeks<br>• Daily or on most days of the week<br>• Symptom free intervals ranging from days to weeks<br>• Eliciting factor | • Spontaneous wheals appearing most days<br>• Spontaneous appearance of wheals |
| *Physical urticaria*: | | |
| • Dermographic urticaria<br>• Delayed pressure urticaria<br>• Cold contact urticaria<br>• Heat contact urticaria<br>• Solar urticaria<br>• Vibratory urticaria/angioedema | • Mechanical shearing forces (wheals arising after 1–5 minutes)<br>• Vertical pressure (wheals arising with a 3–8 hours latency)<br>• Cold air/water/wind<br>• Localized heat<br>• Ultraviolet (UV) and/or visible light<br>• Vibratory forces, e.g., pneumatic hammer | |
| *Special types of urticaria*: | | |
| • Cholinergic urticaria<br>• Adrenergic urticaria<br>• Contact urticaria (allergic or pseudoallergic)<br>• Aquagenic urticaria | | |
| *Different diseases related to urticaria for historical reasons*: | | |
| • Urticaria pigmentosa (mastocytosis)<br>• Urticarial vasculitis<br>• Familial cold urticaria (a vasculitis) | | |

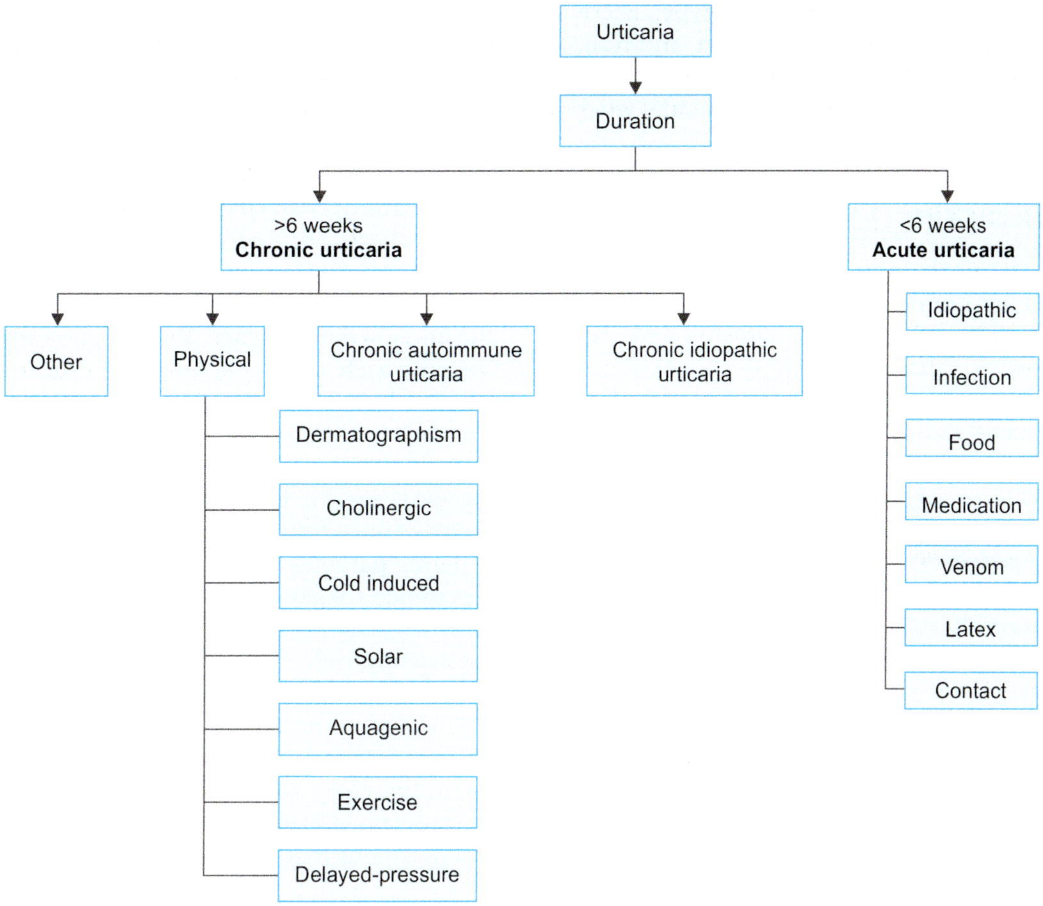


**FLOWCHART 1:** Classification of urticaria based of duration and triggers and frequency.

## Possible Causes of Acute Urticaria

- *Infections*:
    - *Viral*: Upper respiratory infections, viral hepatitis, and infectious mononucleosis.
    - *Bacterial*: Conditions such as dental abscesses, sinusitis, and mycoplasma infections.
- *Allergies*:
    - *Food allergies [immunoglobulin E (IgE)-mediated]*: Common triggers include milk, eggs, peanuts, and shellfish.
    - *Drug allergies (IgE-mediated)*: Often caused by antibiotics.
- *Pseudoallergies*:
    - *Drugs*: Aspirin, nonsteroidal anti-inflammatory drugs (NSAIDs), opiates, and radiocontrast media. These can trigger urticaria without immune activation.
- *Other triggers*:
    - Vaccination
    - *Insect stings*: Bee or wasp stings.
    - *Localized contact urticaria*: For example, rubber latex, which can cause a widespread reaction.

### *Complications*

Severe cases of urticaria can lead to anaphylactic shock, characterized by bronchospasm and collapse.

### *Angioedema without Urticaria*

May occur as a side effect of angiotensin-converting enzyme (ACE) inhibitors, which can cause recurrent episodes of swelling without the typical hives.

Understanding these factors helps in diagnosing and managing acute urticaria effectively.[1,7,8]

## Chronic Urticaria Overview

Recurrence of symptoms beyond 6 weeks. Chronic urticaria can be further divided into chronic spontaneous urticaria (CSU no definite eliciting factor involved) and chronic inducible urticaria (CIU specific definite factor involved). In some cases, angioedema may be the primary or sole manifestation. CSU or CIU can be disabling, impair quality of life, and impact work and school performance. The duration of the disease can vary, and it may persist for several years in CSU cases.[1,3,9]

Proper classification of urticaria subtypes is crucial for accurate diagnosis, effective treatment, and research interpretation. Most subtypes profoundly impact quality of life, making effective management essential when no treatable cause is identified.[10,11]

## URTICARIA DISTINCTIONS

Certain conditions that can present with wheals and/or angioedema are not classified as urticaria due to their distinct pathophysiological mechanisms and clinical presentations.[1,10,11] These include:

- *Urticarial vasculitis*: A form of vasculitis where wheals are associated with inflammation of blood vessels.
- *Maculo-papular cutaneous mastocytosis (formerly known as urticaria pigmentosa)*: Characterized by the presence of mast cell proliferation in the skin.
- *"Indolent systemic mastocytosis" with skin involvement*: A type of mastocytosis where systemic mast cell proliferation affects the skin.
- *Mast cell activation syndrome (MCAS)*: A condition involving episodic mast cell activation with symptoms similar to those of urticaria but driven by different mechanisms.
- *"Autoinflammatory syndromes" (e.g., cryopyrin-associated periodic syndromes or Schnitzler's syndrome)*: Conditions with periodic fever and systemic inflammation that can sometimes mimic urticaria.
- *"Non-mast cell mediator-mediated angioedema" (e.g., bradykinin-mediated angioedema)*: Angioedema caused by factors unrelated to mast cell activation, such as bradykinin.

These conditions are distinct from urticaria due to their unique underlying mechanisms and clinical features.

## EVALUATION AND MONITORING

Wheal size can sometimes indicate the severity of urticaria: larger wheals may signal more severe and difficult-to-treat cases. Wheal color can also aid in diagnosis. Lighter-colored wheals with pink erythema suggest histamine involvement, with the pink hue resulting from the dilation of cutaneous vessels. Conversely, dark red or violaceous wheals are often associated with vascular damage and leakage, which may indicate urticarial vasculitis.[1,12]

It is also essential to monitor disease intensity and wheal appearance throughout treatment. Comparing conditions before and after treatment can provide valuable insights into the disease's underlying course. This evaluation should ideally include assessing the quality of life using specialized instruments for urticaria.

Urticaria is characterized by specific triggers that can induce wheals, angioedema, or both.

These triggers are considered definite because wheals, angioedema, or both consistently occur in their presence and never in their absence. They are also subtype-specific, meaning each subtype of inducible urticaria has its own unique trigger—such as cold for cold urticaria—that does not apply to other forms. In rare cases, certain subtypes of inducible urticaria require a combination of two or more specific triggers to induce wheals or angioedema, such as in cold-induced cholinergic urticaria.[4]

Some patients with spontaneous urticaria may also experience trigger-induced wheals or angioedema, but these triggers are not definite. Their presence does not consistently lead to symptoms, and wheals or angioedema can still occur spontaneously without these triggers.[8]

The spectrum of clinical manifestations of different urticaria subtypes is very wide.

Additionally, some patients may exhibit more than one subtype of urticaria, and each subtype may respond independently to treatment.[1]

## CONCLUSION

Urticaria, commonly known as hives, is a multifaceted condition with a broad range of clinical presentations, including wheals, angioedema, or both. Its impact on patients extends beyond the skin, affecting emotional well-being, quality of life, and daily functioning. Acute urticaria typically resolves within 6 weeks, while chronic urticaria persists longer and may be either spontaneous or induced by specific triggers. Proper classification of urticaria subtypes is essential for effective diagnosis and treatment, as well as for monitoring disease progression. Identifying triggers and understanding underlying mechanisms are key to developing personalized treatment plans. Management of urticaria requires a comprehensive approach to address its diverse manifestations and improve patient outcomes. Given its significant effect on quality of life and potential complications, timely diagnosis and intervention are crucial.

## REFERENCES

1. Zuberbier T, Abdul Latiff AH, Abuzakouk M, Aquilina S, Asero R, Baker D, et al. The international EAACI/GA²LEN/EuroGuiDerm/APAAACI guideline for the definition, classification, diagnosis, and management of urticaria. Allergy. 2022;77(3):734-66.
2. Gonçalo M, Gimenéz-Arnau A, Al-Ahmad M, Ben-Shoshan M, Bernstein JA, Ensina LF, et al. The global burden of chronic urticaria for the patient and society. Br J Dermatol. 2021;184(2):226-36.
3. Zuberbier T, Asero R, Bindslev-Jensen C, Walter Canonica G, Church MK, Giménez-Arnau A, et al. EAACI/GA(2)LEN/EDF/WAO guideline: definition, classification and diagnosis of urticaria. Allergy. 2009;64(10):1417-26.
4. Zuberbier T, Aberer W, Asero R, Bindslev-Jensen C, Brzoza Z, Canonica GW, et al. The EAACI/GA LEN/EDF/WAO Guideline for the definition, classification, diagnosis, and management of urticaria: the 2013 revision and update. Allergy. 2014;69:868-87.
5. Dressler C, Rosumeck S, Werner RN, Magerl M, Metz M, Maurer M, et al. Executive summary of the methods report for 'The EAACI/GA²LEN/EDF/WAO Guideline for the Definition, Classification, Diagnosis and Management of Urticaria. The 2017 Revision and Update'. Allergy. 2018;73(5):1145-6.
6. Kaplan AP. Clinical practice. Chronic urticaria and angioedema. N Engl J Med. 2002;346(3):175-9.
7. Maurer M, Weller K, Bindslev-Jensen C, Giménez-Arnau A, Bousquet PJ, Bousquet J, et al. Unmet clinical needs in chronic spontaneous urticaria. A GA(2)LEN task force report. Allergy. 2011;66(3):317-30.
8. Baiardini I, Braido F, Bindslev-Jensen C, Bousquet PJ, Brzoza Z, Canonica GW, et al. Recommendations for assessing patient-reported outcomes and health-related quality of life in patients with urticaria: a GA(2) LEN taskforce position paper. Allergy. 2011;66(7):840-4.
9. Parisi CA, Ritchie C, Petriz N, Morelo TC. Direct Medical Costs of Chronic Urticaria in a Private Health Organization of Buenos Aires, Argentina. Value Health Reg Issues. 2016;11:57-9.
10. Broder MS, Raimundo K, Antonova E, Chang E. Resource use and costs in an insured population of patients with chronic idiopathic/spontaneous urticaria. Am J Clin Dermatol. 2015;16(4):313-21.
11. Zuberbier T, Aberer W, Asero R, Abdul Latiff AH, Baker D, Ballmer-Weber B, et al. The EAACI/GA²LEN/EDF/WAO guideline for the definition, classification, diagnosis and management of urticaria. Allergy. 2018;73(7):1393-414.
12. Maurer M, Eyerich K, Eyerich S, Ferrer M, Gutermuth J, Hartmann K, et al. Urticaria: collegium internationale allergologicum (CIA) update 2020. Int Arch Allergy Immunol. 2020; 181(5):321-33.

CHAPTER 1.2

# Acute Urticaria

***Michael Rudenko***

## INTRODUCTION

According to the international the European Academy of Allergology and Clinical Immunology (EAACI)/the Global Allergy and Asthma European Network (GA$^2$LEN)/the European Dermatology Forum (EDF; EuroGuiDerm)/the Asia Pacific Association of Allergy, Asthma and Clinical Immunology (APAAACI) guideline, the prevalence of acute urticaria in a lifetime is around 20% ranging between 12 and 23.5% with a cumulative incidence of 18.7%.[1,2] It is a common condition, that can occur in all age groups and can be diagnosed by multiple specialists as a separate nosology or can be accompanied by angioedema.[3] Distinguishing between anaphylaxis and acute urticaria/angioedema can be challenging, especially in emergency and primary care settings where prompt and accurate diagnosis is crucial for appropriate treatment. Both conditions involve mast cell and basophil degranulation, leading to the release of histamine and other inflammatory mediators, which can result in similar skin manifestations and angioedema.[2] Acute urticaria being associated with viral infections or has an immunoglobulin E (IgE)-mediated mechanisms in response to medication, food, or an insect sting usually lasts under 6 weeks and is typically self-healing in a few days or weeks.[2,4]

Urticaria presents with a sudden appearance of erythematous patches with pruritus. The underlying mechanism is associated with degranulation of skin mast cells while the generalized mast cell and basophil degranulation causes anaphylaxis. Besides, acute urticaria and angioedema present as the most prevalent symptoms from the skin in anaphylaxis; thus, in emergencies and in primary healthcare setting the differential diagnosis among anaphylaxis and acute urticaria/angioedema is confusing and puzzling in many cases, leading to errors and delayed treatment as adrenaline is the first-line treatment for anaphylaxis, but not for acute urticaria, where H1-antihistamines are the first choice.[5]

Acute spontaneous urticaria results from hypersensitivity toward the allergens resulting in the formation of IgE antibodies that bind to receptors found on mast cells and basophils.

*This **Box 1** outlines an evaluation process for acute urticaria, emphasizing on the consideration of cofactors, duration, triggers, associated conditions, and management strategies. It serves as a visual aid for understanding the diagnostic approach to this common dermatological condition.*

Physical factors known as cofactors include exercise exceeding the standard daily routine, alcohol, nonsteroidal anti-inflammatory medication, and heat or change in temperature, as well as other factors that can range from increased stress levels, changes in hormonal levels (menstruation), or consequences of an infection. Genetic background may contribute in creating clinically relevant predisposition to particular conditions.[6]

The presence of cofactors may explain why some patients can tolerate an allergen in some circumstances but in others the same patients develop a severe anaphylactic reaction that can appear immediately after a contact with respective allergens and allergy tests may help to avoid re-exposure to relevant causative factors. Cofactors can influence basophils and mast cells, leading to mediator release. In the presence of certain cofactors, less quantity of allergen might be required to cause clinical symptoms.[7]

Cofactors, including exercise and alcohol, might lower the threshold for IgE-mediated mast cell degranulation, increase allergen permeability in the gastrointestinal tract and osmolality, and redistribute blood flow.

**BOX 1 Evaluation process for acute urticaria.**

- *Presenting symptoms*: Sudden onset of erythematous areas with pruritus
- *Co-factors in acute urticaria*:
    - Exercise
    - Alcohol
    - Nonsteroid anti-inflammatory drugs (NSAIDs)
    - Heat or temperature changes
    - Stress
    - Menstruation
    - Infection
- *Duration*: <6 weeks
- *Mechanism*:
    - Mast cell and basophil degranulation due to allergen hypersensitivity
    - Immunoglobulin E (IgE)-mediated response
- *Triggers*:
    - Allergens (e.g., food, medication, and insect stings)
    - Viral and bacterial infections
    - Coronavirus disease 2019 (COVID-19) and other respiratory tract infections
- *Associated conditions*:
    - Angioedema
    - Urticarial vasculitis
    - Delayed anaphylaxis (e.g., α-gal syndrome, ω-5 gliadin sensitivity)
- *Management*:
    - Antihistamines (H1-antihistamines) as first-line treatment
    - Avoidance of triggers, if identified
    - Consideration of additional therapies for refractory cases

We suggested an evaluation process for acute urticaria, emphasizing on the consideration of cofactors, duration, triggers, associated conditions, and management strategies **(Box 1)**.

The best-known mediator contained in mast cells is histamine 2-(4-imidazolyl)-ethylamine, but it is not the only one. The effects of other mediators are significant in mast cell-mediated conditions, and can be future therapeutic targets.[8]

Upon re-exposure, the allergen is recognized by cell-bound specific IgE, leading to receptor crosslinking. This event leads to the release of many immune-mediating enzymes, primarily histamine which causes increased capillary permeability that is presented in the form of swelling on the upper dermal layer of the skin cases of acute urticaria and urticarial vasculitis were reported in association with COVID-19, and influenza A/H1N1 infection.[9,10]

Acute urticaria and angioedema apart from being a symptom of allergic reactions to medications, venoms, and food, can also be present in association with a range of viral and bacterial infections.[3] Acute urticaria and angioedema were reported in addition to respiratory symptoms in COVID-19.[2,4] COVID-19 and other viral infections, in particular, respiratory tract infections can trigger the onset of acute urticaria either occurring concurrently with the infection or in some cases proceeding the infection. Acute urticaria, possibly associated with circulating autoantibodies, was shown to become chronic in 5–39% of the cases.[11]

Urticaria and angioedema were also described as a part of delayed anaphylaxis in people sensitized to galactose-α-1,3-galactose (α-Gal) following tick bites.[12]

Conditional reactions ranging from urticaria and angioedema to even anaphylaxis can occur when sensitized patients to ω-5 gliadin in gluten get exposed to gluten in a presence of a co-factor (stress, exercise, and nonsteroidal anti-inflammatory drugs heat or change of temperature and alcohol).[13,14]

In urticarial vasculitis unlike in urticaria the rash is more persistent (lasting >24 hours) followed by residual bruising.[15,16] Urticarial vasculitis with systemic manifestations can be contributed to presence of circulating anti-C1q autoantibodies and reduction of serum complement levels.[17]

## CONCLUSION

Acute urticaria occurs in up to 20% of individuals. It is a condition characterised by sudden pruritic erythematous lesions, often linked to IgE-mediated triggers or infections. Distinguishing acute urticaria from it being a symptom of anaphylaxis remains critical, as both involve mast cell activation, but later requires urgent intervention. Cofactors like NSAIDs, stress, or infections can lower the stability thresholds, exacerbating symptoms. Management plan can include trigger avoidance, H1-antihistamines, and addressing underlying infections. Emerging associations with COVID-19, urticarial vasculitis, and delayed anaphylaxis (e.g., α-gal syndrome) underscore the need for vigilant evaluation. Future research into the role of non-histamine mediators may refine therapeutic strategies, improving outcomes for this transient yet complex disorder.

## REFERENCES

1. Zuberbier T, Abdul Latiff AH, Abuzakouk M, Aquilina S, Asero R, Baker D, et al. The international EAACI/GA²LEN/EuroGuiDerm/APAAACI guideline for the definition, classification, diagnosis, and management of urticaria. Allergy. 2022;77(3):734-66.
2. Kocatürk E, Muñoz M, Elieh-Ali-Komi D, Criado PR, Peter J, Kolkhir P, et al. How Infection and Vaccination are Linked to Acute and Chronic Urticaria: A Special Focus on COVID-19. Viruses. 2023;15(7):1585.
3. Sabroe RA. Acute urticaria. Immunol Allergy Clin North Am. 2014;34(1):11-21.
4. Caffarelli C, Paravati F, El Hachem M, Duse M, Bergamini M, Simeone G, et al. Management of chronic urticaria in children: a clinical guideline. Ital J Pediatr. 2019;45(1):101.
5. Jadhav R, Alcala E, Sirota S, Capitman J. Risk Factors for Acute Urticaria in Central California. Int J Environ Res Public Health. 2021;18(7):3728.
6. Makris M, Altrichter S, Ensina LF, Kocatürk E, Rudenko M. The complexity of urticaria. Front Allergy. 2023;4:1149540.
7. Allegra A, Asero R, Giovannetti A, Isola S, Gangemi S. Urticaria and coronavirus infection: a lesson from SARS-CoV-2 pandemic. Eur Ann Allergy Clin Immunol. 2021;53(2):51-4.
8. Rudenko M. Central Role of Mast Cells in Mastocytosis, Hereditary α-Tryptasemia, Mast Cell Activation Syndrome, Urticaria, and Angioedema. EMJ. 2022;7(1):90-7.
9. O'Donnell B, Black AK. Urticarial vasculitis. Int Angiol. 1995;14(2):166-74.
10. Najafzadeh M, Shahzad F, Ghaderi N, Ansari K, Jacob B, Wright A. Urticaria (angioedema) and COVID-19 infection. J Eur Acad Dermatol Venereol: JEADV. 2020;34(10):e568-70.
11. Gu SL, Joseph LJ. Urticarial vasculitis. Int J Womens Dermatol 2021;7(3):290-7.
12. Román-Carrasco P, Hemmer W, Cabezas-Cruz A, Hodžić A, de la Fuente J, Swoboda I. The α-Gal Syndrome and Potential Mechanisms. Front Allergy. 2021;2:783279.
13. Rudenko M. The Role of Co-factors in Mast Cell Activation. EMJ Allergy Immunol. 2023.
14. Artunç NY, Çelik M, Rudenko M. Influenza in Children. In: Cingi C, Arısoy ES, Bayar Muluk N (Eds). Pediatric ENT Infections. Cham: Springer; 2022. pp. 723-34.
15. Marzano AV, Maronese CA, Genovese G, Ferrucci S, Moltrasio C, Asero R, et al. Urticarial vasculitis: Clinical and laboratory findings with a particular emphasis on differential diagnosis. J Allergy Clin Immunol. 2022;149(4):1137-49.
16. Lee J, Kim SR, Park JH, Park KH, Jeong KY, Lee JH, et al. Evaluation of Allergenicity on a ω-5 Gliadin-deficient Cultivar in Wheat-Dependent Exercise-induced Anaphylaxis. Allergy Asthma Immunol Res. 2022;14(4):379-92.
17. Konstantinou GN, Konstantinou GN. Psychological Stress and Chronic Urticaria: A Neuro-immuno-cutaneous Crosstalk. A Systematic Review of the Existing Evidence. Clin Ther. 2020;42(5):771-82.

1.3

CHAPTER

# Chronic Urticaria and Its Types

*Andaç Salman*

## INTRODUCTION

Urticaria is a common condition characterized by the presence of wheals and/or angioedema. Wheals typically present as central edema surrounded by reflex erythema, often accompanied by itching or a burning sensation, and individual lesions generally resolve within 24 hours. Angioedema, on the other hand, is marked by swelling that can persist for up to 72 hours and may be associated with pain and burning.

## CLASSIFICATION

Urticaria is classified based on the duration of symptoms: Acute urticaria lasts less than 6 weeks, while chronic urticaria persists for 6 weeks or longer. Chronic urticaria can be further divided into chronic spontaneous urticaria (CSU) and chronic inducible urticaria (CIndU). In CSU, wheals and/or angioedema occur spontaneously, without any identifiable trigger.[1] Conversely, in CIndU, these symptoms arise only after exposure to specific triggering factors, which may include various physical stimuli or specific urticariogenics, as seen in contact urticaria **(Fig. 1 and Flowchart 1)**.[2]

Chronic inducible urticarias encompass a range of conditions, including symptomatic dermographism, cold urticaria, heat urticaria, delayed pressure urticaria, solar urticaria, vibratory angioedema, cholinergic urticaria, aquagenic urticaria, and contact urticaria. It is possible for a patient to experience one or more types of CIndU and/or CSU simultaneously. A thorough medical history, coupled with the question, "Can you provoke your wheals?" is essential for diagnosing CIndUs. To confirm the diagnosis, assess the threshold levels that provoke wheals, and evaluate the response to treatment, standardized provocation tests should be employed.[3]

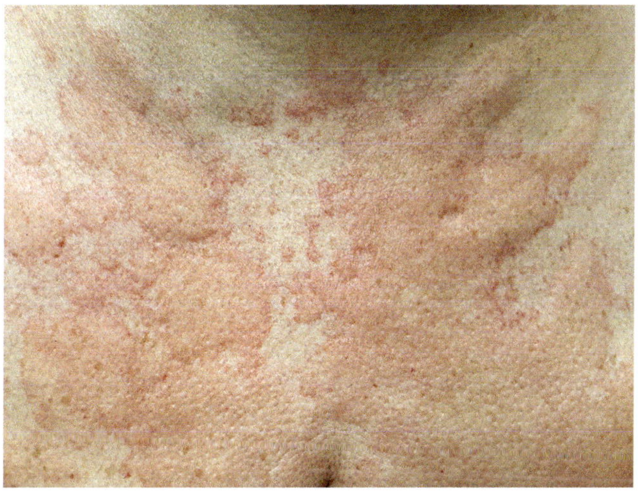

**FIG. 1:** Wheals in a patient with chronic spontaneous urticaria.

## CONCLUSION

Although urticaria is typically a straightforward diagnosis, differential diagnoses should be carefully considered, especially in cases with atypical wheal characteristics. Once urticaria is diagnosed, it should be classified according to the updated nomenclature, which is based on symptom duration and potential triggering factors.

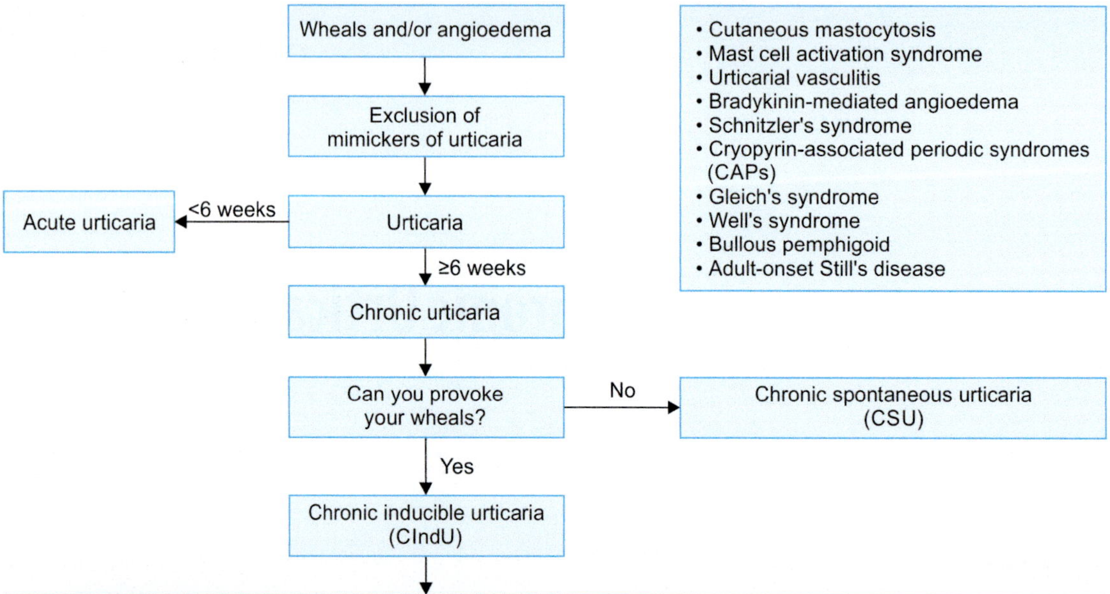


| Type of CIndU | Triggering factor | Provocation test |
|---|---|---|
| Symptomatic dermographism | Shearing forces on the skin | FricTest,® Dermographometer |
| Cold urticaria | Cold air, objects and liquids | Ice cube test, TempTest,® Cold water baths |
| Heat urticaria | Contact heating of the skin | Hot water baths, TempTest® |
| Delayed pressure urticaria | Pressure on the skin | Weighted rods |
| Solar urticaria | Exposure to sunlight | UVA/UVB irradiation, Visible light |
| Vibratory angioedema | Exposure to vibration | Vortex vibrator |
| Cholinergic urticaria | Elevation of body temperature due to exercise or hot bath, etc. | Pulse-controlled ergometry |
| Aquagenic urticaria | Exposure to water | Compress or towel soaked with water 35–37°C |
| Contact urticaria | Various urticariogenics | Open controlled application testing |

**FLOWCHART 1:** Chronic urticaria and its types.

## REFERENCES

1. Zuberbier T, Abdul Latiff AH, Abuzakouk M, Aquilina S, Asero R, Baker D, et al. The international EAACI/GA²LEN/EuroGuiDerm/APAAACI guideline for the definition, classification, diagnosis, and management of urticaria. Allergy. 2022;77(3):734-66.
2. Maurer M, Bonnekoh H, Grekowitz E, Kiefer L, Munoz M, Pereira MP, et al. An algorithm for the diagnosis and treatment of chronic inducible urticaria, 2024 update. Allergy. 2024;79(9):2573-6.
3. Friedman A, Kwatra SG, Yosipovitch G. A Practical Approach to Diagnosing and Managing Chronic Spontaneous Urticaria. Dermatol Ther. 2024;14(6):1371-87.

1.4

CHAPTER

# Angioedema

***Regis A Campos***

## INTRODUCTION

Angioedema (AE) is a paroxysmal, localized, and self-limiting swelling of the subcutaneous and/or submucosal tissue, due to a temporary increase in vascular permeability. The physiological mechanisms that control the endothelial barrier function are abnormal, and therefore the stability of capillaries and small venules are affected. Clinically, AE manifests with recurrent, reversible, swelling episodes of the skin and subcutaneous tissues or submucosal surfaces.

Currently, AE is classified according to the endotype in which there is a distinct functional or pathobiologic mechanism, to form a combination of clinical expression, biomarkers, and genetics. These endotypes are mast cell-mediated (AE-MC), bradykinin-mediated (AE-BK) or due to vascular-endothelium dysfunction (AE-VE). On the other hand, those forms of AE whose mechanisms are yet to be elucidated, such as those caused or aggravated by medications [drug-induced AE (AE-DI)], or AEs with still unknown etiologies (AE-UNK), are designated as subtypes. However, this classification in endotypes and subtypes is not always useful in clinical practice, and AE may be better understood based on specific clinical characteristics.[1,2]

## PATHOGENESIS AND CLINICAL FEATURES

Mast cell-mediated AE refers to the central role played by mast cells, which secrete many proinflammatory products beyond histamine. It can be presented in acute or chronic and recurrent forms and can last from only a few hours up to several days and is often associated with hives, concomitant with or at some distance in time from the AE episode. Therefore, searching for episodes of hives in the patient's medical history is the first step in the AE differential diagnosis. Although a history of hives, or hives concomitant with the AE, points to AE-MC, the absence of these skin lesions poses a dilemma, mainly in chronic and recurrent AE. The acute forms last until 6 weeks and can be due to an immunoglobulin E (IgE)-mediated reaction mostly associated with foods and drugs. However, virus infection is a frequent cause in children. In a large proportion of patients with acute AE-MC, it is not possible to identify a cause. Acute AE-MC also comprises AE in the context of anaphylaxis (AE-ANA), because it may manifest with involvement in various organs carrying the risk of asphyxiation if involving the oropharyngeal area. Chronic AE-MC without hives is considered a form of chronic spontaneous urticaria (CSU) and is not associated with asphyxia risk. Around 30% of the CSU patient increase their symptoms after taking nonsteroidal anti-inflammatories; however, these drugs are also commonly associated with acute AE or recurrent AE when the patient is not aware.

Bradykinin-mediated AE can be associated with hereditary angioedema (HAE) or acquired angioedema (AAE). Although AE-BK is less common than AE-MC, the risk of mortality is 45-fold higher for AE-BK than for AE-MC. The patients have AE affecting different skin sites, mostly the face and extremities but may also involve submucosal surfaces. As a result, involvement of the upper airway may occur, which leads to death by asphyxia if not properly treated. Intestinal wall swelling is associated with abdominal pain, which may progress to obstruction and ascites. AE-BK generally lasts longer than AE-MC, which in contrast does not affect submucosal surfaces and as consequence is not associated with upper airway obstruction or abdominal pain. Also, in AE-MC, the face is the most affected site, whereas the extremities are usually spared except in cases of delayed pressure urticaria, a form of chronic inducible urticaria which frequently manifests as hand and feet AE.[3]

Bradykinin-mediated AE occurs in HAE with or without C1 inhibitor (C1INH) deficiency, AE due to acquired C1INH deficiency (AAE-C1INH), and AE due to drugs that interfere with bradykinin metabolism with angiotensin-converting enzyme inhibitor-associated AE (AE-ACEI) being the most frequent.[4] Most of these diseases are considered rare, except AE-ACEI. HAE due to C1INH deficiency (HAE-C1INH) is the most common form of HAE and results from a quantitative (type1, approximately 85% of patients) or functional (type 2, approximately 15%) deficiency of C1INH. C1INH is the main plasma serine-protease inhibitor of the complement, fibrinolytic, contact, and Kinin–kallikrein systems, which when activated results in BK generation. In HAE-C1INH, the constant autoactivation of the complement system results in low plasma levels of the complement component 4 (C4). Both HAE-C1INH type 1 and type 2 are caused by mutations in the C1INH gene, *SERPING1*, and are inherited as autosomal dominant trait. However, the percentage of new mutations is approximately 20%. The minimal prevalence of HAE-C1INH is 1:67,000 in the general population, without evidence of any gender, ethnic, or racial differences. In HAE with normal C1-INH (HAE-nC1INH), the clinical appearance and genetic inheritance resemble that of HAE-C1INH; however, most patients are female, and their C1INH and plasma complement levels are normal. As of now, mutations in eight genes were found to be pathogenic.[5] Some of these mutations are in the genes of enzymes from contact and Kinin–kallikrein system and included in AE-BK endotype: Factor XII (FXII), plasminogen (PLG), and kininogen-1 (KNG1). Recently, a new variant was described in the gene from carboxypeptidase N (CPN) associated with bradykinin catabolism, which may also be included in the AE-BK endotype.[6] Interestingly, HAE-CPN patients also have hives since CPN also inactivates C3a and C5a, which in turn trigger the mast cells. The other mutations associated with HAE-nC1INH are related to endothelium disfunction and associated with AE-VE endotype: Angiopoietin-1 (ANGPT1), myoferlin (MYOF), heparan sulfate 3-O-sulfotransferase (HS3ST6), and DAB2IP [acts as the key intercellular regulator of the vascular endothelial growth factor receptor 2 (VEGFR2)]. By now, more than 400 patients with HAE-FXII and more than 100 patients with HAE-PLG have been reported. On the other hand, the other HAE-nC1INH were only described in few individuals and families.

In AAE-C1INH, the C1INH deficiency occurs due to increased catabolism of C1INH. Patients with AAE-C1NH often have an underlying disease such as a lymphoproliferative disorder that leads to continuous activation of the classic complement pathway with consequent depletion of C1INH. Some patients may also develop autoantibodies to nC1INH protein, which interferes with its level and activity. Like HAE-C1INH, AE in patients with AAE-C1INH is associated with elevated plasma BK levels.

Angiotensin-converting enzyme (ACE) is a protease that cleaves BK. When ACE is inhibited, BK degradation is impaired, which facilitates the development of AE in some individuals. Indeed, patients with AAE-ACEI have been reported to have increased plasma BK levels. Dipeptidyl peptidase-4 (DPP-4) inhibitors or neprilysin (neutral endopeptidase) inhibitors used in the treatment of diabetes and heart diseases can increase the propensity of AE-DI significantly when combined with ACEI. **Flowchart 1** shows different types of AE.

## DIAGNOSTIC FEATURES

The diagnosis of the different types of AE include a detailed history of the characteristics, localization, duration, family background, and response to treatment used **(Flowchart 1)**. For patients presenting with isolated AE without urticaria that do not respond to fourfold dosage of second generation antihistamines H1, a screening C4 should be obtained, and if low, additional testing should be performed to rule out HAE or AAE. Most HAE patients will have a C4 level less than 50% of normal. A low C4 level should prompt testing for C1INH functional (C1INHf) and quantitative (C1INHq) levels. If the C4 levels are normal, genetic testing of different genes associated with HAE-nC1INH is crucial for the definitive diagnosis. AAE-C1INH is suspected when it occurs in patients older than 40 years old without family in which, besides low C4 and C1INH, there is a reduction in C1q levels. AE due to drugs improves after drug suspension.

## TREATMENT

Most patients with AE-MC improve with H1 antihistamines (up to four times the standard dose), omalizumab (anti-IgE monoclonal antibody) or oral corticosteroids. On the other hand, HAE patients do not respond with these agents. Treatment of HAE can be administered as acute "on-demand" treatment, short-term prophylaxis (STP), and long-term prophylaxis (LTP). Acute treatment is used to ameliorate symptoms of AE. Currently approved treatment for HAE attacks include plasma derived or recombinant intravenous C1INH formulations, subcutaneous kallikrein inhibitor (ecallantide), and a subcutaneous bradykinin receptor antagonist. For LTP, in patients with frequent attacks, regular administered agents are used: Plasma-derived C1INH (intravenous or subcutaneous), kallikrein inhibitors (oral or intravenous), or attenuated androgens. STP is recommended to protect

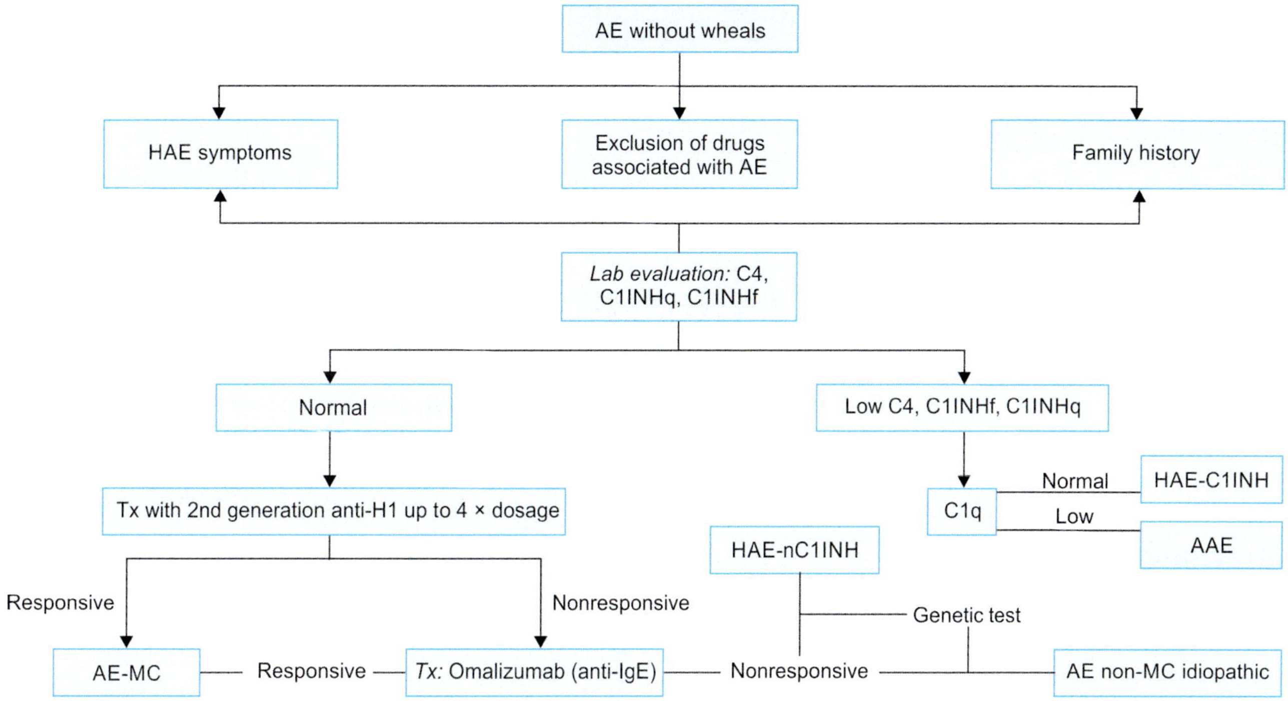


**FLOWCHART 1:** Angioedema (AE) without wheals.

(AAE: acquired angioedema; AE-MC: mast cell-mediated angioedema; C1INHf: C1 inhibitor functional; C1INHq: C1 inhibitor quantitative; nC1INH: normal C1 inhibitor; HAE: hereditary angioedema; IgE: immunoglobulin E; Tx: treatment)

against a likely attack such as dental surgery, intubation, oral surgery, or other stressful events. Medications which can be used for STP include plasma-derived C1INH or recombinant C1INH treatments as first-line treatments, or if neither of the former are available, anabolic androgens or fresh frozen plasma.

## REFERENCES

1. Reshef A, Buttgereit T, Betschel SD, Caballero T, Farkas H, Grumach AS, et al. The Definition, Acronyms, Nomenclature, and Classification of Angioedema: AAAAI, ACAAI, ACARE, and APAACI DANCE Consensus. J Allergy Clin Immunol. 2024;154(2):398-411.e1.
2. Maurer M, Magerl M, Betschel S, Aberer W, Ansotegui IJ, Aygören-Pürsün E, et al. The International WAO/EAACI Guideline for the Management of Hereditary Angioedema-The 2021 Revision and Update. Allergy. 2022;77(7):1961-90.
3. Maurer M, Magerl M. Differences and similarities in the mechanisms and clinical expression of bradykinin-mediated vs. mast cell–mediated angioedema. Clin Rev Allerg Immunol. 2021;61(1):40-9.
4. Cicardi M, Aberer W, Banerji A, Bas M, Bernstein JA, Bork K, et al. Classification, diagnosis, and approach to treatment for angioedema: consensus report from the Hereditary Angioedema International Working Group. Allergy. 2014;69(5):602-16.
5. D'Apolito M, Santacroce R, Vazquez DO, Cordisco G, Fantini CA, D'Andrea G, et al. DAB2IP associates with hereditary angioedema: Insights into the role of VEGF signaling in HAE pathophysiology. J Allergy Clin Immunol. 2024;154(3):698-706.
6. Vincent D, Parsopoulou F, Martin L, Gaboriaud C, Demongeot J, Loules G, et al. Hereditary angioedema with normal C1 inhibitor associated with carboxypeptidase N deficiency. J Allergy Clin Immunol Glob. 2024;3(2):100223.

CHAPTER 1.5

# Differential Diagnosis of Urticaria

*Iman Hamed Nasr, Bushra Al Hinai, Al Baiyan A Al-Wahshi*

## INTRODUCTION

Urticaria is a mast cell-dependent condition, characterized by the presence of itchy wheals (raised areas of reddish or light-colored skin that are itchy), angioedema (submucosal swelling in the face, eyelids, mouth, hands, and/or feet that is nonpitting) or both in the absence of systemic symptoms. Urticaria can be classified as acute and chronic. Acute urticaria is a common skin condition and is usually idiopathic (no trigger identified) and occurs when lesions appear once or on and off for less than 6 weeks. While in chronic urticaria lesions recur for more than 6 weeks. Chronic urticaria (CU) is divided into chronic spontaneous urticaria (CSU) where lesions come and go with no definite trigger and chronic inducible urticaria (CIndU) where lesions appear after certain physical (e.g., heat, vibration and pressure) and nonphysical triggers (e.g., cholinergic, and aquagenic). The wheals are not painful and typically resolve in less than 24 hours. The angioedema on the other hand can last longer than 24 hours but usually resolve within 72 hours.

Several triggers can cause acute urticaria, both allergic and nonallergic such as drugs (antibiotics, nonsteroidal anti-inflammatory drugs, anesthetics, and contrast dyes), insect stings, where urticaria occurs at the site of the sting, food allergies (typically appear within an hour of eating the food and as late as 4 hours as in red meat allergy), physical contact (such as when touching certain substances as in latex and poison ivy), and infections (mainly viral where the urticaria appears around 1 week or more after the illness begins and disappears after 1–2 weeks). Similarly chronic urticaria can be exacerbated by external triggers such as nonsteroidal anti-inflammatory drugs, infections, and stress.

Although urticaria is a straightforward diagnosis, it can be confused with other conditions that can mimic it and should warrant careful investigation, especially when the urticarial lesions are atypical (e.g., lasting longer than 24 hours, purpuric, painful, resolving with hyperpigmentation, associated with systemic symptoms such as fever, malaise, and joint pains). A thorough history and clinical examination are crucial to make the correct diagnosis. Blood investigations and in some cases skin biopsy may be required to help make the diagnosis. We have divided the differential diagnosis of urticaria into those of acute urticaria, chronic urticaria, and angioedema **(Table 1)**.[1]

**TABLE 1: Differential diagnosis of urticaria and angioedema.**

| Acute urticaria | Chronic urticaria | Angioedema |
|---|---|---|
| Anaphylaxis | Urticarial vasculitis | Bradykinin-mediated angioedema (drug-induced, hereditary angioedema, and acquired angioedema) |
| Maculopapular drug exanthem | Autoinflammatory urticarial syndromes:<br>• Cryopyrin-associated periodic syndrome<br>• Schnitzler syndrome<br>• Adult-onset Still disease<br>• Neutrophilic urticarial dermatosis<br>• Gleich syndrome | Allergy |

*Continued*

*Continued*

| Acute urticaria | Chronic urticaria | Angioedema |
|---|---|---|
| Viral exanthem | Hyper eosinophilic syndromes | Granulomatous cheilitis |
| Erythema multiform | | |
| Sweet's syndrome | | |
| Atopic dermatitis | | |
| Contact dermatitis | | |
| Insect bites | | |
| Urticarial dermatitis | | |
| Bullous pemphigoid | | |
| Autoimmune progesterone dermatitis | | |
| Polymorphic light eruption | | |
| Maculopapular cutaneous mastocytosis | | |
| Serum sickness | | |

## DIFFERENTIAL DIAGNOSIS OF ACUTE URTICARIA

- *Anaphylaxis*: A serious systemic hypersensitivity reaction that is usually rapid in onset and may cause death. The usual presentation is sudden onset of generalized wheals and or angioedema accompanied by systemic symptoms such as respiratory, cardiovascular, or gastrointestinal involvement on exposure to an allergen such as food.
- *Maculopapular drug exanthem*: A T cell-mediated cutaneous reaction in exposure to a medication that can occur within a few days to 3 weeks and appears as a symmetrical eruption of small red macules and urticarial papules that become larger and confluent with time and persist for several days unlike urticaria **(Fig. 1)**.
- *Viral exanthem*: Erythematous maculopapular eruptions that appear 1 week or more after the viral illness begins and disappear after 1–2 weeks and are generally nonpruritic. Fever is usually present **(Fig. 2)**.
- *Erythema multiform*: Symmetrical painful or pruritic iris-shaped macules and vesiculobullous lesions with target appearance on extensor surfaces of the extremities lasting several days. Systemic symptoms such as fever and malaise may be present **(Fig. 3)**.
- *Sweet's syndrome (acute febrile neutrophilic dermatosis)*: Recurrent painful chronic inflammatory papules associated with systemic symptoms (fever and arthralgia) **(Fig. 4)**.
- *Atopic dermatitis*: A common skin condition with intensely pruritic erythematous patches lasting days or weeks and have ill-defined borders. The flexural areas are the most commonly affected but can involve the face and wrists. Scaling and xerosis develop with time **(Fig. 5)**.

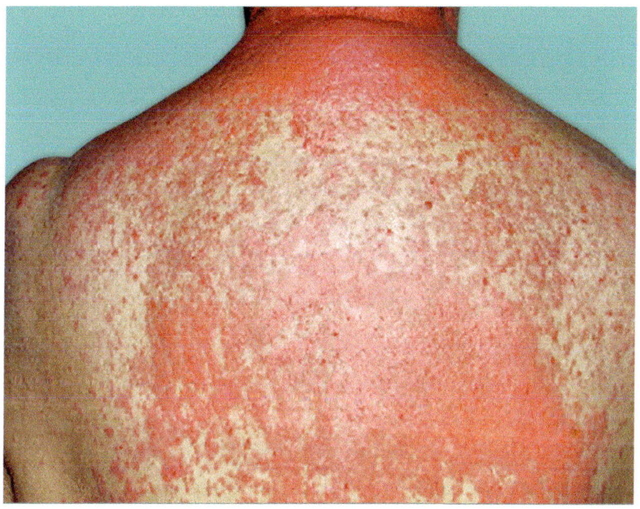

**FIG. 1:** Maculopapular drug exanthem.

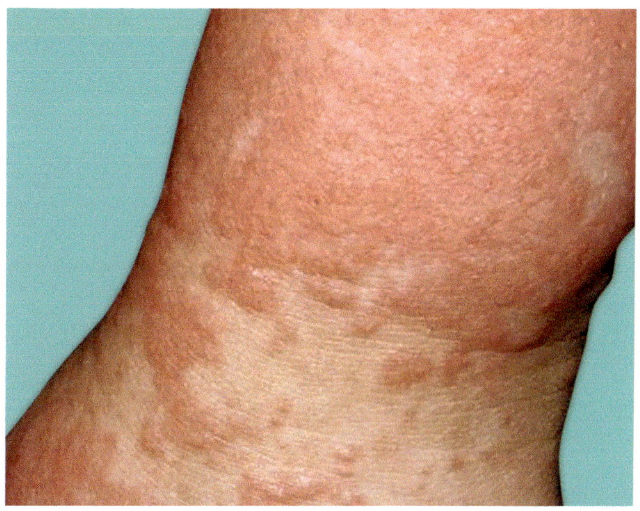

**FIG. 2:** Viral exanthema.

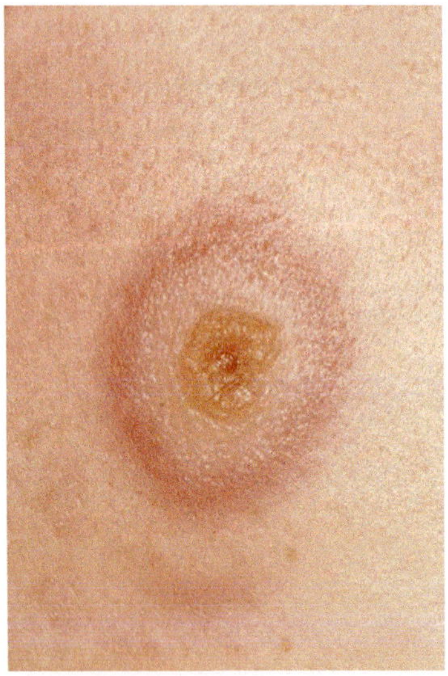

FIG. 3: Erythema multiform.

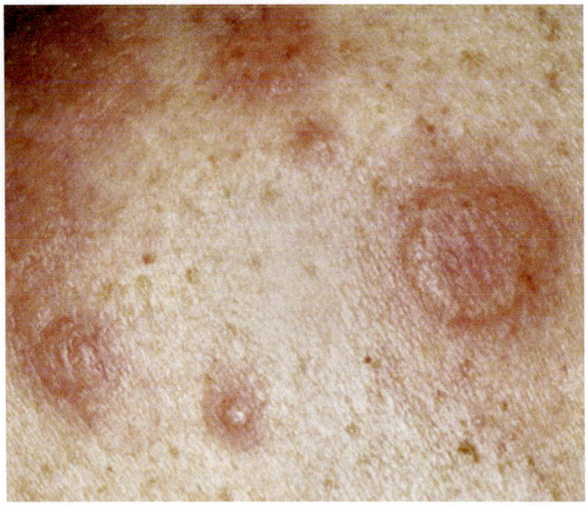

FIG. 4: Sweet's syndrome.

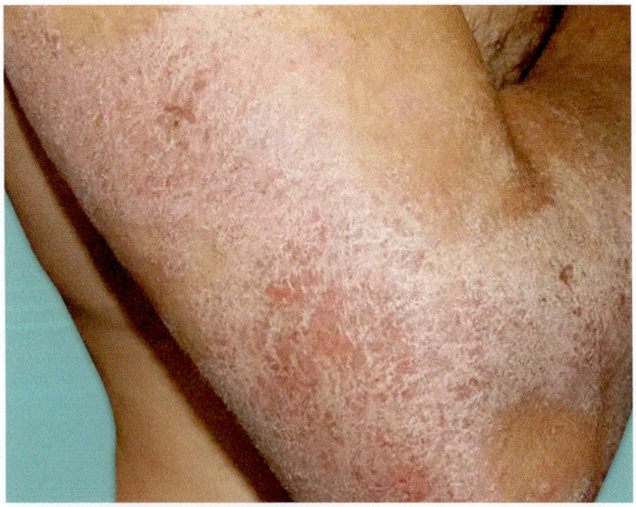

FIG. 5: Atopic dermatitis.

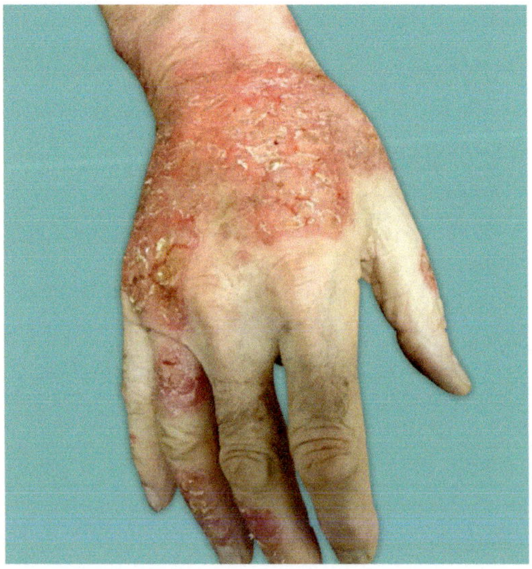

FIG. 6: Contact dermatitis.

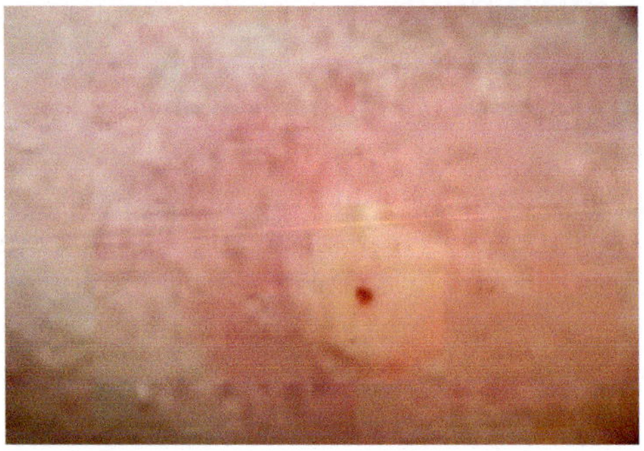

FIG. 7: Insect bite.

- *Contact dermatitis*: Erythematous, pruritic papular lesions with areas of vesiculation on direct skin contact with an allergen or irritant **(Fig. 6)**.
- *Insect bites*: Appear as pruritic lesions at the site of the bite that persist for days. Systemic allergic reaction may occur in allergic individuals **(Fig. 7)**.
- *Urticarial dermatitis*: Intensely pruritic skin eruption resembling urticaria but lasting longer than 24 hours and sometimes accompanied by eczema. It is either idiopathic or represent other skin diseases such as bullous pemphigoid or drug eruptions. This condition may appear acutely or recurrent mimicking chronic urticaria **(Fig. 8)**.
- *Bullous pemphigoid*: May start with pruritus, with or without urticarial lesions that eventually become blisters **(Fig. 9)**.
- *Autoimmune progesterone dermatitis*: It is a rare hypersensitivity reaction to progesterone with variable skin lesions (wheals or eczema) that worsens in the premenstrual period and resolves with menstruation **(Fig. 10)**.

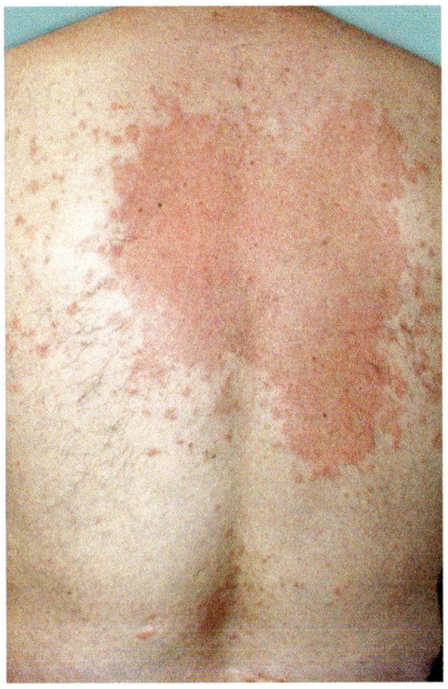

**FIG. 8:** Urticarial dermatitis.

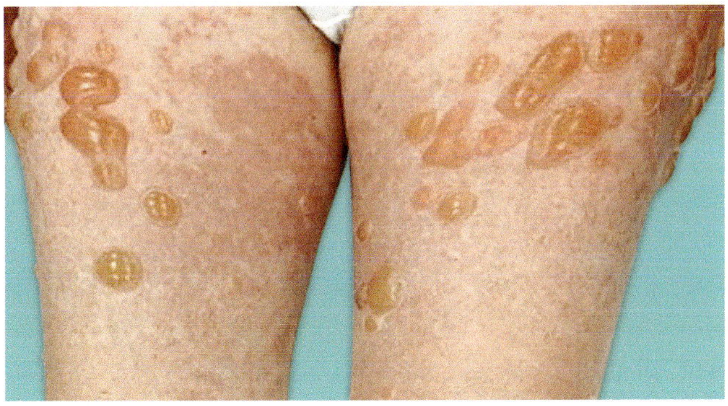

**FIG. 9:** Bullous pemphigoid.

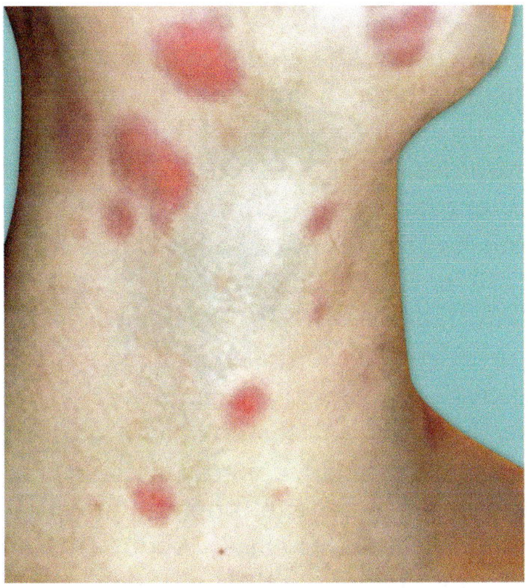

**FIG. 10:** Autoimmune progesterone dermatitis.

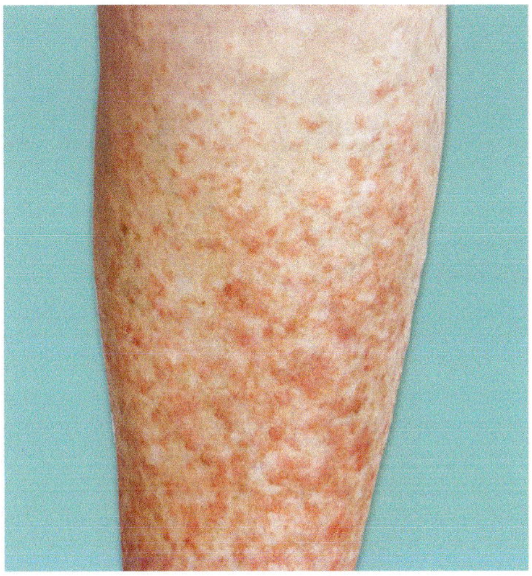

**FIG. 11:** Polymorphic light eruption.

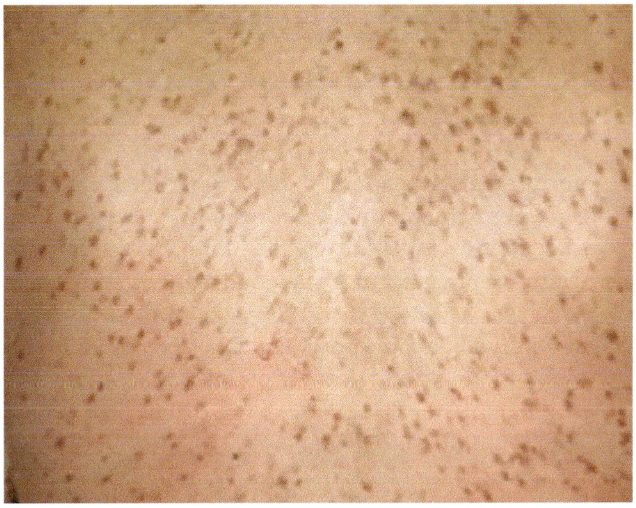

**FIG. 12:** Maculopapular cutaneous mastocytosis.

- *Polymorphic light eruption*: Itchy, polymorphic, erythematous skin lesions that are symmetrical and appear after sun exposure lasting several days **(Fig. 11)**.
- *Maculopapular cutaneous mastocytosis*: Multiple hyperpigmented macular or maculopapular lesions that urticate within a few minutes when rubbed **(Fig. 12)**.
- *Serum sickness*: It may present with an urticarial rash accompanied by fever, polyarthralgias, polyarthritis, and/or lymphadenopathy 1–3 weeks after exposure to exogenous proteins or medications **(Fig. 13)**.

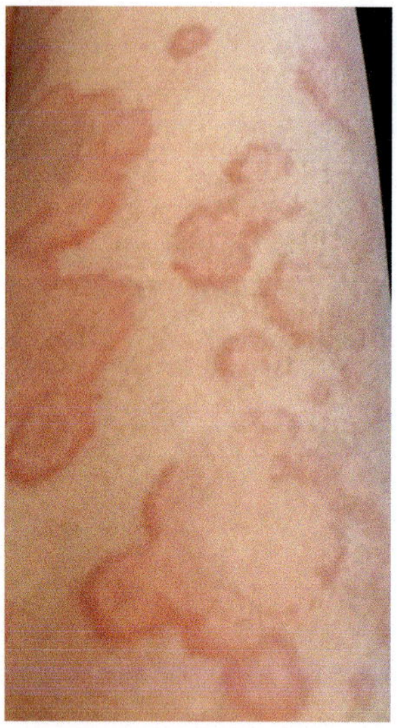

**FIG. 13:** Serum sickness.

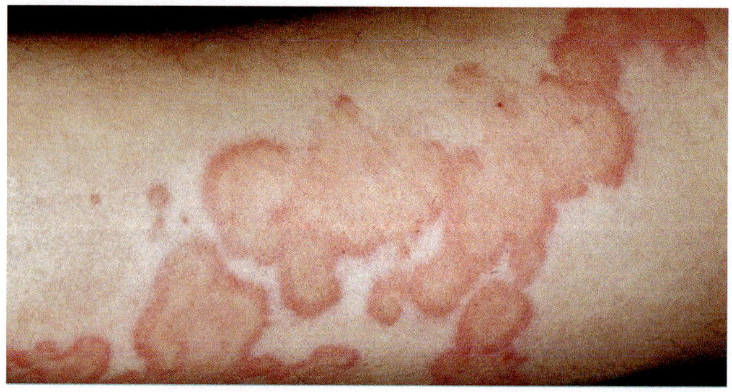

**FIG. 14:** Urticarial vasculitis.

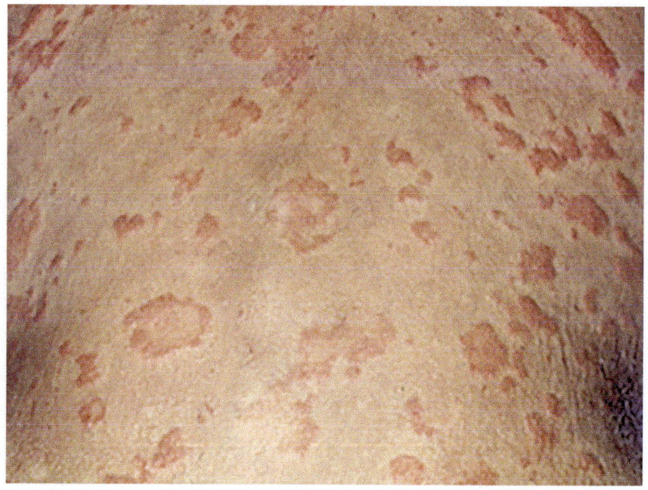

**FIG. 15:** Cryopyrin-associated periodic syndrome.

## DIFFERENTIAL DIAGNOSIS OF CHRONIC URTICARIA

- *Urticarial vasculitis (UV)*: Manifests as painful lesions that are long lasting (>24 hours) and appear purpuric or ecchymotic or leave residual ecchymosis or hyperpigmentation upon resolution. Angioedema may be present. UV is usually limited to the skin but can present with extracutaneous manifestations such as fever, arthralgias, arthritis, lymphadenopathy, abdominal pain, dyspnea, cough, or ocular and renal manifestations. The most common cause is idiopathic but it can be associated with drugs, infections, autoimmunity, and malignancy.

  Based on the levels of serum complements, UV is divided into hypocomplemententemic urticarial vasculitis (HUV), hypocomplemententemic urticarial vasculitis syndrome (HUVS), and normocomplemententemic urticarial vasculitis (NUV). HUV and HUVS are the most severe forms of UV and are often associated with longer disease duration and underlying disorders **(Fig. 14)**.
- *Autoinflammatory urticarial syndromes* are a group of chronic multisystem disorders, resembling chronic urticaria but last longer than 24 hours and are distributed mainly on the trunk and/or extremities and do not respond to antihistamines.[2,3] Pruritus may be absent, and lesions can be painful. Included in this group of disorders are:
  - Cryopyrin-associated periodic syndrome (CAPS): Classified as three distinct entities— (1) Familial cold autoinflammatory syndrome, (2) Muckle-Wells syndrome, and (3) chronic infantile neurological cutaneous and articular syndrome. These are hereditary autoinflammatory diseases that often manifest early in childhood and characterized by episodes of fever, urticaria-like rash, fatigue, headaches, arthralgia, arthritis, myalgia, sensorineural hearing loss, ocular inflammation, and/or bone lesions due to inappropriate activation of the innate immunity and overproduction of the proinflammatory cytokine interleukin 1 (IL-1) **(Fig. 15)**.
  - Schnitzler syndrome: An acquired autoinflammatory disease that usually starts later in life, likely IL-1 mediated and characterized by recurrent fever, urticarial lesions, arthralgia, arthritis, myalgia, lymphadenopathy, hepatosplenomegaly, and monoclonal gammopathy [mostly immunoglobulin M (IgM) class]. About 15% of patients develop a lymphoproliferative disorder **(Fig. 16)**.
  - Adult-onset Still disease: A rare systemic inflammatory disease with fever, arthralgia, an erythematous evanescent rash that accompanies

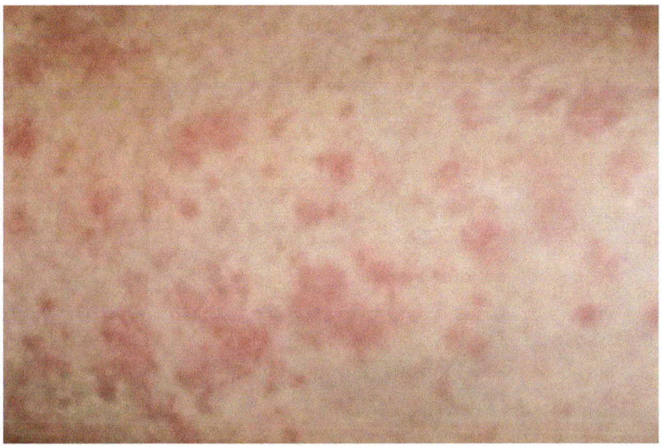

**FIG. 16:** Cryopyrin-associated periodic syndrome.

the fever, leukocytosis, lymphadenopathy, and liver dysfunction. Neutrophilic infiltrates is seen on histopathology in about 22% of the cases. Serum ferritin and other acute inflammatory parameters are significantly elevated. IL-1 has also been implicated in its pathogenesis.

- ◦ Neutrophilic urticarial dermatosis is a rare form of dermatosis and consists of a chronic or recurrent slightly elevated, pink to reddish plaques or macules that last 24–48 hours and resolves without residual pigmentation.[4] Extra-cutaneous signs are common, particularly fever or arthralgia. At histopathology, the dermis contains dense neutrophilic interstitial infiltrate with leukocytoclasis, but without vasculitis and is often associated with other systemic diseases such as adult-onset still disease and CAPS.
- ◦ Gleich syndrome (episodic angioedema with eosinophilia) is characterized by cyclic episodes of angioedema, wheals, fever, weight gain, and marked eosinophilia.

- *Hypereosinophilic syndromes* are a group of disorders characterized by persistent and marked blood eosinophilia associated with tissue infiltration and end organ damage in the absence of other causes (medication and parasitic infection). Cutaneous manifestations are generally urticarial or eczematous.

## DIFFERENTIAL DIAGNOSIS OF ISOLATED ANGIOEDEMA

- *Bradykinin-mediated angioedema*: This type of angioedema is a non-mast cell-mediated angioedema and is triggered by bradykinin released from the vascular endothelial cells and promotes vasodilatation and increases vascular permeability, leading to plasma leakage and edema of the dermis and subcutaneous tissue with no wheals. This type of angioedema lasts up to 3–5 days and may cause life-threating swelling of the larynx and oropharynx leading to asphyxiation. Swelling of the gastrointestinal tract can lead to painful occlusive symptoms mimicking acute abdomen. Causes of this type of angioedema includes:
  - ◦ Drug induced: Such as angiotensin-converting enzyme inhibitors (ACEis), dipeptidyl peptidase 4 (DPP-4) inhibitors, and gliptins. Bradykinin-mediated angioedema does not respond to antihistamines, steroids, and adrenaline (epinephrine). The offending agent must be avoided.
  - ◦ Hereditary angioedema: A condition caused by autosomal dominant mutations in the *SERPING* 1 gene that encodes for the C1 esterase inhibitor enzyme, resulting in low and/or dysfunctional C1 inhibitor (C1INH) levels. C1INH is a crucial enzyme that inhibits steps in the classical and lectin complement pathways, as well as of the intrinsic coagulation (contact system), fibrinolytic, and kinin-generating pathways. Deficiency of this enzyme causes uncontrolled activation of kallikrein and kininogen, which results in bradykinin over-production and subsequent angioedema that can be fatal if the swelling involved the larynx. Other affected sites are the face, hands, feet, genitals, and abdomen. Hereditary angioedema can occur with normal C1INH, due to mutations in other genes involved in bradykinin overproduction, e.g., factor XII (Hageman Factor), plasminogen gene, angiopoeitin-1 gene, and kininogen-1 gene **(Figs. 17A and B)**.
  - ◦ Angioedema due to acquired C1INH deficiency is often accompanied by a lymphoproliferative or autoimmune disorder that leads to continuous activation of the classic complement pathway with consequent depletion of C1INH.
- *Allergy*: Angioedema can be the only manifestation of an allergy with or without no wheals. It is sudden in onset and may last up to 72 hours to resolve.
- *Granulomatous cheilitis* is characterized by intermittent lip swelling, followed by persistent swelling of the lips due to granulomatous inflammation of unknown cause.

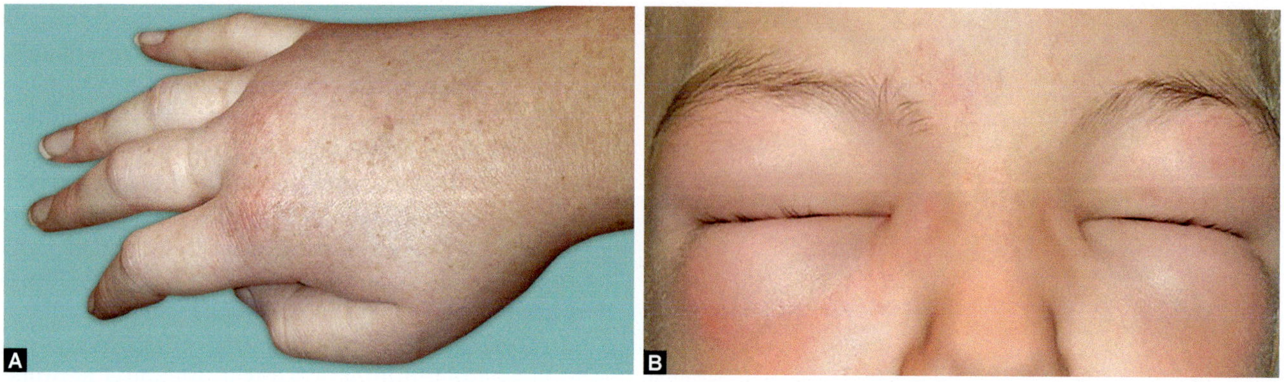

**FIGS. 17A AND B:** (A) Hereditary angioedema of the hand; (B) Hereditary angioedema of the face.
*Courtesy*: (A) LucyHAE/Wikimedia Commons Doc; (B) James Heilman/Wikimedia Commons.

## CONCLUSION

Urticaria is a mast cell-dependent condition, characterized by the presence of itchy wheals (raised areas of reddish or light-colored skin that are itchy), angioedema (submucosal swelling in the face, eyelids, mouth, hands, and/or feet that is nonpitting) or both in the absence of systemic symptoms. Although it is a straightforward diagnosis, it can be confused with other conditions that can mimic it. It should warrant careful investigation, especially when the urticarial lesions are atypical (e.g., lasting longer than 24 hours, purpuric, painful, resolving with hyperpigmentation, associated with systemic symptoms such as fever, malaise, and joint pains) in order to manage it appropriately and avoid possible complications.

## REFERENCES

1. Matos AL, Figueiredo C, Gonçalo M. Differential Diagnosis of Urticarial Lesions. Front Allergy. 2022;3:808543.
2. Davis MDP, van der Hilst JCH. Mimickers of Urticaria: Urticarial Vasculitis and Autoinflammatory Diseases. J Allergy Clin Immunol Pract. 2018;6(4):1162-1170.
3. Saperia C, Kobric D, Barron C, Sussman GL. Autoinflammatory Disease: Presenting As Urticaria. J Allergy Clin Immunol. 2017;139(2):AB272.
4. Gusdorf L, Lipsker D. Neutrophilic urticarial dermatosis: an entity bridging monogenic and polygenic autoinflammatory disorders, and beyond. 2019;34(4).

CHAPTER 1.6

# Diagnostic Approach to Urticaria

***Jorge Sanchez, Claudia Arenas, Elizabeth Garcia***

## INTRODUCTION

The diagnosis of urticaria is based on the presence of hives and angioedema. Although it can be relatively straightforward if the patient comes to the clinic with these lesions, on many occasions, the proper diagnosis of urticaria is not correctly made (underdiagnosis and overdiagnosis). An adequate physical examination and clinical history in addition to a photographic record of the skin will help improve diagnostic accuracy. In this section we provide some key points that may be useful for the correct diagnosis of urticaria.

## HOW IS URTICARIA DIAGNOSED?

Currently, the diagnosis of urticaria is eminently clinical **(Flowchart 1)**. This skin disease is characterized by hives and/or angioedema accompanied by pruritus. According to its duration, it is divided into acute urticaria (<6 weeks) and chronic urticaria (>6 weeks). Being a clinical diagnosis, clinical questions are essential: "*What are the lesions look like? How long have you had this problem? How frequent it appears? How long does each skin lesion last?*". We recommend to confirm the diagnosis with photos, since sometimes the patient does not have hives or angioedema during the medical consultation, additionally, the patient and the doctor may have different concepts of what a hive or angioedema is. Acute and chronic urticaria usually have different causes and prognoses: The acute form usually occurs alongside an infectious process in children. Due to its usually self-limiting nature, generally does not require additional diagnostic studies.[1] Acute urticaria sometimes is the clinical manifestation of a food allergy or drug allergy, which can be suspected when the reaction occurs quickly after exposure to the food/drug exposition (usually within the first 2 hours) and does not occur spontaneously. In these cases, confirmatory tests by an allergist are required **(Fig. 1)**.

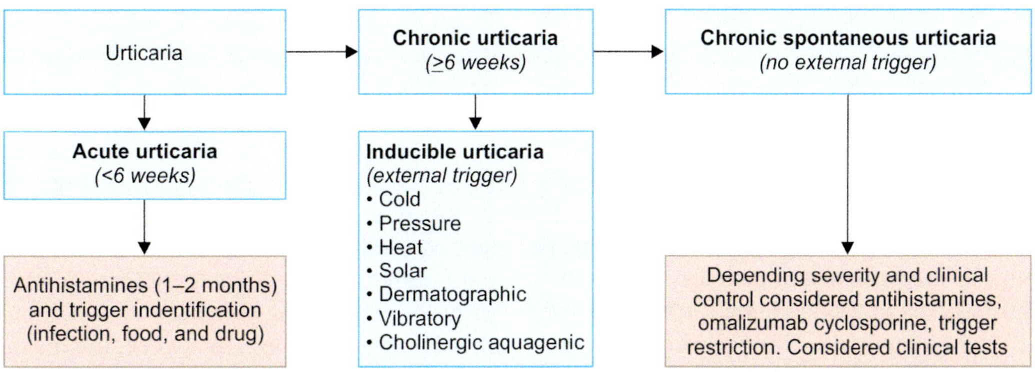


**FLOWCHART 1:** Diagnostic flowchart. With a correct medical examination and the support of photographs, an adequate diagnosis can be made.

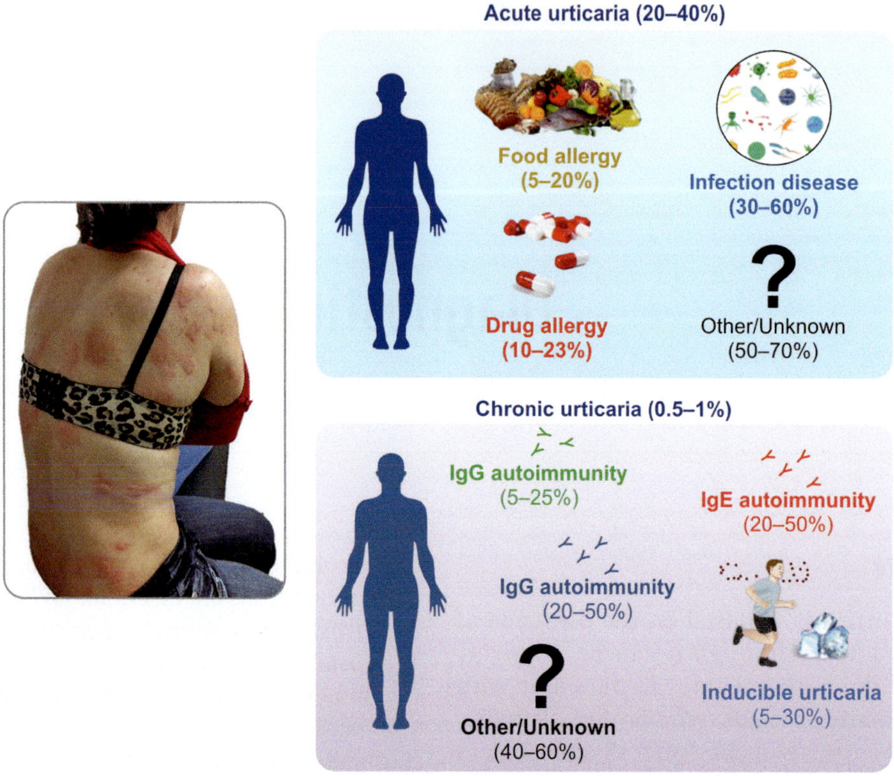


**FIG. 1:** Pathogenesis of urticaria. Chronic and acute urticaria have multiple trigger and pathogenesis pathways. (IgE: immunoglobulin E; IgG: immunoglobulin G)

On the contrary, in chronic urticaria, the causes seem to be mainly self-reactivity mechanisms, and it is divided into two types according to the triggers; chronic spontaneous urticaria (CSU), where the presence of hives is independent of an external stimulus, and chronic inducible urticaria (ICU) where certain physical stimuli can trigger the skin manifestation; cold, water, heat, pressure, friction, vibration, exercise, etc. In 5-30% of patients, both forms of chronic urticaria may occur together (mixed urticaria).[2] Therefore, it is important to ask the patient: "*What do you suspect causes the urticaria? Do the symptoms occur only when there is exposure to that suspect trigger or can they occur spontaneously?*". Because hives and angioedema are not pathognomonic of urticaria, it is necessary to differentiate the disease from other processes such as anaphylaxis, hereditary angioedema, and vasculitic urticaria, among others. This should be suspected when systemic symptoms occur (e.g., fever and joint pain), in the presence of pain lesions or when the resolution of hives or angioedema requires several days. Up to 20% of patients with chronic urticaria may be accompanied by symptoms such as respiratory distress. If these events are repetitive, idiopathic anaphylaxis should be studied. Skin biopsy should be considered when there are atypical or persistent clinical findings, such as painful, ulcerated lesions or lesions that do not respond to conventional treatment.

## HOW TO CLASSIFY URTICARIA ACCORDING TO SEVERITY AND CONTROL?

The severity of chronic urticaria is an important aspect that helps define the level of disease control and the need for changes in management.[3,4] Two simple scales that are easily applicable in clinical appointment allow to get an idea of the severity and response to treatment. The Urticaria Activity Score (UAS) is based on the evaluation of hives and pruritus, which are the key signs and symptoms in urticaria and can be easily documented by the patient.[5,6] The scale evaluates the number of hives (0-3 points) and the intensity of itching (0-3 points) in 24 hours and assigns a score of 0-6 points. This scale can be used during clinical appointment, but ideally the patient should use it for at least 7 consecutive days (UAS7) prior to the medical consultation as it allows to evaluate the changes over time. In a week, the maximum score is 42 points. The minimum clinically relevant difference of the UAS7 is 9 points.

The Urticaria Control Test (UCT) evaluates the control of urticaria according to the response to pharmacological treatment. This scale defined controlled when patients had ≥12 points or uncontrolled when patient had <11 points.[7] The UCT consists of 4 simple questions with a maximum score of 16 points.[8] The minimum relevant clinical difference is 3 points. The lack of control in the UCT or the UAS7 indicates the need to make adjustments in the treatment, which is why it is important to make them in each clinical appointment. To calculate these scales, you can use different web pages available for free (Example CRUSE App).

## WHAT ARE THE MEDICAL TESTS REQUIRED?

In acute urticaria, due to its self-limiting evolution, paraclinical tests are usually not required, unless there is suspicion of a differential diagnosis (infections, vasculitic urticaria, and anaphylaxis) or a causal agent (infections, food allergies, and drug allergy). In chronic urticaria, some international guidelines recommend to perform a complete blood count, acute phase reactants, and total immunoglobulin E (IgE) for all patients.[3] However, its usefulness in daily practice is currently unclear, and its diagnostic or prognostic accuracy appears to be low.[9]

If inducible urticaria is suspected, provocation tests should be considered to avoid unnecessary restrictions. Similarly, action should be taken in the case of chronic urticaria where a food or medication is suspected of aggravating the condition. Due to the high frequency of hypothyroidism, some studies suggest to request a thyroid function test in patients.[10]

## CONCLUSION

An adequate physical examination and clinical history in addition to a photographic record of the skin will help improve diagnostic accuracy. Additionally the correct choice of pharmacological treatment is directly related to the severity of the symptoms, therefore, it is necessary to evaluate the severity of urticaria at baseline and the level of pharmacotherapy control.

Multiple clinical tests are frequently performed in patients with urticaria, which generally do not provide information that leads to changes in management. On the contrary, tests that may be necessary to avoid unnecessary restrictions or make differential diagnoses are not performed.

## REFERENCES

1. Schaefer P. Acute and Chronic Urticaria: Evaluation and Treatment. Am Fam Physician. 2017;95(11):717-24.
2. Sánchez J, Amaya E, Acevedo A, Celis A, Caraballo D, Cardona R. Prevalence of Inducible Urticaria in Patients with Chronic Spontaneous Urticaria: Associated Risk Factors. J Allergy Clin Immunol Pract. 2017;5(2):464-70.
3. Zuberbier T, Abdul Latiff AH, Abuzakouk M, Aquilina S, Asero R, Baker D, et al. The international EAACI/GA²LEN/EuroGuiDerm/APAAACI guideline for the definition, classification, diagnosis, and management of urticaria. Allergy. 2022;77(3):734-66.
4. Sánchez J, Caraballo D, Amaya D. Evaluation of Guideline Line-Care Approach to the Treatment of Chronic Inducible Urticaria. J Allergy Clin Immunol Pract. 2024;12(8):2166-72.
5. Hawro T, Ohanyan T, Schoepke N, Metz M, Peveling-Oberhag A, Staubach P, et al. The Urticaria Activity Score-Validity, Reliability, and Responsiveness. J Allergy Clin Immunol Pract. 2018;6(4):1185-90.e1.
6. Hawro T, Ohanyan T, Schoepke N, Metz M, Peveling-Oberhag A, Staubach P, et al. Comparison and interpretability of the available urticaria activity scores. Allergy. 2018;73(1):251-5.
7. Weller K, Groffik A, Church MK, Hawro T, Krause K, Metz M, et al. Development and validation of the Urticaria Control Test: a patient-reported outcome instrument for assessing urticaria control. J Allergy Clin Immunol. 2014;133(5):1365-72, 72.e1-6.
8. García-Díez I, Curto-Barredo L, Weller K, Pujol RM, Maurer M, Giménez-Arnau AM. Cross-Cultural Adaptation of the Urticaria Control Test from German to Castilian Spanish. Actas Dermosifiliogr. 2015;106(9):746-52.
9. Sanchez J, Lopez JF, Alvarez L. Is anti-TPO IgG and total IgE clinically useful for the detection of autoimmune chronic spontaneous urticaria? J Allergy Clin Immunol Pract. 2022;10(5):1392.
10. Tienforti D, Di Giulio F, Spagnolo L, Castellini C, Totaro M, Muselli M, et al. Chronic urticaria and thyroid autoimmunity: a meta-analysis of case-control studies. J Endocrinol Invest. 2022;45(7):1317-26.

1.7

CHAPTER

# Management of Urticaria

*Maia Gotua*

## INTRODUCTION

The management of urticaria is based on accurate diagnosis to determine whether it is acute urticaria (AU) or chronic urticaria (CU), as well as identifying the role of possible triggers, differentiating with other systemic disorders resembling or involving urticaria, and/or angioedema (AE): Anaphylaxis, urticarial vasculitis, autoimmune and autoinflammatory disorders, mastocytosis and mast cell disorders, malignancies, AE bradykinin-mediated, AE due to intrinsic vascular endothelium dysfunction, AE drug-induced, or AE of unknown cause.[1-5] Urticaria is a mast cell-driven inflammatory disease causing wheals, AE, or both. It is AU if lasting ≤6 weeks and CU if lasting >6 weeks, with subtypes chronic spontaneous urticaria (CSU) or chronic inducible urticaria (CIndU).

## MANAGEMENT OF ACUTE URTICARIA

Management of AU involves several steps, focusing on diagnostic working up and alleviating symptoms, identifying and avoiding triggers, and preventing recurrence. Urticaria mainly is itching. Other pruritic disorders that could be mistaken for AU include insect bites, atopic and contact dermatitis, morbilliform drug eruptions, bullous pemphigoid, erythema multiforme minor, plant-related dermatoses (e.g., poison ivy), while nonpruritic conditions that may resemble acute urticaria include viral exanthems, the skin changes of auriculotemporal syndrome, and Sweet syndrome. Special attention should be given to AU, which might be part of anaphylaxis, including distinguished forms of anaphylaxis like exercise-induced food anaphylaxis and alpha-gal anaphylaxis. Careful history-taking and physical examination are crucial, laboratory tests depend on the severity of the disease and differential diagnosis if needed.[1,3,4,6]

### Components of Management of Acute Urticaria

Identification of comorbidities, etiological and trigger factors, and avoidance of them are very important in the proper management of AU. Infections (viral, bacterial, and parasitic) are considered the most common comorbidities and etiological factors in AU, accounting for approximately 30–40% and even more of cases.[4] This association is particularly prevalent in children (80%) and tends to decrease with age.[4] Potential allergic etiological and nonallergic triggers might be foods, insect stings, medications [nonsteroidal anti-inflammatory drugs (NSAIDs), antibiotics, muscle relaxants, narcotics/opiates, radiocontrast media, etc.], blood transfusions, vaccinations, contact allergy, etc. Generally AU is self-limiting and does not require routine diagnostic tests if not strongly suggested by patient history. In case of severe allergic AU reactions, allergy diagnostics should be performed.[1,4]

Immediate symptom relief can be achieved with first-line treatment using nonsedating second-generation antihistamines (sgAH), which may be increased up to four times the standard dose, considering the potential for increased sedation at higher doses. In some cases, a combination of H1 and H2 antihistamines, along with leukotriene receptor antagonists (LTRA), may be used; however, there is limited high-quality of evidence supporting their use in treating urticaria.[1,3] In patients with persistent symptoms or those with prominent AE, it is suggested to add to antihistamines a short course of oral glucocorticoids: prednisone (30–60 mg daily) in adults or prednisolone (0.5–1 mg/kg/day) in children (maximum 60 mg daily), tapered over 5–7 days, while antihistamines are continued. If AU is a component of anaphylaxis, the first-line treatment is adrenaline (epinephrine), followed by other medication depending on symptoms including oxygen, inhaled bronchodilators for bronchospasm, antihistamines (parenteral first generation H1), vasopressors, vascular filling, and corticosteroids. Referral to allergologist is obligatory. An emergency kit containing an adrenaline autoinjector should be prescribed. Education of patients, and their families is essential for the prevention of anaphylaxis.[1,4]

### Prognosis

Most (two-thirds) cases are self-limited and resolved within days, or 1–3 weeks. *Patient education in case of urticaria becomes persistent and continues for several weeks*; they should be informed to seek re-evaluation in a primary care setting. For those with difficult-to-control symptoms, a referral to an allergy specialist or dermatologist may be necessary.[1,3,4]

## MANAGEMENT OF CHRONIC URTICARIA

Approximately 50% of CU patients experience spontaneous remission within 5 years, although many require long-term treatment.[3] CU is classified as spontaneous (without definite triggers) and inducible (with definite and subtype-specific) triggers; including symptomatic dermographism (SD), cold urticaria (ColdU), cholinergic, delayed pressure, solar, heat, aquagenic, contact, and vibratory urticaria. CU has negative impacts on patients' quality of life (QoL) as well as their performance at work and school.[1,3] The vast majority of patients with CSU present with wheals only (approximately 57%), while around 37% experience both wheals and AE. The occurrence of AE alone is much less common and is about 6%.[4] The primary objective in managing CU should be to achieve complete disease control, allowing patients to remain symptom-free and regain their full QoL. The modern management of CU involves a stepwise approach, tailored to the severity of symptoms and the patient's response to treatment. Management should be started with: *Clinical Assessment and Confirmation of Diagnosis of CU.*

### History and Physical Examination

History and physical examination include detailed history-taking of symptoms to *identify potential triggers* (such as infections, medications, foods, or stress), *differentiating* from other diseases mimicking CU, and identifying *comorbidities* (CIndU, autoimmunity, mental health, allergic diseases) **(Table 1 and Flowchart 1)**.[1-9]

### Laboratory Tests

Basic laboratory tests such as complete blood count (CBC) with differential, erythrocyte sedimentation rate (ESR), C-reactive protein (CRP), immunoglobulin G (IgG) anti-thyroid peroxidase (TPO), and IgE should be done and rule out underlying causes or associated conditions, such as thyroid dysfunction or autoimmune and autoinflammatory diseases, infections, and allergic diseases. Further tests—by indication, skin biopsy if vasculitis suspected. In the case of recurrent AE without wheels, bradykinin-mediated AE including angiotensin-converting enzyme inhibitor-induced AE, hereditary angioedema (HAE), and other forms of AE should be excluded.[1-5] Recommended *seven aims of the diagnostic work-up for patients with CSU*[9] are shown in **Table 1**.

### Evaluation of CU Severity, Disease Control, and Impact on QoL Using Patient-reported Outcome Measures (PROMs) (Table 1)

Current management of CU is based on PROMs, global and validated tools. The Urticaria Activity Score (UAS) is a gold standard to assess disease activity (wheal number and itch intensity) in CSU and is usually used prospectively during seven consecutive days (UAS7). Similarly, the AE Activity Score (AAS) is a prospective, diary-type tool for measuring AE activity in patients with all forms of recurrent AE. In CIndU, the Cholinergic Urticaria Activity Score (CholUAS) and the Cold Urticaria Activity Score (ColdUAS), modified versions of the UAS, collect data daily assessing the intensity of wheals and pruritus as well as the intensity of exposure to specific triggers with a recall period of 24 hours. The Urticaria Control Test (UCT) and the Angioedema Control Test (AECT) are retrospective tools with a recall period of 4 weeks used to assess disease control in all forms of CU. QoL impairment is evaluated with the Chronic Urticaria Quality of Life Questionnaire (CU-Q2oL), Angioedema Quality of Life Questionnaire (AE-Qol), and Dermatology Life Quality Index (DLQI). *Complete control of CU* in clinical practice may be defined as: UAS7 = 0, UCT = 16, and absence of AE (ASS7 or ASS28 = 0) if there is a previous history of AE. Optimal QoL (e.g., DLQI) = 0–1.[1,6-8] *Good control of CU* in clinical practice may be defined as: UAS7 1-6, UCT ≥ 12, and presence of AE (ASS7 or ASS28 > 0) that does *not* interfere with normal activity or does *not* have a high/significant impact on QoL (if there was a previous history of AE). Good QoL (e.g., DLQI) = 2–5.[1,8] *Partial control of CU* in clinical practice may be defined as follows: Despite observing some clinical improvement, the patient continues with active disease by maintaining: UAS7 > 6, UCT < 12, and presence of AE (ASS7 or ASS28 > 0) that interferes with normal activity or has a significant impact on QoL (if there is a previous history of AE). A significant impact on QoL (e.g., DLQI) > 5.[1,8] The time necessary to confirm

**TABLE 1: Management of CU.**

*Assess:* Diagnostic procedures; comorbidities; severity (using PROMs); patient preferences; adverse effects expected[1-9]

*Act:* Start treatment and treat comorbidities; look at nonpharmacological interventions, especially in CIndU; patient education[1]

*Adjust:* Step up if inadequate control; change if adverse effects occur; step down if symptom free for 3–6 months[1]

- *Decision is based on PROMs*: Urticaria and angioedema control tests (UCT and AECT)
- Urticaria and angioedema activity scores (UAS7, AAS7, ColdUAS, and CholUAS)
- Urticaria and angioedema quality of life tools (CU-QoL, AE-QoL, and CholU-QoL)

| Diagnosis with exclusion of mimics[1-5,9] | Diagnostic tests[1-4,7-9] | 7 aims of diagnostic work-up of CSU patients[1,9] | Comorbidities[1,3,4] | CSU endotypes[1-4,6-9] | Biomarkers of treatment response[1,3,4,7,9] |
|---|---|---|---|---|---|
| • Urticarial vasculitis (wheals lasting >24 hours)<br>• Mastocytosis in skin<br>• Schnitzler syndrome<br>• Cryopyrin-associated periodic syndromes, and other autoinflammatory disorders<br>• Erythema multiforme<br>• Erythema marginatum in HAE patient<br>• Figurate and toxic erythema<br>• Bullous pemphigoid (prodromal lesions)<br>• Systemic lupus erythematosus and other autoimmune diseases<br>• In case of recurrent angioedema without wheels bradykinin mediated AE including angiotensin-converting enzyme inhibitor-induced AE, HAE, and other forms of angioedema | CBC with differential, ESR, CRP, IgG anti-TPO, IgE. Further tests by indication<br><br>Provocation tests for CIndU<br><br>*CIndU*: Symptomatic dermo-graphism, cold, cholinergic, delayed pressure, solar, heat, aquagenic, contact, and vibratory | *Confirm*: Rule out differential diagnosis<br>*Cause*: Identify indicators of autoimmune CSU endotypes<br>*Cofactors*: Identify potential triggers<br>*Comorbidities*: For example, identify CIndU, autoimmunity<br>*Consequences*: For example, identify issues with sleep, distress, work/social performance<br>*Components*: Assess potential biomarkers or predictors of treatment response<br>*Course*: Monitor CSU activity, impact, and control<br><br>*Triggers (cofactors) of exacerbation*:<br>• Stress<br>• Foods<br>• Drugs<br>Mostly NSAIDs (mainly COX1 inhibitors)—observed in 30% of CSU and classified as NSAID-exacerbated cutaneous disease | • CSU/CIndU (>10% up to 43%)<br>• *Autoimmune diseases (28%)*: Hashimoto's, thyroiditis, rheumatoid arthritis, type 1 diabetes (1–2%), etc.<br>• Infections<br>• Mental health disorders (up to 60%)<br>• Allergic diseases<br>• *Metabolic syndrome consequences*: Sleep problems, sexual issues work/social performance | • *Autoallergic type I CSU* is 50% of CSU. Type 2 chronic inflammatory diseases (allergic rhinitis, atopic dermatitis, and asthma) are 20% of CU. Th2 cell-derived IL-4, IL-5, IL-13, IL-31, and IgE against autoallergens (auto-IgE-anti-TPO and auto-IgE-anti-IL-24) activate receptors IL-4Rα, IL-5Rα IL-31RA and FcεR1 on mast cells and other target cells. Response to sgAH is higher. High serum total is associated with a complete and early response to omalizumab<br>• *Biomarkers*: High IgE, auto-IgE against TPO, anti-TG, IL-24.<br>• *Autoimmune type IIb CSU* (8–40% of CSU) is linked to high disease activity, autoimmune comorbidities, poor, partial, or no response to increased doses of sgAH, and omalizumab, and a good response to ciclosporin<br>• *Biomarkers*: Low IgE, low FcεR1 expression on basophils, eosinophils, elevated IgG-anti-TPO, positive basophil histamine releasing assay (BHRA) or positive basophil activation test (BAT), positive autologous serum skin test (ASST), positive IgG anti-FceR1, and IgE | • Poor response to sgH1-AHs is associated with elevated CRP and D-dimer<br>• Good response to omalizumab is in patients with autoallergic CSU, CSU with IgE-mediated comorbidities and is associated with high IgE, auto-IgE against autoallergens<br>• Poor response to omalizumab is associated with low total IgE (<40 kU/L), eosinopenia, basopenia, elevated TPO, positive BHRA, BAT, ASST or IgG anti-FcεR1, and IgE and good response to ciclosporine<br><br>CU-treatment adjustments[1] |

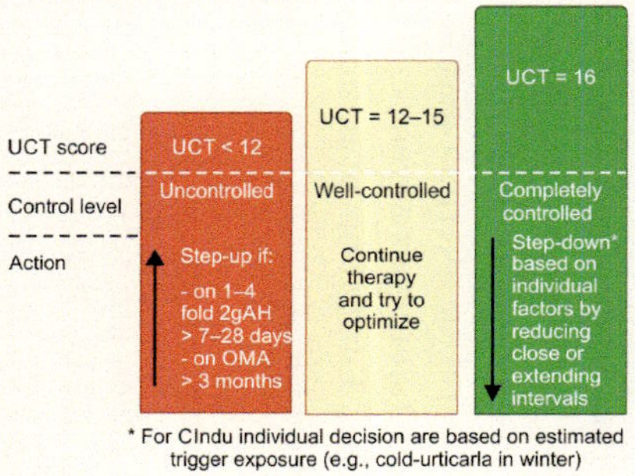


(AE: angioedema; CBC: complete blood count; CU: chronic urticaria; CIndU: chronic inducible urticaria; CRP: C-reactive protein; CSU: chronic spontaneous urticaria; ESR: erythrocyte sedimentation rate; HAE: hereditary angioedema; IgG: immunoglobulin G; IL: interleukin; NSAIDs: nonsteroidal anti-inflammatory drugs; PROMs: patient-reported outcome measures; sgH1-AHs: second-generation H1 antihistamines)

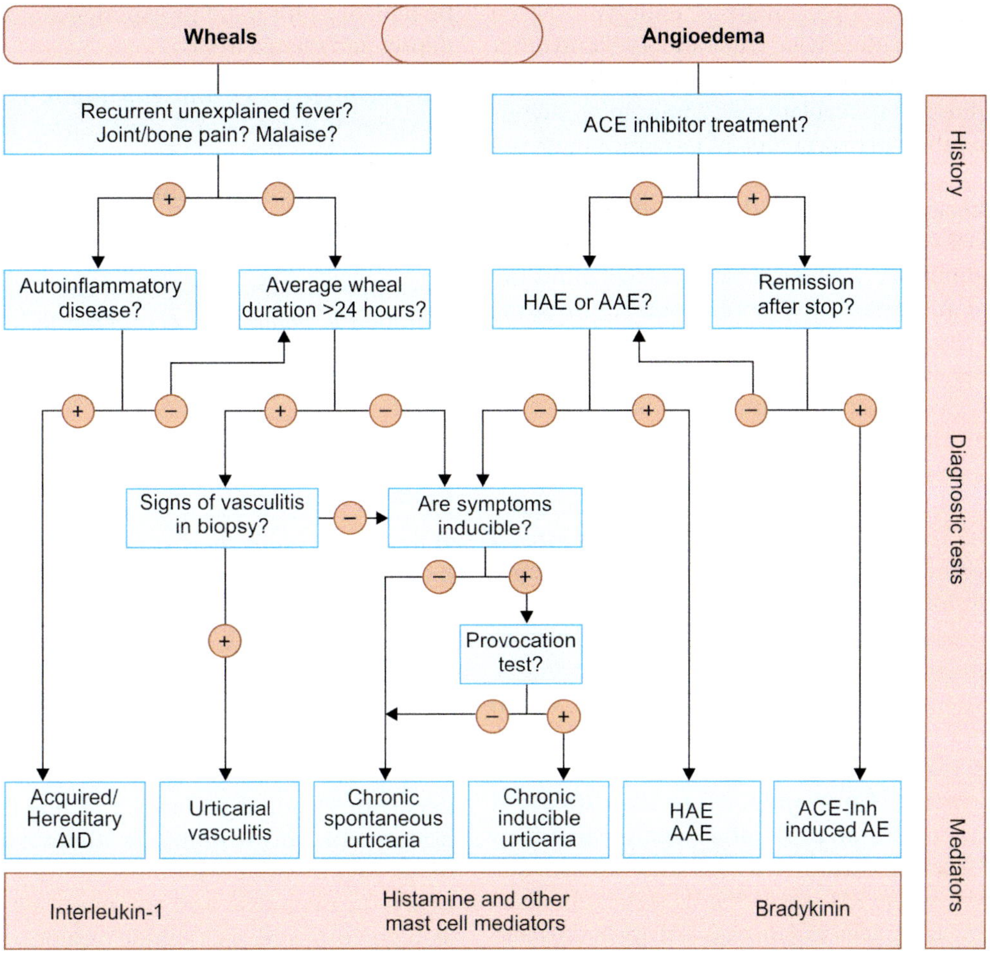


**FLOWCHART 1:** International EAACI/GA$^2$LEN/EuroGuiDerm/APAAACI guideline for the definition, classification, diagnosis, and management of uticrata.[1]

(AE: angioedema; AAE: acquired angioedema; ACE: angiotensin-converting enzyme; AID: autoinflammatory disease; APAAACI: Asia Pacific Association of Allergy, Asthma and Clinical Immunology; EAACI: European Academy of Allergology and Clinical Immunology; GA$^2$LEN: Global Allergy and Asthma European Network; HAE: hereditary angioedema)

the degree of complete, good, or partial control in a patient receiving biological therapy is 3–6 months. The management of CU should aim to completely control the disease, ensuring patients experience no symptoms and enjoy a fully restored QoL. If complete control cannot be achieved despite exhausting all available treatment options, the secondary goal should focus on achieving good control by minimizing symptoms and reducing disease activity to its lowest possible level. However, partial control should not be accepted as a satisfactory outcome, as it still imposes a considerable burden on patients.

## Identification of Indicators of Autoimmune Chronic Spontaneous Urticaria Endotypes

Autoallergic type I CSU and autoimmune type IIb CSU **(Table 1)** are essential for choosing adequate treatment, taking into account effectiveness and side effects.

## Treatment Approaches for Chronic Urticaria

Current guidelines recommend a step-up approach, starting with *sgH1-antihistamines* to fourfold the approved dose. If high-dose antihistamines fail to provide relief after 2–4 weeks (or sooner), the next steps involve adding omalizumab (300 mg every 4 weeks up to 600 mg every 2 weeks) or ciclosporin (up to 5 mg/kg of body weight). Omalizumab has also shown effectiveness in managing CIndU, including subtypes such as cholinergicU, coldU, solarU, heatU, SD, and delayed pressureU. It is safe for long-term use, and successfully treats relapses following discontinuation.[3] Low total IgE level (<40 kU/L) predicted nonresponse to omalizumab. Early responders were associated with a higher initial omalizumab dose (≥300 mg), higher basophil counts, total IgE levels exceeding 798 kU/L, and a lower platelet-to-lymphocyte ratio.[3] However, many patients with CU fail to respond to standard treatments. A personalized, endotype-driven approach focuses on identifying autoantibodies and other underlying drivers of urticaria pathogenesis. This novel approach is directed to regulate type 2 immunity, silence mast cells via inhibitory receptors, or to reduce mast cell numbers.

These therapies include *dupilumab* inhibiting interleukin 4 (IL-4) and IL-13, two key cytokines involved in the inflammatory pathways of type two immune responses in moderate-to-severe atopic dermatitis, asthma, and chronic rhinosinusitis with nasal polyposis. Dupilumab is considered an add-on treatment for patients with CU unresponsive to high doses of second generation H1-antihistamines, with special consideration for a possible positive synergistic effect for the treatment of coexistent diseases associated with type 2 immune dysregulation.[3] *Remibrutinib* is a selective and potent oral Bruton's tyrosine kinase (BTK) inhibitor. By inhibiting BTK, remibrutinib helps reduce the activation of mast cells and the release of histamine and other inflammatory mediators, which are the key drivers of symptoms in CU. It demonstrates a quick onset of symptom relief, which is beneficial for patients suffering from CSU and CIndU. Remibrutinib is recommended as an add-on treatment for patients with CU unresponsive to high doses of second generation H1-antihistamines and omalizumab treatment.[3] *Barzolvolimab* is a humanized anti-KIT antibody that inhibits KIT activation by stem cell factor (SCF), reducing mast cells and disease activity in CSU and CIndU (coldU and SD), showing potential for mast cell-mediated disorders.[3]

*Management of CU consists of long-term management and follow-up of underlying conditions and comorbidities, providing psychiatric support.* Given the significant impact on QoL, psychological support or psychiatric care may be beneficial for patients experiencing stress, anxiety, or depression related to CU.

*Patient preferences and education*: It is important to consider the needs and preferences of patients while educating them about the nature of CU. Emphasizing that CU is often idiopathic and chronic, but not life-threatening, can help patients better understand their condition and manage their expectations. *Further research* is essential to validate the real-world effectiveness of these therapeutic goals and recommendations, which could improve clinical outcomes, personalize treatment plans for individual patients, and enhance the overall quality of care for those with CU.

## CONCLUSION

The modern management of urticaria, particularly CU, follows a structured approach encompassing diagnostic evaluation, symptomatic relief, identification and avoidance of triggers, targeted therapies, and strategies to prevent recurrence. The management of CU should strive for complete disease control, ensuring patients remain entirely symptom-free and achieve a fully restored QoL. Despite significant advancements, several challenges persist in CU management, including limited treatment options for non-responders, the absence of disease-modifying therapies, the need for reliable biomarkers, delays in diagnosis and treatment escalation, as well as high costs and accessibility issues related to biologic therapies. Further research is crucial to validate the real-world effectiveness of current therapeutic strategies and guidelines. This could lead to improved clinical outcomes, more personalized treatment approaches, and an overall enhancement in the quality of care for individuals living with CU.

## REFERENCES

1. Zuberbier T, Abdul Latiff AH, Abuzakouk M, Aquilina S, Asero R, Baker D, et al. The international EAACI/GA²LEN/EuroGuiDerm/APAAACI guideline for the definition, classification, diagnosis, and management of urticaria. Allergy. 2022;77(3):734-66.
2. Kaplan AP, Ferrer M. An algorithm for the diagnosis, pathogenesis and treatment of chronic spontaneous urticaria, 2024 update. Allergy. 2024;79(9):2567-9.
3. Zuberbier T, Ensina LF, Giménez-Arnau A, Grattan C, Kocatürk E, Kulthanan K, et al. Chronic urticaria: unmet needs, emerging drugs, and new perspectives on personalized treatment. Lancet. 2024;404(10450):393-404.
4. Kolkhir P, Giménez-Arnau AM, Kulthanan K, Peter J, Metz M, Maurer M. Urticaria. Nat Rev Dis Primers. 2022;8(1):61.
5. Reshef A, Buttgereit T, Betschel SD, Caballero T, Farkas H, Grumach AS, et al. Definition, acronyms, nomenclature, and classification of angioedema (DANCE): AAAAI, ACAAI, ACARE, and APAAACI DANCE consensus. J Allergy Clin Immunol. 2024;154(2):398-411.e1.
6. Armstrong AW, Soong W, Bernstein JA. Chronic Spontaneous Urticaria: How to Measure It and the Need to Define Treatment Success. Dermatol Ther (Heidelb). 2023;13(8):1629-46.
7. Muñoz M, Kiefer LA, Pereira MP, Bizjak M, Maurer M. New insights into chronic inducible urticaria. Curr Allergy Asthma Reports. 2024;24(8):457-69.
8. Giménez-Arnau AM, Jáuregui I, Silvestre-Salvador JF, Valero A, Ferrer M, Sastre J, et al.; Urticaria Study Group. Consensus on the Definition of Control and Remission in Chronic Urticaria. J Investig Allergol Clin Immunol. 2022;32(4):261-9.
9. Friedman A, Kwatra SG, Yosipovitch G. A Practical Approach to Diagnosing and Managing Chronic Spontaneous Urticaria. Dermatol Ther (Heidelb). 2024;14:1371-87.

1.8

CHAPTER

# Biologicals in Urticaria Management

*Rosana Câmara Agondi, Solange Oliveira Rodrigues Valle*

## INTRODUCTION

Urticaria is a skin disease driven by mast cells, and it is classified into acute and chronic forms based on disease duration. Regarding chronic urticaria, the primary subtype, chronic spontaneous urticaria (CSU), lacks a known trigger, and autoimmunity is thought to play a key role in its pathogenesis.[1] Two autoimmune mechanisms are proposed for CSU, *autoimmune CSU* (aiCSU) where IgG anti-high-affinity immunoglobulin E (IgE) receptors (FcεRI) or IgG anti-IgE, and *autoallergic CSU* (aaCSU) where IgE antiautoantigens are responsible for mast cell degranulation.[1]

Mast cell degranulation releases several mediators, with histamine being a major one. Second-generation antihistamines (sgAH), either at standard licensed dose or up to four times daily, are the first-line treatment for all patients with chronic urticaria. However, they effectively control symptoms in fewer than half of the patients. According to the 2022 International Guidelines for Urticaria Treatment, omalizumab, a monoclonal antibody anti-IgE is recommended as the next treatment step for patients who are refractory to sgAH.[1,2]

Biologicals are large complex glycoproteins that are synthesized by living organisms. Monoclonal antibodies are biological that target a specific antigen or epitope.[3]

Omalizumab is a recombinant humanized monoclonal antibody IgG-anti-IgE, it binds to free IgE exactly to the site where IgE binds to its receptor, reducing free IgE and preventing IgE from binding to its receptor. Consequently, there is no mast cell activation and, further, downregulation of FcεRI is observed. Pivotal and real-life studies showed the effectiveness and safety of omalizumab in antihistamine-unresponsive CSU patients. In 2014, Food and Drug Administration (FDA) and European Medicines Evaluation Agency (EMA) licensed omalizumab for CSU treatment.[4,5]

## EVOLUTION OF CSU TREATMENT WITH OMALIZUMAB IN RECENT YEARS

The introduction of omalizumab has significantly improved the lives of patients with CSU. Its use has been associated with better disease control, reduced reliance on systemic corticosteroids and immunosuppressants, and an enhanced quality of life. Clinical trials have demonstrated omalizumab's efficacy in patients with CSU who do not respond to antihistamines. By reducing free IgE levels and downregulating FcεRI expression on basophils and mast cells, omalizumab decreases cell degranulation and the release of inflammatory mediators central to CSU pathogenesis.[6] Calzari et al. evaluated CSU patients undergoing omalizumab therapy and confirmed the treatment's long-term effectiveness and safety over periods of up to 8 years.[7]

## NEW OPTIONS OF BIOLOGICALS FOR PATIENTS WITH CHRONIC SPONTANEOUS URTICARIA

Other biological drugs than omalizumab have shown promising results in treating CSU.[6] Asero et al. suggested that these emerging treatments offer new options for patients with difficult-to-treat CSU and also that some drugs are designed not only to alleviate symptoms but also to alter the underlying mechanisms driving the disease. Disease modifying therapies (DMTs) aim to prevent or delay disease progression, achieve long-lasting remission without ongoing therapy, and directly target the core disease mechanisms.[8,9]

Monoclonal antibody targeting interleukin (IL)-5 or its receptor may be a potential treatment option for CSU, given the significant interaction between eosinophils and mast cells, there is an important crosstalk between them. However, there are currently no clinical data available on the use of mepolizumab for CSU.[8] Altrichter et al. assessed the clinical efficacy and safety of benralizumab in patients with CSU refractory to antihistamine. They concluded that although benralizumb was effective at reducing blood eosinophils levels, there was no clinical benefit over placebo.[10]

In contrast, dupilumab, a monoclonal antibody targeting IL-4-Rα that blocks the action of IL-4 and IL-13, has demonstrated efficacy in treating CSU. Maurer et al. conducted a two phase three randomized, placebo-controlled, and double-blind trials comparing dupilumab to placebo in patients with symptomatic CSU despite treatment with H1-antihistamines. These trials were part of the LIBERTY-CSU CUPID (NCT04180488). The trial included patients from CUPID Study A, which involved omalizumab-naïve patients with CSU, and CUPID Study B, which included patients who were either omalizumab-intolerant or had an incomplete response to omalizumab.[11] Dupilumab reduced urticaria activity by reducing itch and hives severity in omalizumab-naïve patients with CSU refractory to antihistamines. This study also demonstrated that dupilumab effects were small in patients who were omalizumab-intolerant/incomplete responders.[11] These findings are further supported by a real-life study involving 33 CSU patients treated with dupilumab.[8,9]

Barzolvolimab is a humanized antibody that inhibits the activation of KIT by stem-cell factor (SCF). KIT, a receptor found on mast cells, and its ligand SCF play a critical role in mast cell function. In patients with chronic inducible urticaria (CIndU), including dermographic, cold, and cholinergic urticaria, barzolvolimab demonstrated significant efficacy by leading to marked depletion of skin mast cells, with 95% of patients achieving complete responses.[12] A phase 3 clinical trial (clinicaltrials.gov/study/NCT06445023) is currently underway in patients with CSU, showing rapid and sustained depletion of skin mast cells. Barzolvolimab is generally well-tolerated, though transient adverse effects such as neutropenia and changes in hair color have been observed.[12]

The immunoglobulin superfamily (IgSF) of proteins is defined by the presence of one or more domains that structurally resemble the immunoglobulin (Ig) fold found in Igs. Some IgSF proteins, known as I-type lectins, specifically recognize glycans. Among these, the Siglec family is the largest subgroup of I-type lectins. Siglecs are characterized by sequence similarity, the ability to recognize glycans containing sialic acids (Sias), a conserved Arg residue that engages Sia-bearing ligands, and a distinct arrangement of cysteine (Cys) residues.[13] Siglecs also feature N-terminal binding domains and function as immune checkpoints. They use signaling motifs, such as the intracellular immunoreceptor tyrosine-based inhibitory motif (ITIM), to deliver inhibitory signals that attenuate or terminate activating signals.[14]

Siglecs are expressed on various human cell types, with specific members found on the membranes of different cells, such as, Siglec-2 on B lymphocytes, Siglec-3 on mast cells and macrophages, Siglec-6 on B lymphocytes and mast cells, and Siglec-8 on eosinophils and mast cells. Siglecs recognize and exert biological effects upon binding to clusters of glycans containing Sias.[13] Anti-Siglec agents, known as mast cell silencers, are drugs that regulate the intensity of immune responses to triggers. Lirentelimab, a humanized Siglec-8 agonist antibody, has broad inhibitory effects on several mast cell pathways, including IgE/FcεRI interactions. A phase 2 trial (CURSIG; NCT03436797) in omalizumab-naïve and -refractory CSU patients demonstrated a reduction in urticaria disease activity (UAS7) and an improvement in urticaria control test (UCT) scores after six intravenous doses of the drug.[14]

**Table 1** provides a summary of the biologic treatments for chronic urticaria discussed in this text.

The landscape of urticaria treatments is evolving rapidly. The introduction of emerging targeted therapies for chronic urticaria is paving the way for a more personalized approach to treatment, aiding in endotype characterization and biomarker development. Ultimately, this progress aims to achieve disease modification and long-term remission for patients.[9]

**TABLE 1: Biologicals for the treatment of chronic urticaria.**

| Biological for chronic urticaria | International Guidelines 2022 | Licenced drug (FDA) | Not licenced drug (FDA) |
|---|---|---|---|
| Omalizumab | Yes | Yes | NA |
| Dupilumab | No | Yes | No |
| Mepolizumab/Reslizumab/Benralizumab | No | No | Yes |
| Barzolvolimab | No | No | Yes |
| Anti-Siglec-8 | No | No | Yes |

(FDA: Food and Drug Administration; NA: not applicable)

## CONCLUSION

The treatment landscape for urticaria is rapidly evolving as a deeper understanding of disease mechanisms is being achieved. Therefore, the introduction of new targeted therapies for chronic urticaria is paving the way for a more personalized approach to treatment, aiding in endotype characterization and biomarker development. Ultimately, this progress is aimed at achieving disease modification and long-term remission for patients.

## REFERENCES

1. Kolkhir P, Giménez-Arnau AM, Kulthanan K, Peter J, Metz M, Maurer M. Urticaria. Nat Rev Dis Primers. 2022;8:61.
2. Zuberbier T, Abdul Latiff AH, Abuzakouk M, Aquilina S, Asero R, Baker D, et al. The international EAACI/GA²LEN/EuroGuiDerm/APAAACI guideline for the definition, classification, diagnosis, and management of urticaria. Allergy. 2022;77:734-66.
3. Mustari AP, Bishnoi A, Kumaran MS. Biologicals in treatment of chronic urticaria: a narrative review. Indian Dermatol Online J. 2023;14:9-20.
4. Asero R, Tedeschi A, Cugno M. Treatment of chronic urticaria. Immunol Allergy Clin North Am. 2014;34:105-16.
5. Kaplan AP, Popov TA. Biologic agents and the therapy of chronic spontaneous urticaria. Curr Opin Allergy Clin Immmunol. 2014;14:347-53.
6. Manti S, Giallongo A, Papale M, Parisi GF, Leonardi S. Monoclonal antibodies in treating chronic spontaneous urticarial: new drugs for an old disease. J Clin Med. 2022;11:4453.
7. Calzari P, Gallo AC, Barei F, Bono E, Cugno M, Marzano AV, et al. Omalizumab for the treatment of chronic spontaneous urticaria in adults and adolescents: an eight-year real-life experience. J Clin Med. 2024;13:5610.
8. Asero R, Calzari P, Vaienti S, Cugno M. Therapies for chronic spontaneous urticarial: present and future developments. Pharmaceuticals (Basel). 2024;17:1499.
9. Zuberbier T, Ensina LF, Gimenez-Arnau AM, Grattan C, Kocatürk E, Kulthanan K, et al. Chronic urticaria: unmet needs, emerging drugs, and new perspectives on personalised treatment. Lancet. 2024;404:393-404.
10. Altrichter S, Gimenez-Arnau AM, Bernstein JA, Metz M, Bahadori L, Berquist M, et al. Benralizumab does not elicit therapeutic effect in patients with chronic spontaneous urticaria: results from the phase IIb multinational randomized double-blind placebo-controlled ARROYO trial. Br J Dermatol. 2024;191:187-99.
11. Maurer M, Casale TB, Saini SS, Ben-Shoshan M, Gimenez-Arnau AM, Bernstein JA, et al. Dupilumab in patients with chronic spontaneous urticaria (LIBERTY-CSU CUPID): Two randomized, double-blind, placebo-controlled, phase 3 trials. J Allergy Clin Immunol. 2024;154:184-94.
12. Muñoz M, Kocatürk E, Maurer M, Kolkhir P. Emerging therapeutics in chronic urticaria. Immunol Allergy Clin North Am. 2024;44: 517-28.
13. Angata T, Varki A. Discovery, classification, evolution and diversity of siglecs. Mol Aspcts Med. 2023;90:101117.
14. Metz M, Kolkhir P, Altrichter S, Siebenhaar F, Levi-Schaffer F, Youngblood BA, et al. Mast cell silencing: a novel therapeutic approach for urticaria and other mast cell-mediated diseases. Allergy. 2024;79:37-51.

CHAPTER 1.9

# Approach to Chronic Spontaneous Urticaria

*Subhajit Sadhukhan, Indrashis Podder*

## INTRODUCTION

Chronic spontaneous urticaria (CSU) is characterized by unpredictable and sudden onset of transient (<24 hours) itchy wheals, angioedema, or both for >6 weeks. Notably, wheals disappear by 24 hours, but angioedema may take 48–72 hours for resolution.[1] Clinical history and physical examination alone are usually sufficient to establish the diagnosis.

## HISTORY

In most cases, a thorough medical history is necessary to determine the kind of urticaria and its diagnosis. Firstly, one must enquire about the duration of individual wheals. Drawing a fresh lesion and noting how long it takes for it to go away can be helpful for patients who are unable to estimate how long the lesion has been present. If the duration of individual wheal exceeds 24 hours, urticarial vasculitis must be considered and a skin biopsy must be done for diagnostic confirmation. If the patient complains of concomitant systemic symptoms such as fever and arthralgia, one must rule out autoinflammatory syndromes.[1]

Once the diagnosis of urticaria is confirmed by ruling out the aforementioned differentials, it needs to be categorized into acute (<6 weeks) and chronic (≥6 weeks) variants based on duration.[1] Chronic urticaria can be further classified into spontaneous or inducible subtypes based on the absence or presence of inducible triggers respectively. Different aggravating factors such as heat, cold, pressure, etc. can induce urticaria and these questions should be asked to rule out chronic inducible urticaria.

In this chapter, we are dealing with the approach to CSU, which accounts for almost 70–80% of all chronic urticaria. In these patients, no identifying trigger can be established. It is now established that CSU can either be autoallergic [mediated by immunoglobulin (Ig)-E autoantibodies against autoallergens, e.g., thyroid peroxidase (TPO), interleukin (IL)-24] or autoimmune [mediated by IgG autoantibodies against IgE receptor high-affinity IgE receptor (FcεR1) or IgE].[2] In both pathways, the final common outcome is activation and degranulation of mast cells to release histamine and other inflammatory mediators.

Chronic spontaneous urticaria is often associated with autoimmune disorders, most commonly hypothyroidism, but also celiac disease, systemic lupus erythematosus (SLE) and type 1 diabetes mellitus.[3] Personal and family history of autoimmune disorders is necessary to explore this link. Patients with autoimmune chronic urticaria have been found to have a more aggressive disease course and are resistant to treatment.[2] The association between chronic urticaria and malignancy is unclear. Urticarial vasculitis is, however, associated with malignancy.[4]

### Drug History

Urticaria can be caused on by a variety of medications, such as nonsteroidal anti-inflammatory drugs (NSAIDs), opioids, antibiotics, antidepressants, antihypertensives, antifungals, angiotensin-converting enzyme (ACE) inhibitors, and cyclooxygenase (COX)-2 inhibitors.[2] The condition can manifest months or even years after the onset of the medication. Thus, eliciting the proper drug history is of utmost importance. NSAID-mediated urticaria can either be induced (appearing after medication) or exacerbated (flare-up of preexisting urticaria).

### Burden of Disease

After establishing the diagnosis of CSU, one must assess the disease burden in every patient, as recommended by the current international guidelines. Disease burden includes disease activity, disease control, and impact on quality of life. There are validated patient reported outcome measures (PROMs) to evaluate these disease characteristics—urticaria activity score (UAS) = 7 for disease activity, urticaria control test (UCT) for disease control, and chronic urticaria quality of life (CU-QoL) questionnaire to assess the disease impact on patient's quality of life.[1]

## PHYSICAL EXAMINATION

Urticaria appears as pink or white well-defined elevated wheals surrounded by an erythematous halo and center pallor. These wheals may coalesce into large plaques. Urticarial lesions can vary in size and form, with annular to serpiginous borders with sizes ranging from millimeters to a few centimeters. Wheals may be associated with angioedema, a nonpitting asymmetric swelling that affects the lips, cheeks, limbs, genitals, and periorbital region.

## DIFFERENTIAL DIAGNOSES

There are several underlying conditions that may cause urticaria. Urticaria is a nonspecific cutaneous manifestation in SLE.[5] Cryopyrin-associated periodic syndromes (e.g., Muckle-Wells syndrome) are inherited autoinflammatory disorders characterized by periodic urticaria, fever, conjunctivitis, and muscle and skin sensitivity. They may also be linked to sensorineural hearing loss and arthritis. Mastocytosis causes wheals and, in rare occasions, bulla to form following extremely slight physical stress.[1,2] The clinical history and physical examination results may give information about these differentials. A skin biopsy might be conducted if the diagnosis is uncertain.

## INVESTIGATIONS

Laboratory tests are usually not necessary to diagnose chronic urticaria, and most tests will be normal. The current guidelines recommend complete blood count (CBC) with erythrocyte sedimentation rate (ESR)/C-reactive protein (CRP), total serum IgE, and anti-TPO IgG estimation in all patients with CSU.[1] CRP/ESR levels are often normal in chronic urticaria or slightly raised. If either CRP or ESR levels are significantly elevated, one must consider investigating systemic illnesses such as urticarial vasculitis and autoinflammatory syndromes. If there is eosinophilia, additional testing for atopic disorders and parasite infections may be performed. Polycythemia vera can be linked to aquagenic urticaria, a type of chronic inducible urticaria (CIndU). Thyroid function tests may be considered in individuals who do not respond adequately to antihistamines or have a personal/family history of autoimmune disorders. Skin prick testing (SPT) for aeroallergens and/or food allergens is not recommended in CSU as there is very little clinical relevance of these tests in CSU.[6]

Skin biopsies are usually not required for chronic urticaria. However, if the diagnosis is in question, particularly if there is suspicion of urticarial vasculitis, then a biopsy can be performed.[2] Usually, mild dermal edema with dilated and congested capillaries and mild perivascular inflammatory infiltrate composed of lymphocytes and few eosinophils can be noted in most cases.

**Flowchart 1** provides a schematic algorithm for approach to chronic spontaneous urticaria (CSU).

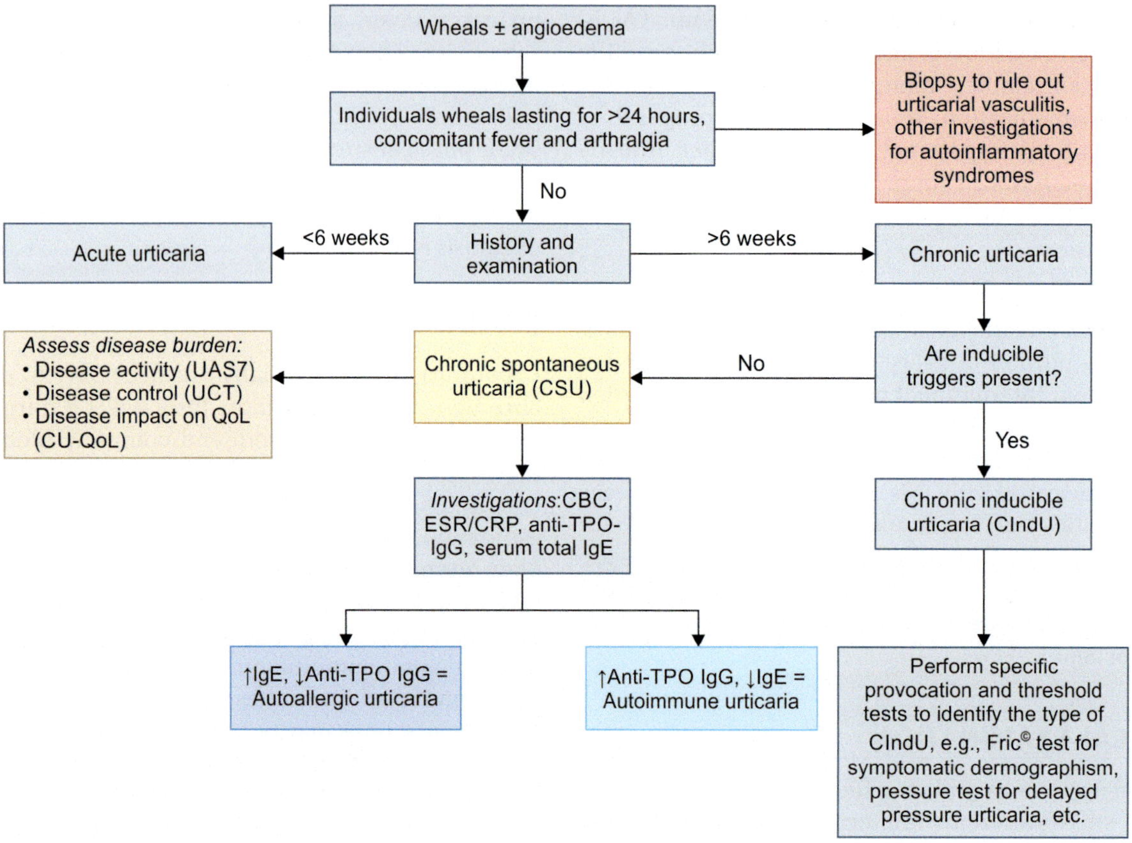


**FLOWCHART 1:** Schematic diagram showing approach to chronic urticaria.

(CBC: complete blood count; CRP: C-reactive protein; ESR: erythrocyte sedimentation rate; Ig: immunoglobulin; QoL: quality of life; TPO: thyroid peroxidase; UAS7: urticaria activity score 7; UCT: urticaria control test)

## CONCLUSION

A patient-centered holistic approach is needed for the proper approach to CSU including detailed history taking and necessary investigations to rule out differentials. Specialized investigations like serum IgE and anti-TPO IgG antibodies may be undertaken to identify the endotype of CSU, which may be useful in predicting treatment course and therapeutic response. All patients must be evaluated for disease activity, disease control and impact of disease on quality of life, for proper counseling and monitoring.

## REFERENCES

1. Zuberbier T, Abdul Latiff AH, Abuzakouk M, Aquilina S, Asero R, Baker D, et al. The international EAACI/GA²LEN/EuroGuiDerm/APAAACI guideline for the definition, classification, diagnosis, and management of urticaria. Allergy. 2022;77:734-66.
2. Kolkhir P, Giménez-Arnau AM, Kulthanan K, Peter J, Metz M, Maurer M. Urticaria. Nat Rev Dis Primers. 2022;8:61.
3. Murdaca G, Paladin F, Borro M, Ricciardi L, Gangemi S. Prevalence of Autoimmune and Autoinflammatory Diseases in Chronic Urticaria: Pathogenetic, Diagnostic and Therapeutic Implications. Biomedicines. 2023;11:410.
4. Calvo-Romero J. Diffuse large B cell lymphoma in a patient with hypocomplementemic urticarial vasculitis. J Postgrad Med. 2003;49:252.
5. Kolkhir P, Pogorelov D, Olisova O, Maurer M. Comorbidity and pathogenic links of chronic spontaneous urticaria and systemic lupus erythematosus–a systematic review. Clin Exper Allergy. 2016;46:275-87.
6. Kulthanan K, Wachirakaphan C. Prevalence and clinical characteristics of chronic urticaria and positive skin prick testing to mites. Acta Derm Venereol. 2008;88:584-8.

# 1.10

CHAPTER

# Approach to Chronic Inducible Urticaria

*Andaç Salman*

## INTRODUCTION

Chronic inducible urticaria (CIndU) is a form of chronic urticaria characterized by the development of pruritic wheals and/or angioedema in response to specific triggers. CIndUs constitute 20–30% of chronic urticaria cases and may coexist with chronic spontaneous urticaria. The triggers for CIndU can be either physical or nonphysical.[1]

Chronic inducible urticaria caused by physical stimuli include:[1]

- Symptomatic dermographism, triggered by shearing forces or friction on the skin **(Fig. 1)**
- Cold urticaria, resulting from exposure to cold temperatures
- Heat urticaria, induced by exposure to heat
- Delayed pressure urticaria, caused by pressure on the skin
- Solar urticaria, triggered by exposure to sunlight
- Vibratory angioedema, brought on by exposure to vibration

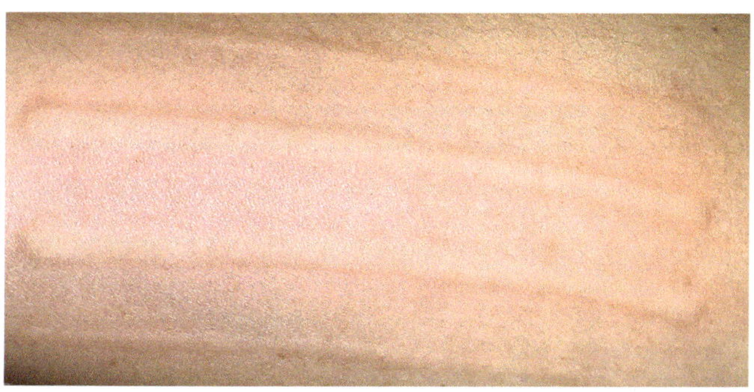

**FIG. 1:** Linear wheals in a patient with symptomatic dermographism following FricTest.

Nonphysical stimuli can trigger CIndUs such as:

- Cholinergic urticaria, associated with exercise
- Aquagenic urticaria, triggered by contact with water
- Contact urticaria, caused by specific allergens (urticariogens)

Diagnosing CIndU requires a detailed patient's history, supported by the key question, "Can you provoke your wheals?" Standardized provocation tests are also crucial for confirming the diagnosis, determining the threshold levels that provoke wheals, and assessing the response to treatment.[2]

The primary approach to managing CIndU involves avoiding the triggers **(Flowchart 1)**. However, complete avoidance may not always be practical, especially if it interferes with daily activities. Medical treatment typically includes second-generation nonsedating H1-antihistamines, administered at standard doses or, if necessary, at higher doses (up to four times the standard amount). In some cases, off-label use of omalizumab and other treatments may be considered, depending on the specific type of CIndU.[3]

## CONCLUSION

The presence of CIndUs should be assessed in all patients with chronic urticaria, as it can coexist with CSU. A key diagnostic question—"Can you make your wheals appear?"—should be included in the evaluation of patients with urticarial lesions.

While avoidance of triggers is an important aspect of management, it is often impractical in many cases. Given the significant impact of CIndUs on quality of life, effective medical treatment options are essential, with an expanding range of therapeutic choices available.

Can you provoke your wheals? → No → Chronic spontaneous urticaria (CSU)

↓ Yes

Chronic inducible urticaria (CIndU)

↓

| Type of CIndU | Triggering factor | Provocation test |
|---|---|---|
| Symptomatic dermographism | Shearing forces on the skin | FricTest,® Dermographometer |
| Cold urticaria | Cold air, objects, and liquids | Ice cube test, TempTest,® Cold water baths |
| Heat urticaria | Contact heating of the skin | Hot water baths, TempTest® |
| Delayed pressure urticaria | Pressure on the skin | Weighted rods |
| Solar urticaria | Exposure to sunlight | UVA/UVB irradiation, visible light |
| Vibratory angioedema | Exposure to vibration | Vortex vibrator |
| Cholinergic urticaria | Elevation of body temperature due to exercise or hot bath, etc. | Pulse-controlled ergometry |
| Aquagenic urticaria | Exposure to water | Compress or towel soaked with water 35–37°C |
| Contact urticaria | Various urticariogenics | Open controlled application testing |

↓

Treatment → Avoidance of triggering factors

↓

Nonsedating second generation H1-antihistamines (Up to four-fold of standard doses)

Omalizumab

*Other treatments:*
- Symptomatic dermographism (Phototherapy and cyclosporine)
- Cold urticaria (Desensitization, penicillin, doxycycline, cyclosporine, and danazol)
- Heat urticaria (Desensitization)
- Delayed pressure urticaria (Sulfasalazine, dapsone, chloroquine, and tranexamic acid)
- Solar urticaria (Phototherapy, IVIG, and α-MSH analogs)
- Vibratory angioedema (Amitriptyline)
- Cholinergic urticaria (Desensitization and β-blockers)
- Aquagenic urticaria (Phototherapy and barrier creams)

**FLOWCHART 1:** Approach to chronic inducible urticaria.

(IVIG: intravenous immunoglobulin; MSH: melanocyte stimulating hormone; UVA: ultraviolet A; UVB: ultraviolet B)

## REFERENCES

1. Zuberbier T, Abdul Latiff AH, Abuzakouk M, Aquilina S, Asero R, Baker D, et al. The international EAACI/GA²LEN/EuroGuiDerm/APAAACI guideline for the definition, classification, diagnosis, and management of urticaria. Allergy. 2022;77(3):734-66.
2. Maurer M, Bonnekoh H, Grekowitz E, Kiefer L, Munoz M, Pereira MP, et al. An algorithm for the diagnosis and treatment of chronic inducible Urticaria, 2024 update. Allergy. 2024;79(9):2573-6.
3. Muñoz M, Kiefer LA, Pereira MP, Bizjak M, Maurer M. New insights into chronic inducible urticaria. Curr Allergy Asthma Rep. 2024;24(8):457-69.

CHAPTER 1.11

# Urticaria in Children

*Roy Khalaf, Carly Sillcox, Adnan Al Ali, Sofianne Gabrielli, Moshe Ben-Shoshan*

## INTRODUCTION

Urticaria, a frequently encountered skin disorder, exhibits a diverse clinical presentation, encompassing both acute and chronic forms. Acute forms may develop due to an IgE-mediated degranulation of mast cells triggered by an allergen such as food, drug, or venom. In the most severe forms of IgE-mediated mast cell degranulation, the reaction will not be limited to the skin and anaphylaxis, a life-threatening reaction, may develop.[1] Viral infection is a potential trigger and sometimes is the main etiologic agent in causing acute urticaria when no trigger is identified, and symptoms are limited to the skin.[2] This chapter will focus on chronic urticaria (CU) in children. CU in children is defined similarly to adults by the presence of hives **(Fig. 1)** or angioedema or both for at least 6 weeks most days of the week.

## CLINICAL PRESENTATION, INVESTIGATION, AND MANAGEMENT OF URTICARIA IN CHILDREN

Epidemiological investigations have provided valuable insights into urticaria prevalence, with a meta-analysis of 11 studies involving 86,000 participants revealing an increasing trend in point prevalence over time. Geographic variations have been observed, with rates ranging from 0.1 to 0.7% in North America, 0.2 to 1.0% in Europe, 0.6 to 0.6% in Latin America, and 0.5 to 2.9% in Asia.[3] Notably, children under 15 years of age exhibit a higher prevalence in Europe and North America compared to other regions.[4] The prevalence of urticaria varies across studies, with children displaying prevalence rates ranging from 0.73 to 1.97%, while rates in adults fluctuate more widely, ranging from 0.21 to 3.44%. The pooled prevalence of CU in children in contrast to previously held premises is similar to adults and the pooled estimates are reported to be 1.4%.[4]

The median age of CU in children is 5–9 years.[5] Urticaria classification in children mirrors that in adults and encompasses chronic spontaneous urticaria (CSU), chronic inducible urticaria (CIndU) triggered by specific stimuli (e.g., aspirin, physical factors, or contact), and urticaria-related diseases such as urticaria vasculitis, urticaria pigmentosa, Schnitzler's syndrome, and cryopyrin-associated periodic fever (CAPS).[5] CSU represents the most common form, accounting for 78% of cases.[6] Notably, children with CSU exhibit a heightened rate of healthcare utilization, leading to increased inpatient and outpatient visits, as well as emergency department visits, resulting in elevated per-patient-per-year (PPPY)

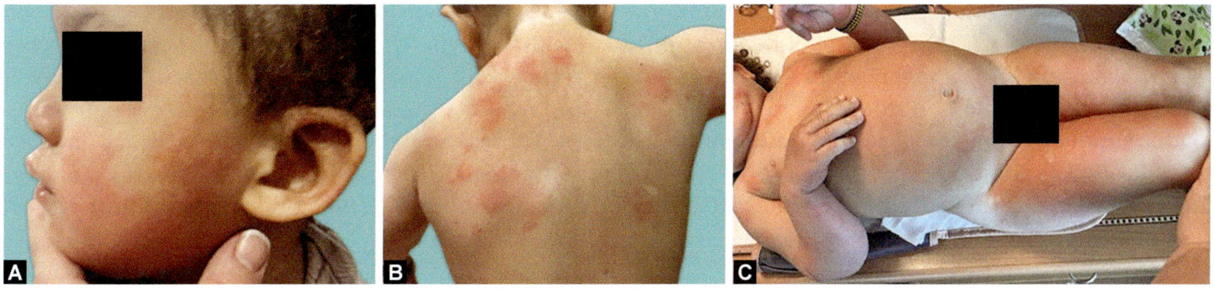

**FIGS. 1A TO C:** Common clinical presentation of pediatric urticaria, visible as urticarial lesions (hives) throughout the body.

healthcare costs in both inpatient settings [incidence rate ratio (IRR) = 2.05], outpatient settings (IRR = 2.20), and emergency department (IRR = 1.64) visits ($p \leq 0.05$).[7]

Some clinical characteristics of CU in children are reported to differ from adults. Angioedema occurrence and atopy are more prevalent in adult CU cases. It is reported that concomitant angioedema presents in only 5–20% of children although it is seen in up to 50% of adult cases with CU.[8]

Laboratory data indicates disparities between children and adults with CU, including higher median IgG-anti-thyroid peroxidase (TPO) levels in adults. A retrospective study by Özçeker et al. (2023) examined 751 patients with CSU, including 162 patients from the pediatric population and 589 adults. Adult CU patients displayed a higher IgG-anti-TPO positivity rate, elevated C-reactive protein (CRP) levels, eosinopenia, and skin prick test positivity which are less frequent in children. Additionally, the prevalence of comorbid autoimmune thyroiditis was higher in adults with CU.[8] Laboratory biomarkers for moderate and severe forms of CSU in children included thyroid-stimulating hormone (TSH), CD63, and total IgE while adjusting for age and sex.[9]

The pathogenesis of CSU involves mast cells and basophils which act as primary effectors of CU.[10] Mast cells and basophils highly express high-affinity IgE receptor (FcεRI) on their cell surfaces, which is further upregulated by interactions between IgE and FcεRI.[10] Studies in adults reveal that the main mechanism underlying mast cell degranulation is related to cross-linking of IgE with a self-antigen [e.g., interleukin (IL)-24] while a smaller proportion of cases is related to the presence of IgG against the constant region of IgE or the IgE receptor.[11] The origin of CSU in children is speculated to be similar. Children commonly exhibit positive CD63 basophil activation tests (BAts), (58% in a Canadian pediatric CSU cohort), suggestive of autoimmune urticaria.[12] Furthermore, a positive autologous serum skin test was observed with similar frequency in the population of both children and adults (40–45%). Comparing CSU in children with the general pediatric population reveals a higher prevalence of autoimmune diseases within the CSU group, including hypothyroidism, lupus, juvenile arthritis, and type I diabetes mellitus, suggesting an autoimmune or autoallergic etiology. This is in line with the shift of paradigm regarding the pathogenesis of CSU suggesting that it is an autoimmune or autoallergy rather than an idiopathic condition. However, no specific autoantibodies were established as pathogenic in children.[13]

The resolution rate for CU is approximately 10.3% per year, with patients demonstrating positive BAT results, being twice as likely to experience resolution after 1 year. Conversely, a higher presence of basophils correlates with a reduced likelihood of resolution.[6] Pediatric inducible forms are reported to have a lower resolution rate compared to spontaneous forms. In a study by Prosty et al., the annual rate of resolution of cold-induced urticaria was approximately half of the resolution rate of CSU.[14] Resolution rate was 13.8–26.5% at 5 years and 24.5–44.5% at 10 years, with CSU cases significantly hindering resolution.[14]

Patient-reported outcome measures (PROMs) have been used frequently in adults to assess disease activity and guide management. The major PROMs used in CU are the urticaria activity score 7 (UAS7), a simple score that ranks the extent of hives and itchiness over 7 days, and the urticaria control test (UCT). The UCT is a retrospective assessment tool used according to the European Academy of Allergology and Clinical Immunology (EAACI)/the Global Allergy and Asthma European Network (GA$^2$LEN)/the European Dermatology Forum (EDF: EuroGuiDerm)/Asia Pacific Association of Allergy, Asthma and Clinical Immunology (APAAACI) international urticaria guidelines to determine if treatment for CU is sufficient to control symptoms. The use of UAS7 in children with CSU has recently been validated by a prospective cohort study of 53 pediatric patients which correlated UAS7 with children's dermatology life quality index (CDLQI) scores. A partial correlation was found between UAS7 and the CDLQI scores in children while adjusting for age and sex ($r = 0.42$, $p = 0.002$).[15] Furthermore, UAS7 was able to discriminate between groups with different CDLQI scores. A UAS7 cutoff ≤ 31.50 was shown to be of fair accuracy in defining well-controlled disease (sensitivity: 57.1% and specificity: 91.4%).[15] The use of UCT in children was recently validated in a prospective study of 52 children with CU. UCT scores were found to be strongly correlated with CDLQI scores in children with CU ($r = -0.67$; $p < 0.01$).[14] Significantly different UCT scores were demonstrated among different strata of disease severity, as established by CDLQI for children with CU. For CU generally and the CSU subtype, UCT cutoff of ≤10 showed excellent screening accuracy for defining poorly controlled disease (CU: sensitivity 95.5%, 63.3%; CSU: sensitivity 100%, specificity 65.0%).[14] For the CIndU subtype, UCT ≤ 10 showed an acceptable screening accuracy for poorly controlled disease (sensitivity: 95.5% and specificity: 60.0%).[14]

At present, data concerning the efficacy and safety of managing CU in children are sparse and management is extrapolated from the management algorithm in adults. Primary management of CU in children

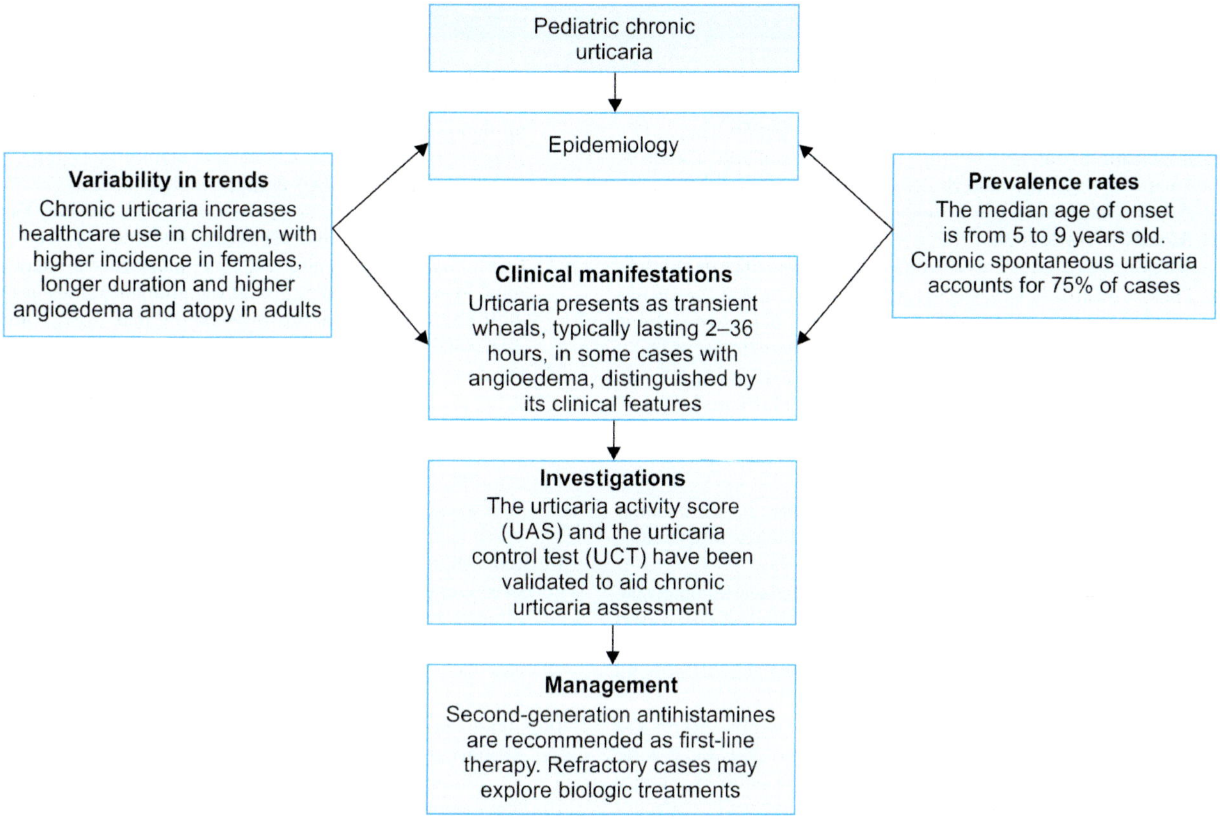


**FLOWCHART 1:** Epidemiology, clinical presentation, investigations, and treatment of chronic urticaria in children.

should involve second-generation antihistamines, potentially increasing the dosage fourfold if symptoms persist beyond 2–4 weeks.[16] Avoiding the use of first-generation antihistamines is recommended due to reported increased risks of attention, working memory, vigilance and speed disorders.[17] In children, hydroxyzine increased somnolence compared to baseline ($p < 0.05$), with a similar trend for diphenhydramine ($p = 0.07$).[18] In contrast, there were no significant differences in behavior and cognition between cetirizine and placebo over 18 months treatment period in a double-blind, randomized, and placebo-controlled trial.[19] If the child presents severe flares, a short course of oral corticosteroids could be considered. In contrast to adults, studies in children suggest that most cases of CU could be controlled with standard doses of second-generation antihistamines and 10% or less will require treatment with omalizumab. A Canadian study spanning from April 2013 to January 2019 and involving 175 pediatric patients with CU revealed that daily second-generation antihistamine usage effectively controlled symptoms in 92% of the population. Only 17 children (9.7%) experienced refractory CU necessitating treatment with omalizumab. Similarly in a recent Turkish study, most cases were well-controlled with standard doses of antihistamines mainly in children younger than 7 years and none in that age group required treatment with omalizumab. Small-scale nonrandomized controlled studies report on the effectiveness of cyclosporin at a dosage of 2.5–5 mg/kg/day for refractory cases of CU in children.[20] **Flowchart 1** summarizes epidemiology, clinical presentation, investigations and treatment of CU in children.

## CONCLUSION

In conclusion, studies suggest that epidemiology, clinical presentation, and management response differ between pediatric and adult CU. Large scale studies are required to establish the pathogenic mechanisms and best management strategies of pediatric CU and whether a modified treatment algorithm should be applied to better manage children with CU.

## REFERENCES

1. Hourihane JO, Byrne AM, Blümchen K, Turner PJ, Greenhawt M. Ascertainment Bias in Anaphylaxis Safety Data of COVID-19 Vaccines. J Allergy Clin Immunol Pract. 2021;9(7):2562-6.
2. Imbalzano E, Casciaro M, Quartuccio S, Minciullo PL, Cascio A, Calapai G, et al. Association between urticaria and virus infections: A systematic review. Allergy Asthma Proc. 2016;37(1):18-22.
3. Ban GY, Ye YM. Real-World Disease Burden of Chronic Urticaria and Vaccine Hesitancy. Allergy Asthma Immunol Res. 2023;15(1):1-3.
4. Fricke J, Ávila G, Keller T, Weller K, Lau S, Maurer M, et al. Prevalence of chronic urticaria in children and adults across the globe: Systematic review with meta-analysis. Allergy. 2020;75(2):423-32.
5. Zuberbier T, Abdul Latiff AH, Abuzakouk M, Aquilina S, Asero R, Baker D, et al. The international EAACI/GA$^2$LEN/EuroGuiDerm/APAAACI guideline for the definition, classification, diagnosis, and management of urticaria. Allergy. 2022;77(3):734-66.
6. Netchiporouk E, Sasseville D, Moreau L, Habel Y, Rahme E, Ben-Shoshan M. Evaluating Comorbidities, Natural History, and Predictors of Early Resolution in a Cohort of Children with Chronic Urticaria. JAMA Dermatol. 2017;153(12):1236-42.
7. Williams PV, Kavati A, Pilon D, Xiao Y, Zhdanava M, Balp MM, et al. Treatment Patterns, Healthcare Resource Utilization, and Spending among Medicaid-Enrolled Children with Chronic Idiopathic/Spontaneous Urticaria in the United States. Dermatol Ther (Heidelb). 2018;8(1):69-83.
8. Özçeker D, Can PK, Terzi O, Ornek SA, Degirmentepe EN, Kiziltac K, et al. Differences between adult and pediatric chronic spontaneous urticaria from a cohort of 751 patients: Clinical features, associated conditions and indicators of treatment response. Pediatr Allergy Immunol. 2023;34(2):e13925.
9. Zhang L, Le M, Gabrielli S, Netchiporouk E, Gooding G, Shand G, et al. Biomarkers associated with chronic spontaneous urticaria severity in 108 children. Pediatr Allergy Immunol. 2022;33(2):e13727.
10. Bracken SJ, Abraham S, MacLeod AS. Autoimmune theories of chronic spontaneous urticaria. Front immunol. 2019;10:627.
11. Kolkhir P, Muñoz M, Asero R, Ferrer M, Kocatürk E, Metz M, et al. Autoimmune chronic spontaneous urticaria. J Allergy Clin Immunol. 2022;149(6):1819-31.
12. Netchiporouk E, Moreau L, Rahme E, Maurer M, Lejtenyi D, Ben-Shoshan M. Positive CD63 Basophil Activation Tests are Common in Children with Chronic Spontaneous Urticaria and Linked to High Disease Activity. Int Arch Allergy Immunol. 2016;171(2):81-8.
13. Le M, Zhang L, Gabrielli S, Prosty C, Miles LM, Netchiporouk E, et al. Increased prevalence of autoimmune diseases in children with chronic spontaneous urticaria. Pediatr Allergy Immunol. 2022;33(2):e13736.
14. Prosty C, Gabrielli S, Mule P, Noorah N, Baum S, Greenberger S, et al. Validation of the Urticaria Control Test (UCT) in children with chronic urticaria. J Allergy Clin Immunol Pract. 2022;10(12):3293-8.
15. Gabrielli S, Mulé P, Prosty C, Gooding G, Le M, Zhang L, et al. Validation of UAS7 among children with chronic spontaneous urticaria. J Allergy Clin Immunol Pract. 2022;10(7):1927-9.e1.
16. Gabrielli S, Le M, Netchiporouk E, Miedzybrodzki B, Baum S, Greenberger S, et al. Chronic urticaria in children can be controlled effectively with updosing second-generation antihistamines. J Am Acad Dermatol. 2020;82(6):1535-7.
17. Kay GG. The effects of antihistamines on cognition and performance. J Allergy Clin Immunol. 2000;105(6 Pt 2):S622-7.
18. Simons FE, Fraser TG, Reggin JD, Roberts JR, Simons KJ. Adverse central nervous system effects of older antihistamines in children. Pediatr Allergy Immunol. 1996;7(1):22-7.
19. Stevenson J, Cornah D, Evrard P, Vanderheyden V, Billard C, Bax M, et al. Long-term evaluation of the impact of the h1-receptor antagonist cetirizine on the behavioral, cognitive, and psychomotor development of very young children with atopic dermatitis. Pediatr Res. 2002;52(2):251-7.
20. Ben-Shoshan M, Grattan CE. Management of Pediatric Urticaria with Review of the Literature on Chronic Spontaneous Urticaria in Children. J Allergy Clin Immunol Pract. 2018;6(4):1152-61.

CHAPTER 1.12

# Urticaria in Pregnancy and Lactation

*Salma Rashid Al Abri, Iman Hamed Nasr, Bushra Al Hinai*

## INTRODUCTION

Chronic urticaria (CU) is a condition characterized by the presence of wheals, angioedema, or both for longer than weeks.[1] It is further subdivided into chronic spontaneous urticaria (CSU), which occurs briefly with no definite triggers, and chronic inducible urticaria (CIndU), triggered by certain types of physical stimulation such as heat, vibration, and pressure. It is estimated that 1% of the adult population develops CSU. Its unpredictable nature can be extremely stressful for patients and may lead to decrements of daily functions and activities with absenteeism from work or school.[2] Although there is better understanding of CU in the general population, less is known about it in pregnancy and lactation. Here, we summarize what is known so far about CU in pregnancy and lactation.

## EPIDEMIOLOGY

A study by Fricke J et al. showed that CSU has a prevalence of 1.3% in women compared to 0.8% in men and CIndU shows a female:male ratio of 2:1 to 3:1[3] and since there is no gender difference in younger children with CU, female hormones were suggested to have a disease-modifying role.[3,4]

In addition to CU being more common in females, it is associated with more severe disease, angioedema, higher disease activity, and refractoriness to maximum doses of antihistamines. It also tends to have a longer disease course.[5-9]

In the PREG-CU international multicenter study by Kocatürk E et al., 50% of the women reported improvement of their symptoms during pregnancy, while one-third of the patients had worsening of the symptoms and 20% remained as unchanged.[10] Of the 50% who reported improvement of CU during pregnancy, half of them reported worsening of urticaria after delivery. Those whose CU worsened during prernancy did not change after delivery. The increase in CU disease activity was observed mostly during the first and third trimester.

The associated risk factors for worsening of CU during pregnancy were:

- Having mild disease before pregnancy.
- Not being on treatment before pregnancy.
- Absence of angioedema before pregnancy.
- Need for treatment during pregnancy.
- Having CIndU.
- History of worsening CU in previous pregnancies.

Stress as well as nonsteroidal anti-inflammatory medications are significant triggers for urticaria exacerbations. It was found that patients who showed improvement during their pregnancy had type IIb autoimmune CSU which is T-helper 1 and T-helper 17 driven (Th1 and Th17) driven), while those with worsening of their symptoms had type I autoallergic CSU [T helper 2 (Th2) driven].[4]

## DIFFERENTIAL DIAGNOSIS OF URTICARIA IN PREGNANCY (FLOWCHART 1)[10]

Most cases of pruritus can be attributed to dry skin; however, certain conditions are unique to pregnancy being pruritus as a leading symptom. Up to 20% of pregnant woman can be affected by pruritus and can be severe enough to affect sleep and quality of life.[10] **Flowchart 1** illustrates the approach to pruritus in pregnancy.

## DIAGNOSIS

Chronic spontaneous urticaria is a diagnosis of exclusion, with history being the most important diagnostic tool in

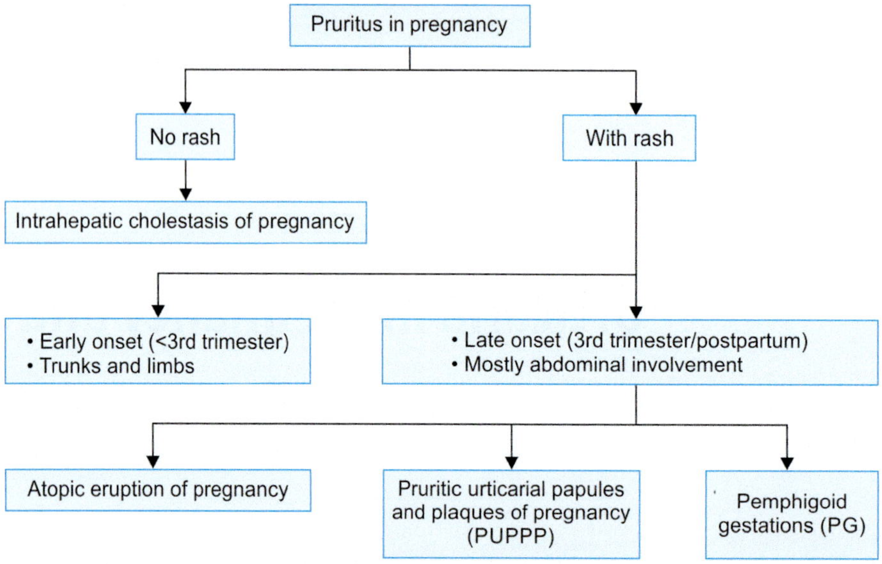


**FLOWCHART 1:** Approach to pruritus in pregnancy. (1) Intrahepatic cholestasis of pregnancy; (2) Atopic eruption of pregnancy; (3) Polymorphic eruption of pregnancy; and (4) Gestational pemphigoid.

addition to laboratory tests and skin biopsy if the diagnosis remains unclear. The work-up is practically the same as nonpregnant CU patients with basic workup including full blood count, renal function tests, liver function tests, erythrocyte sedimentation rate, and C-reactive protein. Additional investigations include thyroid function tests, thyroid peroxidase antibody, and immunoglobulin E if thyroid disease is suspected. Stool microscopy and cultures are required to rule out parasitic infection. Autoimmune serological workup such as antinuclear antibodies (ANA), anticytoplasmic antibodies (ANCA), complements, rheumatoid factor (RF), anticitrullinated C peptide (anti-CCP) can be done if the patient's history or symptoms suggest an autoimmune disease.

Provocation tests can be done in inducible urticarias. It is crucial to exclude mimickers of CU including those that occur during pregnancy as illustrated in **Flowchart 1**.

## MANAGEMENT OF CHRONIC URTICARIA IN PREGNANCY AND LACTATION

Avoidance of possible triggers (such as stress or medications such as nonsteroidal anti-inflammatory agents) is important.

The international European Academy of Allergology and Clinical Immunology (EAACI)/the Global Allergy and Asthma European Network (GA²LEN)/the European Dermatology Forum (EDF; EuroGuiDerm)/the Asia Pacific Association of Allergy, Asthma, and Clinical Immunology (APAAACI) guideline advises following the same urticaria treatment algorithm for pregnant and lactating women but with caution and a thorough risk-benefit assessment.[1] The safety of CU medications in pregnancy and lactation as well as their effect on pregnancy outcome has not been thoroughly studied. This is also the case with lactating women and the effect of medications on their babies. Therefore, treatment for this population should involve the minimal amount of medication necessary.[1]

Currently, there are no reports of birth defects in women who have used modern second-generation H1-antihistamines during pregnancy. Most patients can be treated with these second-generation H1-antihistamines alone, but short courses of steroids may be considered for severe flare-ups. The International guidelines recommend loratadine and cetirizine as the preferred antihistamines followed by desloratadine and levocetirizine. First-generation antihistamines should be avoided due to their sedative effects, which can be transmitted via breast milk during lactation.

The use of omalizumab as a second-line therapy for pregnant and lactating women who do not respond to maximum doses of antihistamines has not been studied in humans but appears to be safe in pregnancy and breastfeeding. In the prospective and observational pregnancy registry study (EXPECT) where 250 pregnant women with asthma exposed to omalizumab had a similar prevalence of major congenital anomalies (8.1% vs. 8.9%).[11] In the same study, 154 infants who had been exposed to omalizumab during pregnancy and throughout breastfeeding did not show adverse effects on the breastfed infant.[11] The lowest effective dose should be used.

Ciclosporin is the third-line therapy after omalizumab. Although not teratogenic, the international guidelines advise against its use during pregnancy due to embryotoxic effects demonstrated in animal models. It is associated with preterm delivery and low birth weight in human infants.

Close monitoring and follow-up by the obstetrician and allergist are very important to keep urticaria under control and/or adjust the medications to avoid exacerbations. The stress of pregnancy and the physical discomfort of CU can have significant psychological effects. Providing support and considering the mental health aspect both are essential.

## CONCLUSION

Chronic urticaria in pregnancy and lactation has significant challenges and requires a careful personalized approach to diagnosis and management. Most cases are effectively controlled on second generation antihistamines, however treatment options should carefully balance symptom control with fetal and maternal safety. Ongoing research and multidisciplinary approach are essential to achieve the most effective yet safest disease control for this special population.

## REFERENCES

1. Zuberbier T, Abdul Latiff AH, Abuzakouk M, Aquilina S, Asero R, Baker D, et al. The International EAACI/Ga2Len/EuroGuiDerm/APAAACI guideline for the definition, classification, diagnosis, and management of urticaria. Allergy. 2022;77(3):734-66.
2. Saini S. Chronic spontaneous urticaria: Clinical manifestations, diagnosis, pathogenesis, and natural history. UpToDate. 2024.
3. Fricke J, Ávila G, Keller T, Weller K, Lau S, Maurer M, et al. Prevalence of chronic urticaria in children and adults across the globe: Systematic review with meta-analysis. Allergy. 2020;75(2):423-32.
4. Weller K, Maurer M, Bauer A, Wedi B, Wagner N, Schliemann S, et al. Epidemiology, Comorbidities, and healthcare utilization of patients with chronic urticaria in Germany. J Eur Acad Dermatol Venereol. 2021;36(1):91-9.
5. Maurer M, Ortonne JP, Zuberbier T. Chronic urticaria: an internet survey on health behaviours, symptom patterns and treatment needs in European adult patients. Br J Dermatol. 2009;160:633-41.
6. Ue AP, Souza PK, Rotta O, FurlaniWde J, Lima AR, Sabbag DS. Quality of life assessment in patients with chronic urticaria. An Bras Dermatol. 2011;86:897-904.
7. Gregoriou S, Rigopoulos D, Katsambas A, Katsarou A, Papaioannou D, Gkouvi A, et al. Etiologic aspects and prognostic factors of patients with chronic urticaria: nonrandomized, prospective, descriptive study. J Cutan Med Surg. 2009;13:198-203.
8. Sánchez Borges M, Tassinari S, Flores A. Epidemiologic features in patients with antihistamine-resistant chronic urticaria. Rev Aler México. 2015;62:279-86.
9. Kocatürk E, Al-Ahmad M, Krause K, Gimenez-Arnau AM, Thomsen SF, Conlon N, et al. Effects of pregnancy on chronic urticaria: Results of the preg-cu UCARE study. Allergy. 2021;76(10):3133-44.
10. Bergman H, Melamed N, Koren G. Pruritus in pregnancy. Canad Fam Phys. 2013;59:1290-4.
11. Namazy J, Cabana MD, Scheuerle AE, Thorp JM Jr, Chen H, Carrigan G, et al. The Xolair Pregnancy Registry (EXPECT): the safety of omalizumab use during pregnancy. J Allergy Clin Immunol. 2015;135(2):407-12.

CHAPTER 1.13

# Urticaria in Elderly

*Mona Al-Ahmad*

## INTRODUCTION

Urticaria is identified by itchy, red, raised patches, typically caused by mast cell degranulation in the top layer of skin and typically disappears within a day.[1]

Urticaria can be categorized into acute and chronic forms. Acute urticaria is characterized by symptoms lasting 6 weeks or less, while chronic urticaria is identified by lesions appearing most days of the week for over 6 weeks.

Our knowledge of the immunopathogenesis at the core has greatly advanced recently, encompassing the categorization of urticaria in various groups and age ranges.

With changes in population demographics, the number of people aged 65 years and older is gradually growing.[2] Chronic urticaria has a lifetime prevalence rate of 4.4%.[3]

The existing recommendations for the diagnosis and treatment of acute and chronic urticaria provide guidelines for adults.[1] Children and pregnant women are recognized as special populations according to the international guidelines. Irrespective of age, experts suggest using the same initial treatment algorithm for children, the elderly, and pregnant women due to consensus expert opinion and medication safety in treating chronic spontaneous urticaria (CSU).

## DIAGNOSIS OF URTICARIA IN ELDERLY

Diagnosing CSU in older individuals is comparable in diagnosis to younger patients. Presently, the recommendations advise conducting a comprehensive history and physical evaluation.[1] It is crucial to carefully examine all medications the patient is using, including aspirin (acetylsalicylic acid) and other nonsteroidal anti-inflammatory drugs, as these commonly used medications among the elderly can exacerbate or trigger urticaria **(Table 1)**.

Other possible diagnoses to think about in older individuals during the first assessment, particularly if the hives do not respond to high doses of systemic glucocorticosteroids, are urticarial vasculitis, lymphoproliferative disease, Schnitzler syndrome, adult-onset Still's disease, bullous pemphigoid, and eosinophilic cellulitis.[4,5]

## TREATMENT OF URTICARIA IN ELDERLY

The elderly receive the same CSU treatment guidelines as other groups. Nevertheless, it is crucial to take into account the comorbid conditions, medication interactions, existing organ impairment, and potential side effects that may

**TABLE 1: Current knowledge and future needs of elderly with chronic urticaria.**

| | Elderly |
|---|---|
| Current knowledge | Almost no studies |
| | CSU may be more common than in younger adults |
| | Treatments complicated by comorbid disease, polypharmacy, and organ insufficiency |
| | Side effects of antihistamines more pronounced |
| | Differential diagnoses include urticarial vasculitis and Schnitzler syndrome |
| Future needs | Efficacy and safety data for treatments |
| | Improved prevalence data for CSU and CIndU |

(CIndU: chronic inducible urticaria; CSU: chronic spontaneous urticaria)

*Source*: Adapted from Saini S, Shams M, Bernstein JA, Maurer M. Urticaria and Angioedema Across the Ages. J Allergy Clin Immunol Pract. 2020;8(6):1866-74.

lead to sedation and cognitive issues when developing a treatment plan for these patients.[1]

According to the treatment guidelines and when antihistamines fail to treat CSU, omalizumab or cyclosporine may be the options to consider. At present, omalizumab is highly recommended in the guidelines for treating CSU and is approved by the Food and Drug Administration (FDA) for use in patients who are 12 years old and above.[1] Nevertheless, the available data suggest that omalizumab can be safely used in elderly patients.[4]

Trials with cyclosporine have demonstrated effectiveness in treating chronic spontaneous urticaria in older patients; however, careful monitoring is required for potential renal toxicity, worsening of hypertension, and hyperlipidemic disorders.[4]

## CONCLUSION

The diagnosis and management of chronic urticaria in older individuals is similar to those younger ones. However, an emphasis should be given to the presence of comorbid diseases and the polypharmacy that is commonly present in elderly patients. There is a growing need for more research in this field among elderly population as the global population demogroaphics are changing.

## REFERENCES

1. Zuberbier T, Abdul Latiff AH, Abuzakouk M, Aquilina S, Asero R, Baker D, et al. The International EAACI/GA2LEN/EuroGuiDerm/APAAACI guideline for the definition, classification, diagnosis, and management of urticaria. Allergy. 2022;77(3):734-66.
2. Caplan Z. (2023). U.S. Older Population Grew From 2010 to 2020 at Fastest Rate Since 1880 to 1890. [online] Available from https://www.census.gov/library/stories/2023/05/2020-census-united-states-older-population-grew.html [Last accessed January, 2025].
3. Kolkhir P, Gimeenez-Arnau AM, Kulthanan K, Peter J, Metz M, Maurer M. Urticaria. Nat Rev Dis Prim. 2022;8(1):61.
4. Patruno C, Fabbrocini G, Cillo F, Torta G, Stingeni L, Napolitano M. Chronic urticaria in older adults: treatment considerations. Drugs Aging. 2023;40(3):165-77.
5. Robson M, Bernstein JS, Bernstein JA. Chronic urticaria in special population: Pediatric, Pregnancy, and the Elderly. Immunol Allergy Clin North Am. 2024;44(3):469-81.

CHAPTER 1.14

# Urticaria and Comorbidities

***Mona Al-Ahmad***

## INTRODUCTION

While chronic urticaria (CU) affects all age groups, it is more frequent in patients aged 30–50 years and, thus, influences mostly young and middle-aged women.[1]

The pathophysiology underlying the disease is still not clear, but some studies have suggested autoimmunity mechanisms such as type I (autoallergy by means of autoantibodies to self-antigens) and type IIb (autoimmunity).[2,3]

Atopic diseases, autoimmune disorders, and psychiatric illnesses are common comorbid diseases associated with chronic spontaneous urticaria (CSU) in both children and adults. Also, various other studies have reported malignancies, cardiovascular diseases among others as comorbidities of CSU patients but these data are rare.[2]

Specific endotypes of CSU are linked to comorbid autoimmune diseases. Therefore, early diagnosis and therapeutic intervention of associated diseases may be beneficial in the multidisciplinary therapeutic approach as suggested by EAACI/GA$^2$LEN/EuroGuiDerm/APAAACI guidelines.[4]

Chronic spontaneous urticaria is an autoimmune skin disorder that often occurs alongside other autoimmune diseases.[5] About 30% of CSU patients have at least one autoimmune disorder, and 2% may have two or more autoimmune disorders. Hashimoto's disease and vitiligo are among the most common coexistent diseases **(Figs. 1A to C)**.

Additionally, it is well known that urticarial rash is common in patients with systemic lupus erythematosus (SLE), with prevalence ranging from 0.4 to 27.5% in adults and 4.5 to 12% in children as shown in the meta-analysis by Kolkhir et al.[5]

Regarding the associated allergic diseases, it has been shown that atopic diseases are commonly reported in patients with CU.[6] The results from the Scandinavian arm of the AWARE (A World-wide Antihistamine-Refractory chronic urticaria patient Evaluation) study showed that atopic diseases are the most frequent comorbidities in a cohort of 158 adult patients with CU. Specifically, asthma was reported in 19.6% of the patients, allergic rhinitis in 16.5%, atopic dermatitis in 6.3%, and food allergy in 8.2%.[6]

Psychiatric and mental disorders are commonly reported among patients with CU in the literature. A recent systematic review and meta-analysis found that nearly one-third of CU patients have at least one underlying psychiatric disorder.[7]

Sleep-wake disorders, along with anxiety and mood disorders, including depression, are commonly identified (with a pooled prevalence of 36.7, 30.6, and 29.4%, respectively). Additionally, trauma and stressor-related disorders, somatic symptom and related disorders, obsessive-compulsive and related disorders and substance-related and addictive disorders were also reported.[7]

Other systemic comorbid diseases have also been linked with CU, such as cardiovascular diseases. The Scandinavian arm of the AWARE study reported a prevalence of obesity at 7% and hypertension at 1.9%, among an adult CU population. Half of the patients were overweight, with a body mass index (BMI) > 25 kg/m$^2$.[6]

Similarly, metabolic syndrome was reported in 29.8% of patients with CU compared to 17.8% in a matched control group ($p = 0.001$) in a Korean cohort study and was independently correlated with uncontrolled urticaria, as assessed by total urticaria activity score (UAS).[8] Moreover, hyperlipidemia has been identified as a risk factor for CU development (OR: 1.97; 95% CI: 1.85–2.09).[8]

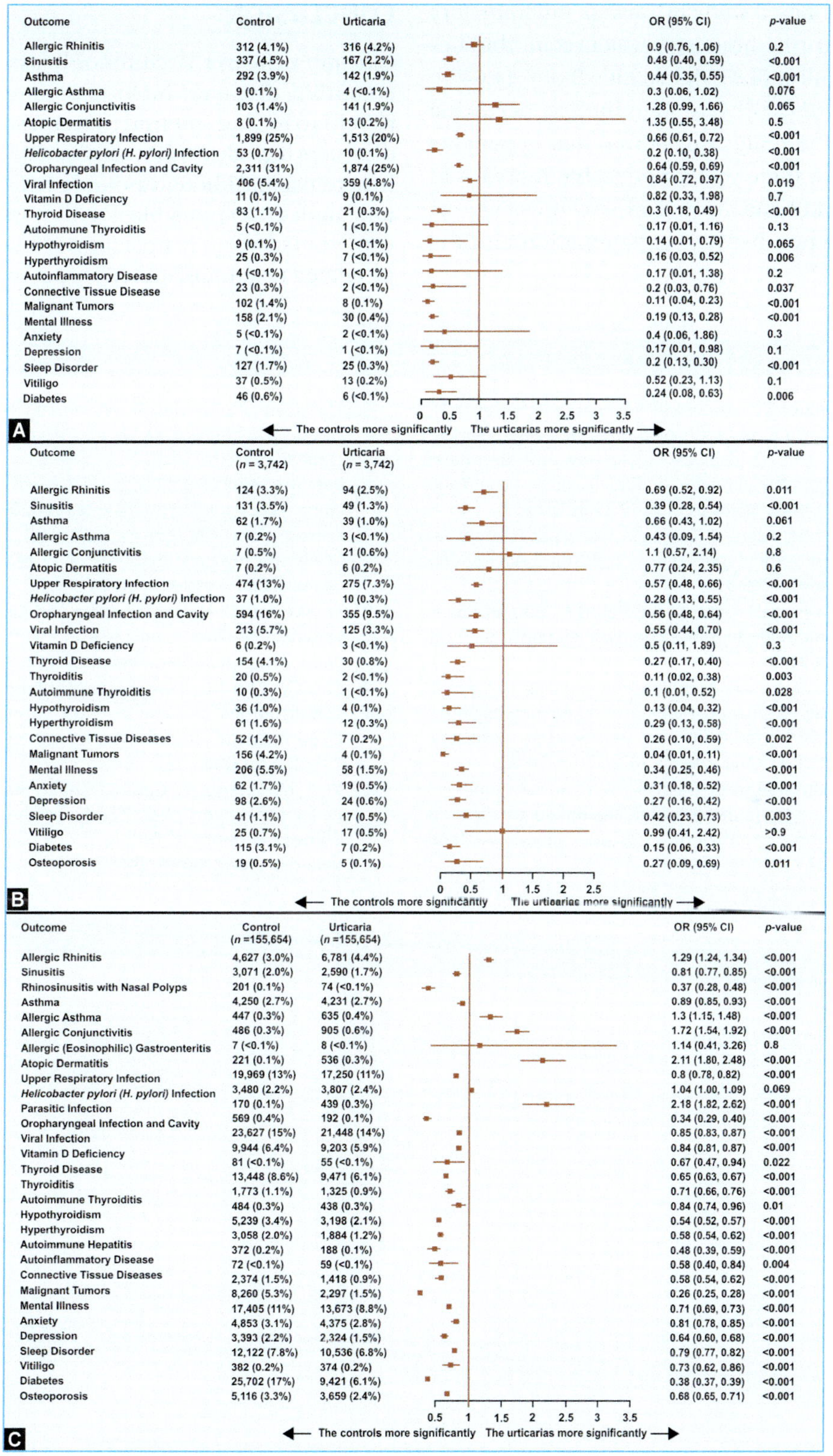


| Outcome | Control | Urticaria | OR (95% CI) | p-value |
|---|---|---|---|---|
| Allergic Rhinitis | 312 (4.1%) | 316 (4.2%) | 0.9 (0.76, 1.06) | 0.2 |
| Sinusitis | 337 (4.5%) | 167 (2.2%) | 0.48 (0.40, 0.59) | <0.001 |
| Asthma | 292 (3.9%) | 142 (1.9%) | 0.44 (0.35, 0.55) | <0.001 |
| Allergic Asthma | 9 (0.1%) | 4 (<0.1%) | 0.3 (0.06, 1.02) | 0.076 |
| Allergic Conjunctivitis | 103 (1.4%) | 141 (1.9%) | 1.28 (0.99, 1.66) | 0.065 |
| Atopic Dermatitis | 8 (0.1%) | 13 (0.2%) | 1.35 (0.55, 3.48) | 0.5 |
| Upper Respiratory Infection | 1,899 (25%) | 1,513 (20%) | 0.66 (0.61, 0.72) | <0.001 |
| *Helicobacter pylori (H. pylori)* Infection | 53 (0.7%) | 10 (0.1%) | 0.2 (0.10, 0.38) | <0.001 |
| Oropharyngeal Infection and Cavity | 2,311 (31%) | 1,874 (25%) | 0.64 (0.59, 0.69) | <0.001 |
| Viral Infection | 406 (5.4%) | 359 (4.8%) | 0.84 (0.72, 0.97) | 0.019 |
| Vitamin D Deficiency | 11 (0.1%) | 9 (0.1%) | 0.82 (0.33, 1.98) | 0.7 |
| Thyroid Disease | 83 (1.1%) | 21 (0.3%) | 0.3 (0.18, 0.49) | <0.001 |
| Autoimmune Thyroiditis | 5 (<0.1%) | 1 (<0.1%) | 0.17 (0.01, 1.16) | 0.13 |
| Hypothyroidism | 9 (0.1%) | 1 (<0.1%) | 0.14 (0.01, 0.79) | 0.065 |
| Hyperthyroidism | 25 (0.3%) | 7 (<0.1%) | 0.16 (0.03, 0.52) | 0.006 |
| Autoinflammatory Disease | 4 (<0.1%) | 1 (<0.1%) | 0.17 (0.01, 1.38) | 0.2 |
| Connective Tissue Disease | 23 (0.3%) | 2 (<0.1%) | 0.2 (0.03, 0.76) | 0.037 |
| Malignant Tumors | 102 (1.4%) | 8 (0.1%) | 0.11 (0.04, 0.23) | <0.001 |
| Mental Illness | 158 (2.1%) | 30 (0.4%) | 0.19 (0.13, 0.28) | <0.001 |
| Anxiety | 5 (<0.1%) | 2 (<0.1%) | 0.4 (0.06, 1.86) | 0.3 |
| Depression | 7 (<0.1%) | 1 (<0.1%) | 0.17 (0.01, 0.98) | 0.1 |
| Sleep Disorder | 127 (1.7%) | 25 (0.3%) | 0.2 (0.13, 0.30) | <0.001 |
| Vitiligo | 37 (0.5%) | 13 (0.2%) | 0.52 (0.23, 1.13) | 0.1 |
| Diabetes | 46 (0.6%) | 6 (<0.1%) | 0.24 (0.08, 0.63) | 0.006 |

| Outcome | Control (n = 3,742) | Urticaria (n = 3,742) | OR (95% CI) | p-value |
|---|---|---|---|---|
| Allergic Rhinitis | 124 (3.3%) | 94 (2.5%) | 0.69 (0.52, 0.92) | 0.011 |
| Sinusitis | 131 (3.5%) | 49 (1.3%) | 0.39 (0.28, 0.54) | <0.001 |
| Asthma | 62 (1.7%) | 39 (1.0%) | 0.66 (0.43, 1.02) | 0.061 |
| Allergic Asthma | 7 (0.2%) | 3 (<0.1%) | 0.43 (0.09, 1.54) | 0.2 |
| Allergic Conjunctivitis | 7 (0.5%) | 21 (0.6%) | 1.1 (0.57, 2.14) | 0.8 |
| Atopic Dermatitis | 7 (0.2%) | 6 (0.2%) | 0.77 (0.24, 2.35) | 0.6 |
| Upper Respiratory Infection | 474 (13%) | 275 (7.3%) | 0.57 (0.48, 0.66) | <0.001 |
| *Helicobacter pylori (H. pylori)* Infection | 37 (1.0%) | 10 (0.3%) | 0.28 (0.13, 0.55) | <0.001 |
| Oropharyngeal Infection and Cavity | 594 (16%) | 355 (9.5%) | 0.56 (0.48, 0.64) | <0.001 |
| Viral Infection | 213 (5.7%) | 125 (3.3%) | 0.55 (0.44, 0.70) | <0.001 |
| Vitamin D Deficiency | 6 (0.2%) | 3 (<0.1%) | 0.5 (0.11, 1.89) | 0.3 |
| Thyroid Disease | 154 (4.1%) | 30 (0.8%) | 0.27 (0.17, 0.40) | <0.001 |
| Thyroiditis | 20 (0.5%) | 2 (<0.1%) | 0.11 (0.02, 0.38) | 0.003 |
| Autoimmune Thyroiditis | 10 (0.3%) | 1 (<0.1%) | 0.1 (0.01, 0.52) | 0.028 |
| Hypothyroidism | 36 (1.0%) | 4 (0.1%) | 0.13 (0.04, 0.32) | <0.001 |
| Hyperthyroidism | 61 (1.6%) | 12 (0.3%) | 0.29 (0.13, 0.58) | <0.001 |
| Connective Tissue Diseases | 52 (1.4%) | 7 (0.2%) | 0.26 (0.10, 0.59) | 0.002 |
| Malignant Tumors | 156 (4.2%) | 4 (0.1%) | 0.04 (0.01, 0.11) | <0.001 |
| Mental Illness | 206 (5.5%) | 58 (1.5%) | 0.34 (0.25, 0.46) | <0.001 |
| Anxiety | 62 (1.7%) | 19 (0.5%) | 0.31 (0.18, 0.52) | <0.001 |
| Depression | 98 (2.6%) | 24 (0.6%) | 0.27 (0.16, 0.42) | <0.001 |
| Sleep Disorder | 41 (1.1%) | 17 (0.5%) | 0.42 (0.23, 0.73) | 0.003 |
| Vitiligo | 25 (0.7%) | 17 (0.5%) | 0.99 (0.41, 2.42) | >0.9 |
| Diabetes | 115 (3.1%) | 7 (0.2%) | 0.15 (0.06, 0.33) | <0.001 |
| Osteoporosis | 19 (0.5%) | 5 (0.1%) | 0.27 (0.09, 0.69) | 0.011 |

| Outcome | Control (n =155,654) | Urticaria (n =155,654) | OR (95% CI) | p-value |
|---|---|---|---|---|
| Allergic Rhinitis | 4,627 (3.0%) | 6,781 (4.4%) | 1.29 (1.24, 1.34) | <0.001 |
| Sinusitis | 3,071 (2.0%) | 2,590 (1.7%) | 0.81 (0.77, 0.85) | <0.001 |
| Rhinosinusitis with Nasal Polyps | 201 (0.1%) | 74 (<0.1%) | 0.37 (0.28, 0.48) | <0.001 |
| Asthma | 4,250 (2.7%) | 4,231 (2.7%) | 0.89 (0.85, 0.93) | <0.001 |
| Allergic Asthma | 447 (0.3%) | 635 (0.4%) | 1.3 (1.15, 1.48) | <0.001 |
| Allergic Conjunctivitis | 486 (0.3%) | 905 (0.6%) | 1.72 (1.54, 1.92) | <0.001 |
| Allergic (Eosinophilic) Gastroenteritis | 7 (<0.1%) | 8 (<0.1%) | 1.14 (0.41, 3.26) | 0.8 |
| Atopic Dermatitis | 221 (0.1%) | 536 (0.3%) | 2.11 (1.80, 2.48) | <0.001 |
| Upper Respiratory Infection | 19,969 (13%) | 17,250 (11%) | 0.8 (0.78, 0.82) | <0.001 |
| *Helicobacter pylori (H. pylori)* Infection | 3,480 (2.2%) | 3,807 (2.4%) | 1.04 (1.00, 1.09) | 0.069 |
| Parasitic Infection | 170 (0.1%) | 439 (0.3%) | 2.18 (1.82, 2.62) | <0.001 |
|  | 569 (0.4%) | 192 (0.1%) | 0.34 (0.29, 0.40) | <0.001 |
| Oropharyngeal Infection and Cavity | 23,627 (15%) | 21,448 (14%) | 0.85 (0.83, 0.87) | <0.001 |
| Viral Infection | 9,944 (6.4%) | 9,203 (5.9%) | 0.84 (0.81, 0.87) | <0.001 |
| Vitamin D Deficiency | 81 (<0.1%) | 55 (<0.1%) | 0.67 (0.47, 0.94) | 0.022 |
| Thyroid Disease | 13,448 (8.6%) | 9,471 (6.1%) | 0.65 (0.63, 0.67) | <0.001 |
| Thyroiditis | 1,773 (1.1%) | 1,325 (0.9%) | 0.71 (0.66, 0.76) | <0.001 |
| Autoimmune Thyroiditis | 484 (0.3%) | 438 (0.3%) | 0.84 (0.74, 0.96) | 0.01 |
| Hypothyroidism | 5,239 (3.4%) | 3,198 (2.1%) | 0.54 (0.52, 0.57) | <0.001 |
| Hyperthyroidism | 3,058 (2.0%) | 1,884 (1.2%) | 0.58 (0.54, 0.62) | <0.001 |
| Autoimmune Hepatitis | 372 (0.2%) | 188 (0.1%) | 0.48 (0.39, 0.59) | <0.001 |
| Autoinflammatory Disease | 72 (<0.1%) | 59 (<0.1%) | 0.58 (0.40, 0.84) | 0.004 |
| Connective Tissue Diseases | 2,374 (1.5%) | 1,418 (0.9%) | 0.58 (0.54, 0.62) | <0.001 |
| Malignant Tumors | 8,260 (5.3%) | 2,297 (1.5%) | 0.26 (0.25, 0.28) | <0.001 |
| Mental Illness | 17,405 (11%) | 13,673 (8.8%) | 0.71 (0.69, 0.73) | <0.001 |
| Anxiety | 4,853 (3.1%) | 4,375 (2.8%) | 0.81 (0.78, 0.85) | <0.001 |
| Depression | 3,393 (2.2%) | 2,324 (1.5%) | 0.64 (0.60, 0.68) | <0.001 |
| Sleep Disorder | 12,122 (7.8%) | 10,536 (6.8%) | 0.79 (0.77, 0.82) | <0.001 |
| Vitiligo | 382 (0.2%) | 374 (0.2%) | 0.73 (0.62, 0.86) | <0.001 |
| Diabetes | 25,702 (17%) | 9,421 (6.1%) | 0.38 (0.37, 0.39) | <0.001 |
| Osteoporosis | 5,116 (3.3%) | 3,659 (2.4%) | 0.68 (0.65, 0.71) | <0.001 |

**FIGS. 1A TO C:** Differences in comorbidities of patients with and without urticaria at different ages using a logistic regression model. (A) Differences in comorbidities of patients with and without urticaria at ages 6–11 years using a logistic regression model; (B) Differences in comorbidities of patients with and without urticaria at ages 12–17 years using a logistic regression model; (C) Differences in comorbidities of patients with and without urticaria at age >18 years using a logistic regression model.

In a population-based study in Taiwan, inflammatory diseases were found to be the most prevalent comorbidities specifically peptic ulcer (4.83%), hepatitis B or C (1.64%), and periodontitis (2.82%) were identified as occurring more frequently. The study also showed that in patients with persistent CU, there was a noticeable increase in the prevalence of inflammatory diseases. This suggests a potential connection between inflammation and the persistence of CU.[9,10]

## CONCLUSION

Chronic urticaria is commonly associated with many comorbid diseases, including autoimmune disorders, psychiatric and mental illnesses. Other associated disorders include cardiovascular diseases like obesity and hypertension. Although the underlying pathophysiological mechanism responsible for the associated metabolic comorbid diseases in not known, however, this link might be related to autoinflammatory pathways.

## REFERENCES

1. Thomsen SF, Pritzier EC, Anderson CD, Vaugelade-Baust N, Dodge R, Dahlborn AK, et al. Chronic urticaria in the real-life clinical practice setting in Sweden, Norway and Denmark: baseline results from the non-interventional multicentre AWARE study. J Eur Acad Dermatol Venereol. 2017;31(6):1048-55.
2. Kolkhir P, Muñoz M, Asero R, Ferrer M, Kocatürk E, Metz M, et al. Autoimmune chronic spontaneous urticaria. J Allergy Clin Immunol. 2022;149(6):1819-31.
3. Papapostolou N, Xepadaki P, Katoulis A, Makris M. Comorbidities of chronic urticaria: Aglimse into a complex relationship. Front Allergy. 2022;3:1008145.
4. Zuberbier T, Abdul Latiff AH, Abuzakouk M, Aquilina S, Asero R, Baker D, et al. The international EAACI/GA²LEN/EuroGuiDerm/APAAACI guideline for the definition, classification, diagnosis, and management of urticaria. Allergy. 2022;77(3):734-66.
5. Kolkhir P, Altrichter S, Asero R, Daschner A, Ferrer M, Giménez-Arnau A, et al. Autoimmune diseases are linked to type IIb autoimmune chronic spontaneous Urticaria. Allergy Asthma Immunol Res. 2021;13(4):545-59.
6. Thomsen SF, Pritzier EC, Anderson CD, Vaugelade-Baust N, Dodge R, Dahlborn AK, et al. Chronic urticaria in the real-life clinical practice setting in Sweden, Norway and Denmark: baseline results from the non-interventional multicentre AWARE study. J Eur Acad Dermatol Venereol. 2017;31(6):1048-55.
7. Konstantinou GN, Konstantinou GN. Psychiatric comorbidity in chronic urticaria patients: a systematic review and meta-analysis. Clin Transl Allergy. 2019;9:42.
8. Ye YM, Jin HJ, Hwang EK, Nam YH, Kim JH, Shin YS, et al. Co-existence of chronic urticaria and metabolic syndrome: clinical implications. Acta Derm Venereol. 2013;93(2):156-60.
9. Chu CY, Cho YT, Jiang JH, Lin EI, Tang CH. Epidemiology and comorbidities of patients with chronic urticaria in Taiwan: a nationwide population-based study. J Dermatol Sci. 2017;88(2):192-8.
10. Xiao M, Zhang X, Guo A, Zhang K, Zhao Q, Fan L, et al. A Retrospective Cohort Study on the Comorbidity in 19,264 Chinese Patients of Different Ages with Urticaria. Acta Derm Venereol. 2024;104:adv24050.

SECTION

2

# Atopic Dermatitis

**Section Editors:** Abhishek De and Disha Chakraborty

2.1

CHAPTER

# Clinical Features and Classification of Atopic Dermatitis

***Disha Chakraborty, Shrayan Pal***

## INTRODUCTION

Atopic dermatitis (AD), also known as atopic eczema (AE), is a disorder that is challenging to describe accurately due to its varied clinical symptoms and absence of a diagnostic test.

Atopic eczema is a skin condition characterized by itching, chronic inflammation, or recurrent inflammation that typically begins in early childhood, usually before the age of two **(Table 1)**.

Other associated features seen are:
- Macular erythema
- Papules or papulovesicles as a hallmark feature of eczema

**TABLE 1: Hallmark essential feature of atopic dermatitis (AD).**

| Symptom | Description | Factors influencing the symptoms and essential features |
|---|---|---|
| *Primary symptom/first necessary component* | | |
| Itching, or pruritus | • Rubbing and scratching make the patient's itching worse<br>• During the night it aggravates, but scratching while sleeping has no conscious control, which makes AD worse | Factors that increase worsen or trigger the itching:<br>• Heat and sweat (96%)<br>• Wool clothings (91%)<br>• Emotional stress (81%)<br>• Specific foods (44%)<br>• Upper respiratory illnesses (36%)<br>• House dust mites (>35%) |
| *Additional components/symptoms* | | |
| Sensitivity of surrounding skin | The skin areas all over the body, independent of inflammation | Reflexively reacting (alloknesis) to external stimuli like light, may lead to the polymorphic light eruption (PMLE) |
| Pityriasis alba | Red, scaly patches that eventually disappear and leave behind areas of hypopigmentation, usually at the face, upper limbs, and trunk | It may become more noticeable when exposed to sunlight as the surrounding skin tans |
| Keratosis pilaris | Dead skin cell plugs cause small bumps on the skin—"plucked chicken skin"—looking skin on their thighs, buttocks, cheeks, and upper arms | |
| Ichthyosis vulgaris | They look like "fish scales," typically observed on the lower limbs; however, they can also affect other areas | • 50% association with AD<br>• Linked to an earlier onset and more severe AD |
| Dermatographism | Scratching the skin causes a crimson, elevated wheal that develops five minutes after stimulation and can last up to thirty minutes | Can be a part of inducible urticaria associated with AD |

- Eczematous areas with crusting
- Lichenification and excoriation
- Hyper- or hypopigmentation followed by the chronic inflammatory response
- Dryness of the skin due to impaired barrier function
- *Secondary infection*: Usually, precipitated by repeated itching causing inoculation of infections and damage of the skin, along with an already damaged barrier function of the skin.

## CLASSIFICATION BASED ON CLINICAL PHASES OF ATOPIC DERMATITIS

The wide range of symptoms associated with AD varies based on the patient's age. It is separated into stages: infancy, childhood, and adolescence/adulthood. Every stage of the condition can cause individuals to acquire extremely itchy and frequently excoriated acute, subacute, and chronic eczematous lesions. Acute lesions, more commonly seen in infantile AD, are characterized by erythematous, edematous papules and plaques that may include serous crusting, vesiculation, or oozing. Lesions with subacute eczema exhibit varied crusting, scaling, and erythema. Adolescent and adult AD are characterized by chronic lesions that appear as thicker plaques with lichenification and scale; prurigo nodule-like lesions can also form. Patients with African or Asian ancestry are more likely to get papular eczema, which is characterized by tiny, flat-topped papules and perifollicular accentuation. The most severely affected patients in any stage of AD may develop a generalized exfoliative erythroderma **(Table 2)**. After resolution, lesions of any kind including AD might result in postinflammatory hyper-, hypo-, or sporadically depigmentation.[1,2]

## SUBTYPES BASED ON DISEASE PERSISTENCE PATTERN[4]

The disease course of AD is characterized by a pattern rather than being static in addition to the clinical phases.

**TABLE 2: Classification of atopic dermatitis according to age.[5,6]**

| Phase | Clinical features | Associations |
|---|---|---|
| Infantile phase (<2 years) | • Usually starting at the second month of life<br>• Most commonly begin on the face (>90% of children with AD had facial involvement during the first 6 months of life),[3] and usually spares the napkin area<br>• Exposed surfaces, particularly the extensor portion of the knees and elbows, are most affected as the kid starts to crawl<br>• Erythema and discrete or confluent edematous, very inflamed papules seen with oozing and crusting in the lesions<br>• Protracted, fluctuating course that is influenced by things, such as teething, respiratory infections, emotional disturbances, and humidity fluctuations[2] | • Lymphadenopathy<br>• Secondary infection |
| Childhood phase (2–12 years) | • Reticulate pigmentation on the sides of the neck can be rather noticeable; this condition is frequently called "atopic dirty neck"<br>• Even after extended rubbing, some AE patients may not lichenify<br>• Patients who develop eczema in later childhood with an extensor distribution are rare and may require more time for remission[1]<br>This distribution is more prevalent in children who are Asian or Black | |
| Adult phase (>12 years) | • Lichenified appearance particularly on the hands and flexures<br>• Isolated patches of AE on the nipples, especially in young and adolescent females<br>• Vermilion of the lips and surrounding skin involvement<br>• Follicular lichenified papules (Blacks and Japanese people are more likely to have)<br>• Hands often develop a more diffuse, chronic lichenified eczema. Foot involvement is also typical[2] | Photosensitivity |
| Senile phase (>60 years) | • Distinguished by pronounced xerosis<br>• The majority of these individuals lack the lichenified flexural lesions that are typical of AD in younger people and children<br>• Severe negative effects on their quality of life, including sleep difficulties, psychological discomfort, social isolation, disruptions in family relations, and decreased functioning at work or school due to extreme pruritus and stigmatization[1] | |

In a 2004 study, the illness course was examined, and AD fit into one of three disease patterns:

1. Remission (43%; no AD after the age of 2 years)
2. Intermittent (38%; early AD not meeting persistent or remission criteria)
3. Persistent (19%; AD at every follow-up until age 7 years).[5]

The clinical phenotypes and their corresponding AD subtypes are outlined in **Table 3**.[5-7]

## ROLE OF FOOD ALLERGY

The intricate relationship between food allergies and AD is evident in the shifting perspectives on the function of foods in the disease. A third to half of kids with moderate-to-severe AD have dietary sensitivities.

However, 85% of children with AD will have raised immunoglobulin E (IgE) to food or inhalant allergens, and because of the high false-positive rate of testing, diagnosing food allergy with serum or prick tests alone can be difficult. Treatment for AD should be optimized before testing for food allergies. When a child's AD may be treated with the right topical treatments, parents frequently look for a "cause" for it. Food restriction diets can be challenging, put the child in danger of malnutrition, and may even cause the development of an allergy, and should never be followed without the supervision of a nutritionist and allergist to guarantee enough nutrition. Only younger children with moderate-to-severe AD who have not responded to traditional therapies should have their food allergies investigated. Additionally, there should be a history of food exposures that may have contributed to the development of AD in these kids. If testing is done, it should focus on foods that the kid is likely to be exposed to; the most relevant foods to AD have historically been found to be wheat, eggs, soy, cow's milk, and peanuts.

A child's AD is most likely not causally related to a positive skin prick or RAST test result for food that the youngster consumes infrequently or never. Greater susceptibility to responding to these foods when challenged is linked to higher blood IgE levels and larger wheal diameters (>8–10 mm). Only a few items, as follows, are responsible for about 90% of food allergies:

- *Infants and children < 2 years old*: Eggs, soybeans, wheat, and cow's milk.
- *Children (2–10 years old)*: Fish, crustacean shellfish, sesame, kiwi fruit, peanuts, tree nuts, and cow's milk.
- *Older children (>10 years)*: Meals containing peanuts, tree nuts, seafood, shellfish, sesame, and pollen.[6]

In **Table 4** we have described the atypical forms of AD.[7-20]

**TABLE 3: Clinical phenotypes and related atopic dermatitis (AD) subtypes (extrinsic/intrinsic).[5-7]**

| Clinical manifestations | Related subtypes (mostly extrinsic/intrinsic) |
|---|---|
| Ichthyosis vulgaris | Mostly extrinsic |
| Palmar hyperlinearity | Mostly extrinsic |
| Hand eczema/Paronychia | Mostly extrinsic |
| Hertoghe's sign | Mostly extrinsic |
| Dennie–Morgan folds | Mostly intrinsic |
| Lichen amyloidosis | Mostly extrinsic |
| Vitiligo (leukoderma) | Mostly extrinsic |
| Chondrodermatitis of auricle | Mostly extrinsic |
| Angiohistiocytoid papule | Mostly extrinsic |
| Metal allergy | Mostly intrinsic |
| Food allergy | Mostly extrinsic |
| Cutaneous infection | Mostly extrinsic |
| Senior (asteatotic) eczema | Mostly extrinsic |

**TABLE 4: Atypical forms of atopic dermatitis.[7-20]**

| Atypical form | Salient features | Associations |
|---|---|---|
| Lichenoid atopic dermatitis | • Erythematous, flat-topped, itchy, heavily pigmented, and nonviolaceous papules that frequently occur along the upper and lower extremities, at extensor aspects<br>• To differentiate it from lichen planus, a biopsy could be needed[7] | |
| Juvenile plantar dermatosis | The presence of glossy, erythematous, intensely itchy plaques on the toes' soles and plantar surfaces (particularly the first toe) in school-going children[7] | Coexistence of hyperhidrosis and/or the use of occlusive footwear, such as plastic shoes, which can aggravate the condition and/or cause flare-ups[8] |

*Continued*

*Continued*

| Atypical form | Salient features | Associations |
|---|---|---|
| Nummular eczema | • Red, oozing, nummular, or annular plaques with excoriations and studded pustules across the extensor extremities, particularly the wrists and ankles[7]<br>• Hyperpigmentation may be seen<br>• Commonly noticed over the hands, feet, and over face less frequently<br>• This condition, only in the context of more typical atopic dermatitis symptoms, can be classified as nummular type atopic dermatitis[8] | • Frequently observed in individuals of color<br>• Childhood nummular dermatitis can be triggered by molluscum[9] and/or allergic contact dermatitis.[10] |
| Follicular atopic dermatitis | Parents report that their child is extremely itchy without any eczematous changes. However, on examination, the child has bilateral follicular prominence over their entire chest, back, abdomen, and proximal extremities, covering a significant amount of their body surface area[8] | This has been connected to adult-onset intrinsic type atopic dermatitis (also known as atopiform dermatitis)[9] |
| Alopecia associated with atopic dermatitis | This is usually on the edges of the scalp and happens when there is concomitant xerosis of the hair shaft, a frequent childhood symptom, and scalp atopic dermatitis or other dermatoses[11,12] | Observed in children with Netherton's disease in the context of atopic dermatitis because of the fragility of the bamboo hairs (trichorrhexis invaginata)[13] |
| Eczema coxsackium | • Eczema coxsackium is characterized by eczematous plaques studded with pustules and erosions. Pseudocubital and popliteal fossae, as well as the areas above the extremities, are common locations<br>• A diffuse vesiculobullous eruption will also be experienced by the patients<br>• There are palmoplantar purpuric papules, and acral illness is more common in children under two[15] | It is observed in children with AD who get coxsackie infections[14] |
| Psoriasiform atopic dermatitis | This condition, which affects 5% of children, is known as psoriasiform atopic dermatitis. Alternatively, it may be psoriasiform contact dermatitis in the context of atopic dermatitis (often identified by biopsying a case of atopic dermatitis that is resistant to treatment). When diagnosed, psoriasiform involvement is frequently observed in the diaper area and scalp, and it may run in the family. Asian children and/or adults are frequently diagnosed with psoriasiform atopic dermatitis. Similar to atopic dermatitis, psoriasiform dermatitis may be linked to a decrease in the skin's production of ceramides.[16] Basic science studies have recently shown that these people truly have TH17 and TH2 signaling,[17] which plays a role in the development of both disorders. Topical therapies are not effective in treating these people[16] | |
| Perianal bacterial dermatitis | Diaper-covered areas of the buttocks and perianal area are known as perianal bacterial dermatitis, which is a kind of atopic dermatitis. A number of factors, including xerosis, discomfort from leftover stool, forceful cleaning, and contact with staph and strep in a group or school environment, can cause children to experience this eruption during potty training. Reports have been made of adult instances. Unlike group A strep or *Staphylococcus aureus*, which have been reported in childhood, cases are typically linked to group B strep in adults. In the perianal region, the surrounding buttocks, and the inside parts of the thighs, the condition manifests as erythematous plaques. There are visible excoriations, erosions, and maceration[18] | |
| Lip licker's dermatitis | When atopic dermatitis manifests in the lips and surrounding skin, perioral lesions can be observed (Hanifin and Rajka minor criteria include cheilitis). Lip licking exacerbates the latter, resulting in a well-marginated plaque with lichenification and dermatitis on the lips and surrounding skin. Frequently, the patient is not aware of the habit, which arises when they perceive dryness in their lips. Clearance may be accelerated by generous use of petrolatum-based emollient and a few weeks of midpotency topical corticosteroid treatment twice daily. After lesional clearing, postinflammatory pigmentary change may continue in patients of African American or Black heritage | Food allergies and/or contact dermatitis may be linked to chronic, unrelenting atopic dermatitis, often known as lip licker's dermatitis. Testing appropriateness could be required[19] |

*Continued*

*Continued*

| Atypical form | Salient features | Associations |
|---|---|---|
| Beekeeper distribution | Atopic dermatitis on the head and neck, extending to the V of the chest and back, is known as the "beekeeper distribution" | This distribution is consistent with aeroallergens, such as dust mites, and/or allergies to *Malassezia* species, which colonize the skin of the scalp, face, neck, upper chest, and back. It is linked to head and neck atopic dermatitis, which is more frequently observed in boys. It could be necessary to investigate the allergy status and practice proper dust avoidance[20] |

(TH2: T helper 2; Th17: T helper 17)

## CONCLUSION

Atopic dermatitis presents with a heterogeneous clinical spectrum, influenced by age, genetics, immune dysregulation, and environmental factors. The dynamic interplay of acute flares, chronic lichenification, and site-specific variations underscores the need for a well defined classification system. Emerging phenotypic and endotypic frameworks attempt to bridge clinical presentation with underlying pathophysiology, paving the way for precision medicine approaches. While traditional classifications rely on morphology and distribution, newer paradigms integrate immune signatures, filaggrin mutations, and barrier dysfunction. Recognizing these evolving patterns is crucial for tailoring therapeutic strategies, improving disease stratification, and refining prognostic insights in atopic dermatitis.

## REFERENCES

1. McAleer MA, O'Regan GM, Irvine AD. Atopic Dermatitis. In: Bolognia JL, Schaffer JV, Cerroni L (Eds). Dermatology, 4th edition. Edinburgh: Elsevier; 2018. pp. 208-24.
2. Ardern-Jones MR, Flohr C, Reynolds NJ, Holden CA. Atopic Eczema. In: Griffiths C, Barker J, Bleiker T, Chalmers R, Creamer D (Eds). Rook's Textbook of Dermatology, 9th edition. West Sussex: Wiley-Blackwell; 2016. pp. 41.1-41.34.
3. Eller E, Kjaer HF, Høst A, Andersen KE, Bindslev-Jensen C. Development of atopic dermatitis in the DARC birth cohort. Pediatr Allergy Immunol. 2010;21(2 Pt 1):307-14.
4. Tokura Y, Hayano S. Subtypes of atopic dermatitis: From phenotype to endotype. Allergol Int. 2022;71(1):14-24.
5. Illi S, von Mutius E, Lau S, Nickel R, Grüber C, Niggemann B, et al. The natural course of atopic dermatitis from birth to age 7 years and the association with asthma. J Allergy Clin Immunol. 2004;113(5):925-31.
6. James WD, Elston DM, Treat JR, Rosenbach MA, Neuhaus IM. Eczema, Atopic Dermatitis, and Noninfectious Immunodeficiency Disorders. In: James WD, Elston DM, Treat JR, Rosenbach MA, Neuhaus IM (Eds). Andrew's diseases of the skin, 13th edition. Edinburgh: Elsevier; 2020. pp. 63-73.
7. Julián-Gónzalez RE, Orozco-Covarrubias L, Durán-McKinster C, Palacios-Lopez C, Ruiz-Maldonado R, Sáez-de-Ocariz M. Less common clinical manifestations of atopic dermatitis: prevalence by age. Pediatr Dermatol. 2012;29(5):580-3.
8. Zagne V, Fernandes NC, Cuzzi T. Histopathological aspects of juvenile plantar dermatosis. Am J Dermatopathol. 2014;36(4):359-61.
9. Seize MB, Ianhez M, Cestari Sda C. A study of the correlation between molluscum contagiosum and atopic dermatitis in children. An Bras Dermatol. 2011;86(4):663-8.
10. Bonamonte D, Foti C, Vestita M, Ranieri LD, Angelini G. Nummular eczema and contact allergy: a retrospective study. Dermatitis. 2012;23(4):153-7.
11. Silverberg NB: Chapter 8. Eczematous Eruptions in Atlas of Pediatric Cutaneous Biodiversity. New York; Springer 2004.
12. Kulthanan K, Boochangkool K, Tuchinda P, Chularojanamontri L. Clinical features of the extrinsic and intrinsic types of adult-onset atopic dermatitis. Asia Pac Allergy. 2011;1(12):80-6.
13. Silverberg NB, Silverberg JI, Wong ML. Trichoscopy using a handheld dermoscope: an in-office technique to diagnose genetic disease of the hair. Arch Dermatol. 2009;145(5):600-1.
14. Horsten HH, Fisker N, Bygum A. Eczema Coxsackium Caused by Coxsackievirus A6. Pediatr Dermatol. 2016;33(3):e230-1.
15. Neri I, Dondi A, Wollenberg A, Ricci L, Ricci G, Piccirilli G, et al. Atypical Forms of Hand, Foot, and Mouth Disease: A Prospective Study of 47 Italian Children. Pediatr Dermatol. 2016;33(4):429-37.
16. Kapila S, Hong E, Fischer G. A comparative study of childhood psoriasis and atopic dermatitis and greater understanding of the overlapping condition, psoriasis-dermatitis. Australas J Dermatol. 2012;53(2):98-105.
17. Noda S, Suárez-Fariñas M, Ungar B, Kim SJ, de Guzman Strong C, et al. The Asian atopic dermatitis phenotype combines features of atopic dermatitis and psoriasis with increased TH17 polarization. J Allergy Clin Immunol. 2015;136(5):1254-64.
18. Heath C, Desai N, Silverberg NB. Recent microbiological shifts in perianal bacterial dermatitis: *Staphylococcus aureus* predominance. Pediatr Dermatol. 2009;26(6):696-700.
19. Watt CJ, Hong HC. Dermacase. Lip licker's dermatitis. Can Fam Physician. 2002;48:1051-9.
20. Brodská P, Panzner P, Pizinger K, Schmid-Grendelmeier P. IgE-mediated sensitization to malassezia in atopic dermatitis: more common in male patients and in head and neck type. Dermatitis. 2014;25(3):120-6.

# Clinical Criteria of Atopic Dermatitis Diagnosis

*Disha Chakraborty, Shrayan Pal*

## INTRODUCTION

Atopic dermatitis (AD) is still predominantly diagnosed clinically, using a variety of clinical signs and symptoms such as pruritus, the presence and location of skin lesions, and a personal or family history of atopic diseases to aid in the diagnosis. Several well-respected sets of criteria have been developed in recent decades to facilitate diagnosis. There is a need to refine our understanding of AD's clinical features and further clarify and solidify the current diagnostic criteria in light of the condition's rising awareness and the recent development of systemic immunomodulators as a treatment.

## HANNIFIN AND RAJKA CRITERIA

The 1980 Hanifin and Rajka criteria, which demand that three of the four major criteria and three of the twenty-three minor criteria be satisfied, are among the oldest and most well-known sets of diagnostic criteria **(Table 1)**.[1]

## UK REFINEMENT OF HANIFIN AND RAJKA'S DIAGNOSTIC CRITERIA OF ATOPIC DERMATITIS

In order to qualify as a case of AD (eczema) with the UK diagnostic criteria,[2] the child must have:

- An itchy skin condition (or parental report of scratching or rubbing in a child)
- Plus, three or more of the following:
  i. Onset below the age of 2 years (not used if a child is under 4 years)
  ii. History of skin crease involvement (including cheeks in children under 10 years)
  iii. History of a generally dry skin

**TABLE 1: Hannifin and Rajka criteria.**

| | |
|---|---|
| Major features (three out of four required) | Pruritus |
| | Typical morphology and distribution:<br>• Flexural lichenification or linearity in adults<br>• Facial and extensor involvement in infants and children |
| | Chronic or chronically relapsing dermatitis |
| | Personal or family history of atopy, such as asthma, allergic rhinitis, and atopic dermatitis |
| | Xerosis |
| Minor features (three out of 23 required) | Ichthyosis/palmar hyperlinearity/keratosis pilaris |
| | Immediate (type 1) skin test reactivity |
| | Elevated serum immunoglobulin E |
| | Early age of onset |
| | A tendency toward cutaneous infections (*Staphylococcus aureus* and Herpes simplex virus)/impaired, cell-mediated immunity |
| | A tendency toward nonspecific hand or foot dermatitis |
| | Nipple eczema |
| | Recurrent conjunctivitis |
| | Dennie–Morgan infraorbital fold |
| | Anterior subcapsular cataract |
| | Orbital darkening and keratoconus |
| | Facial pallor/facial erythema |
| | Pityriasis alba |
| | Anterior neck fold |
| | Itch when sweating |

*Continued*

*Continued*

| | |
|---|---|
| Minor features (three out of 23 required) | Intolerance to wool and lipid solvents |
| | Perifollicular accentuation |
| | Food intolerance |
| | Course influence by environmental/ emotional factors |
| | White dermographism/delayed blanch |

iv. Personal history of other atopic diseases (or history of any atopic disease in a first-degree relative in children under 4 years)
v. Visible flexural dermatitis (or dermatitis of cheeks/ forehead and outer limbs in children under 4 years)

## MILLENNIUM CRITERIA

To further streamline and reduce the Hanifin and Rajka as well as the UK Working Party criteria into a set that would identify and diagnose patients with actual AD, Bos and colleagues initially presented the Millennium criteria in 1998. It was the initial criterion to incorporate allergen-specific immunoglobulin E (IgE) as a diagnostic characteristic.[3]

The Millennium criteria, which were further improved and validated by Schram and associates in 2011, state that five factors:

- Typical morphology
- Early age of onset
- Dennie–Morgan infraorbital skin fold
- History of flexural involvement
- Visible flexural eczema

These must be met to correctly identify AD patients.

The authors conducted a comparison between their improved criteria and the UK Working Party and Hanifin and Rajka criteria in a group of 210 outpatients for whom an AD diagnosis was taken into consideration throughout the differential diagnostic process. Compared to the Hanifin and Rajka criteria, which are 100% and 48.8%, respectively, and the UK criteria, which are 97.7% and 72.9%, the Millennium criteria demonstrated a sensitivity of 81.8% and a specificity of 98.8%.[4]

## CONCLUSION

The clinical diagnosis of atopic dermatitis hinges on well-defined yet evolving criteria, balancing specificity and sensitivity across diverse patient populations. Traditional frameworks, such as the Hanifin and Rajka criteria, remain foundational, yet refinements incorporating age-dependent manifestations, ethnic variations, and biomarker-driven insights enhance diagnostic precision. The integration of minor features, comorbidities, and disease chronicity into newer models reflects a shift toward holistic patient assessment. As understanding of the disease advances, refining clinical criteria to align with emerging immunophenotypes and predictive markers will be pivotal in optimizing diagnosis, guiding treatment decisions, and improving patient outcomes.

## REFERENCES

1. Dutta A, De A, Das S, Banerjee S, Kar C, Dhar S. A Cross-sectional Evaluation of the Usefulness of the Minor Features of Hanifin and Rajka Diagnostic Criteria for the Diagnosis of Atopic Dermatitis in the Pediatric Population. Indian J Dermatol. 2021;66(6):583-90.
2. Rudzki E, Samochocki Z, Rebandel P, Saciuk E, Gałecki W, Rączka A, et al. Frequency and significance of the major and minor features of Hanifin and Rajka among patients with atopic dermatitis. Dermatology. 1994;189(1):41-6.
3. Bos JD, Van Leent EJ, Smitt SJH. The millennium criteria for the diagnosis of atopic dermatitis. Exp Dermatol. 1998;7(4):132-8.
4. Schram ME, Leeflang MM, DEN Ottolander JP, Spuls PI, Bos JD. Validation and refinement of the millennium criteria for atopic dermatitis. J Dermatol. 2011;38(9):850-8.

CHAPTER 2.3

# Differential Diagnosis in Atopic Dermatitis

*SK Shahriar Ahmed, Disha Chakraborty*

## INTRODUCTION

Atopic dermatitis exhibits broad clinical variability, often overlapping with other inflammatory, infectious, and genetic dermatoses, making accurate diagnosis a challenge. The differentiation from psoriasis, seborrheic dermatitis, contact dermatitis, immunodeficiencies, and rare genodermatoses requires a comprehensive assessment of morphology, distribution, chronicity, and patient history. Advancements in biomarkers, immunophenotyping, and genetic profiling are refining diagnostic precision, yet clinical acumen remains central. A systematic approach integrating cutaneous findings, systemic associations, and response to treatment is essential to distinguish atopic dermatitis from its mimickers, ensuring timely and appropriate management.

## DIFFERENTIAL DIAGNOSIS IN ATOPIC DERMATITIS

Atopic dermatitis can have a variable range of clinical presentation. The differential diagnosis of each presentation is listed in **Table 1**.[1]

### Differential Diagnosis of Eczematous Rash All Over the Body

- *Allergic contact dermatitis (CD)*: There could be a generalized or localized itchy rash along with dry, cracked, scaly skin with poorly defined borders and sometimes bumps and blisters, oozing, and crusting. A patch test is the most reliable investigation for the identification of the compound.
- *Irritant contact dermatitis*: The usual symptoms of acute irritant CD include erythema, blisters, pustules, hemorrhage, crusts, scales, erosions, and even pruritus or discomfort. The majority of skin lesions in

**TABLE 1: Differential diagnosis of different presentations in atopic dermatitis.**

| Presentation | Differential diagnosis |
|---|---|
| Eczematous rash all over the body | • Allergic contact dermatitis<br>• Irritant contact dermatitis<br>• Photoallergic contact dermatitis<br>• Seborrheic dermatitis<br>• Id reaction<br>• Scabies<br>• Erythroderma<br>• Disseminated dermatophytosis<br>• Dermatomyositis<br>• Viral exanthem<br>• Drug rash |
| Flexural lichenification | • Inverse psoriasis<br>• Seborrheic dermatitis<br>• Candidiasis<br>• Intertrigo<br>• Allergic/irritant contact dermatitis<br>• Langerhans cell histiocytosis<br>• Perianal dermatitis<br>• Tinea cruris<br>• Diaper dermatitis<br>• Erythrasma |
| Discoid eczema/ Nummular eczema | • Dyshidrotic eczema/a steatotic eczema<br>• Lichen simplex chronicus<br>• Chronic plaque psoriasis<br>• Stasis dermatitis<br>• Lichen aureus<br>• Tinea corporis<br>• Impetigo<br>• Granuloma annulare |

*Continued*

*Continued*

| | |
|---|---|
| Generalized xerosis | • Leprosy<br>• Sarcoidosis<br>• Hypothyroidism<br>• Hypopituitarism<br>• Cutaneous T-cell lymphoma<br>• Drugs (hypolipidemic drugs, clofazimine, and INH)<br>• HIV infection<br>• Malnutrition<br>• Essential fatty acid deficiency<br>• Graft-versus-host disease<br>• Scleroderma<br>• Ichthyosis |
| Pityriasis Alba | • Vitiligo<br>• Tuberculoid leprosy<br>• Seborrheic dermatitis<br>• Polymorphous light eruption<br>• Pityriasis versicolor<br>• Postinflammatory hypopigmentation<br>• Nevus depigmentosus<br>• Nevus anemicus |
| Keratosis pilaris | • Follicular lichen planus<br>• Pityriasis rubra pilaris<br>• Lichen spinulosus<br>• Lichen scrofulosorum<br>• Lichen nitidus<br>• Phrynoderma |
| Hand/Foot eczema | • Allergic/cumulative irritant contact dermatitis<br>• Psoriasis<br>• Lichen planus<br>• Pityriasis rubra pilaris<br>• Scabies<br>• Tinea manuum/pedis<br>• Pompholyx<br>• Id reaction<br>• Palmoplanter pustulosis |
| Associated with systemic disease/syndrome | • Wiscott–Aldrich syndrome<br>• Agammaglobulinemia<br>• Job's syndrome<br>• Omenn syndrome<br>• Leiner's disease<br>• Acrodermatitis enteropathica<br>• Phenylketonuria<br>• Hartnup disease<br>• Hurler syndrome |

(INH: isoniazid; HIV: human immunodeficiency virus)

cases of acute irritant CD are asymmetric and have strong borders around the sites of contact; distant dissemination is not common.

- *Photoallergic/phototoxic contact dermatitis*: Erythema, itching, pain, burning sensation, and blisters can be present. Phototoxic dermatitis is confined only to photoexposed sites having a well-defined sharp margin, unlike photoallergic dermatitis.
- *Seborrheic dermatitis*: Commonly presents as patches of greasy skin covered with flaky white or yellow scales or crust on the scalp, hair, eyebrows, beard or mustache, sides of the nose, ears, eyelids, chest, armpits, groin area, or under the breasts. Extensive generalized seborrheic dermatitis could be a feature of immunodeficiency.
- *Id reaction*: It is a type of secondary inflammatory reaction that develops from a remote localized immunological insult. It presents as acute onset of an extremely pruritic, erythematous, morbilliform, or papulovesicular eruption that occurs 1–2 weeks after primary infection along with vesicles that may be present on the hands or feet.
- *Scabies*: It may present as a generalized rash along with papules, nodules, oozing, crusting, and secondary impetiginization. Classical distribution is along the circle of Hebra. The itching is often severe and usually worse at night.
- *Erythroderma*: Erythema and scaling that covers > 90% of the body. Psoriasis (23%), atopic dermatitis, CD, pityriasis rubra pilaris, drug reaction, dermatophytosis, scabies, human immunodeficiency virus (HIV), and idiopathic are the most common causes of erythroderma.
- *Disseminated dermatophytosis*: Due to certain host and environmental factors dermatophytosis may present as multiple plaques with extensive involvement of skin with scaling and erythema. Few lesions could be found with classical central clearing and peripheral extension.
- *Dermatomyositis*: The classical rash is confluent macular violaceous erythema that may be missing in Indian skin. Gottron's sign, V sign, shawl sign, heliotrope rash, and Holster sign could be present along with variable degrees of muscle weakness.
- *Viral exanthem*: Generalized morbilliform rash along with fever and enanthem could be present in different viral infections such as measles, dengue, coronavirus disease 2019 (COVID-19), and HIV infection. Mostly the rash starts from the face and the palm/sole remains uninvolved.
- *Drug rash*: Itchy morbilliform rash that starts mostly from the acral part of the body. The face generally remains uninvolved unless DRESS.[1,2]

## Differential Diagnosis of Flexural Lichenification

- *Inverse psoriasis*: At the groin, it presents mostly a confluent patch. Due to moisture, the classical scaling may be absent. Searching for psoriatic plaque in other parts of the body is important.
- *Seborrheic dermatitis*: In infants, it can present at the groin and is very difficult to differentiate from candidiasis or dermatitis.
- *Candidiasis*: It is very common in neonates and infants. It mostly occurs over the neck, groin, or axillary area. Multiple pustules, satellite lesions, and fringing of scale can provide clues.
- *Intertrigo*: It is an inflammatory dermatosis affecting the flexural areas, aggravated by high temperatures, dampness, friction, maceration, and inadequate ventilation. Often it becomes secondarily infected by bacteria or fungus.
- *Langerhans cell histiocytosis*: Skin rash along with crusted or scaly nodules and papules, blisters which can affect the intertriginous areas in infants and children. Purpuric spots are the clue for suspicion. Examination of bones and lymph nodes is very important.
- *Perianal dermatitis*: It is a superficial inflammation of the perianal skin caused by group A beta-hemolytic streptococci among infants and children. It presents as perianal pain, painful defecation with consequent retentive constipation, blood-streaked stools anal fissures.
- *Tinea cruris*: A definite border with peripheral papules could provide a clue unless the morphology is not altered by the application of topical steroids. A family history of dermatophytosis is crucial.
- *Diaper dermatitis*: It is an inflammatory reaction of the skin of the perineal and perianal areas that occurs due to increased moisture, and prolonged contact with urine or feces. Whereas, atopic rash generally does not involve the groin due to increased moisture.
- *Erythrasma*: It presents as brown hyperpigmented asymptomatic patches over flexural areas. The lesion is mostly confluent and coral-pink fluorescence during Wood lamp examination is confirmatory.[3]

## Differential Diagnosis of Discoid Eczema/ Nummular Eczema

- *Dyshidrotic eczema/asteatotic eczema*: It presents as circumscribed plaque along with scaling, fissuring, and crusted vesicles in between. Xerosis over the surrounding area could be an important clue.
- *Lichen simplex chronicus*: The classical triad of skin thickening, increased skin marking, and hyperpigmentation is a classical presentation along with a history of severe itching.
- *Chronic plaque psoriasis*: It presents as a well-defined plaque with classical silvery scaling and erythema. Clinically Auspitz's sign and Grattage test will be positive.
- *Stasis dermatitis*: It presents over the lower limb along with varicose veins and lipodermatosclerosis.
- *Lichen aureus*: It is a subtype of pigmented purpuric dermatosis. It presents as persistent asymptomatic rust-colored plaques or patches over the lower extremities in children or young adults.
- *Impetigo*: The honey-colored crust or the ruptured bulla sometimes forms an annular configuration which builds confusion.
- *Granuloma annulare*: It presents as an infiltrated plaque with no scaling at the center and beaded papules at the periphery. Necrobiotic palisading granuloma in histopathology confirms the diagnosis.[3-5]

## Differential Diagnosis of Pityriasis Alba

- *Vitiligo*: It presents as milky-white depigmented patches with sharp borders, whereas Pityriasis alba is characterized by ill-defined patches, typically circular or oval, often with mild scaling and occasional pruritus.
- *Tuberculoid leprosy*: The lesion may be hypopigmented with xerosis, loss of hair, and loss of sensation. So, checking sensation is very important for any hypopigmented lesion.
- *Seborrheic dermatitis*: It could also present as hypopigmented scaly patches over the face. It generally occurs in infants from 2 weeks to 2 years. Checking of cradle cap and other seborrheic areas of the face such as over the eyebrows, side of the nose, and mouth is also important.
- *Polymorphous light eruption*: It has a variable presentation. But if presented as a hypopigmented patch over the face it would be itchy, and scaly with ill-defined borders.
- *Pityriasis versicolor*: It could be hypopigmented with well-defined circular macules over the face, and few of them coalesce to form a polycyclic lesion. Involvement of the angle of the nose is very common.
- *Postinflammatory hypopigmentation*: It presents as hypopigmented patches with no scaling and itching, which generally occurs after certain inflammatory dermatosis.

- *Nevus depigmentosus*: It is a congenital, nonprogressive, hypopigmented macule or patch with a serrated margin that remains relatively constant in terms of size and distribution throughout a lifetime.
- *Nevus anemicus*: It is a congenital hypopigmented cutaneous macules and/or patches. Reactive erythema is typically not produced by lesional skin in reaction to trauma, heat, or cold. Diascopy can be carried out by applying pressure to the lesion's edge with a glass slide, which will make the lesion's edge blend in with the surrounding skin.[6]

## Differential Diagnosis of Keratosis Pilaris

- *Follicular lichen planus*: It is a variant of lichen planopilaris (LP) involving the hair follicles with a lichenoid hue. When it involves the scalp it is called lichen planopilaris. It can also present as Graham Little–Piccardi–Lassueur syndrome. Scalp, oral mucosa, axilla, and nail are the important sites to be examined.
- *Pityriasis rubra pilaris*: It is characterized by waxy yellow follicular hyperkeratotic papules with palmoplantar keratoderma and erythroderma with islands of sparing.
- *Lichen spinulosus*: It is most common among children and adolescents. It presents as multiple tiny skin-colored follicular papules with keratotic horny rough spines of 1–3 mm in size with a sandpaper-like appearance grouped within a plaque of 2–5 cm in diameter.
- *Lichen scrofulosorum*: It is a type of tuberculid clinically characterized by multiple asymptomatic, closely clustered, skin-colored to reddish-brown mostly extrafollicular papules primarily distributed on the back, abdomen, chest, and proximal limbs.
- *Lichen nitidus*: It presents as asymptomatic, shiny, flat-topped, fleshy pink to dark brown papules of 1–2 mm in diameter. Among males, the most common site is the penile shaft. It can also be present over the neck, trunk, limbs, abdomen, mucosa, and palm sole. Koebner phenomenon is a clinical hallmark and "ball-in-clutch" appearance is a histopathological hallmark of lichen nitidus.
- *Phrynoderma*: It is due to nutritional deficiency which presents as red-brown follicular papules with a central keratotic spine. Lesions tend to be distributed symmetrically and are often localized to the elbows, knees, extensor extremities, and/or buttocks.
- *Keratosis pilaris*: It presents as multiple discrete noninflammatory tiny shiny follicular papules present on the upper thighs and arms with little to no tendency to group.[3,4]

## Differential Diagnosis Palmoplantar Eczema

When presents as palmoplantar keratoderma:

- *Allergic/cumulative irritant CD*: Generally, presents with ill-defined border confined to palm-sole; along with more history of itching and oozing with vesicle formation than scaling and fissuring.
- *Psoriasis*: It presents mostly with well dry scaly demarcated plaque with fissuring and no history of oozing. Involvement of other parts of the body along with knuckles is characteristic.
- *Lichen planus*: Palmoplantar LP is very difficult to diagnose unless LP presents to another part of the body as it does not present with any classical morphology or color of LP. Histopathology should clinch the diagnosis.
- *Pityriasis rubra pilaris*: It presents primarily as palmoplantar erythema, then it forms keratoderma. Yellowish follicular papules at another part of the body along with the involvement of the elbow and knee are characteristic.
- *Tinea manuum/pedis*: Asymmetric involvement over one palm or sole or involvement of two feet and one hand is the clue. We have to look for fringing of scales at the border, and involvement of tinea at other places along with onychomycosis.

*When presents as papules/vesicles/pustules:*

- *Crusted scabies*: Classical distribution is along the circle of Hebra and borrows are very important for diagnosis.
- *Pompholyx*: It presents as crops of clear itchy fluid-filled vesicles or bulla that with symmetrical distribution over the palm and sole as well as the lateral aspects of fingers and toes. Vesicles typically resolve without rupturing, followed by desquamation.
- *Palmoplantar pustulosis*: It presents as bilateral, symmetric dermatosis that consists of pustular lesions typically limited to the palms and/or soles that appear on an erythematous-squamous background.

Atopic dermatitis with syndromes are discussed in **Table 2.**[6,7]

**TABLE 2: Atopic dermatitis with syndromes.[6,7]**

| | Inheritance pattern | Gene responsible | Clinical features other than eczema |
|---|---|---|---|
| Wiscott–Aldrich syndrome | X-linked recessive | *WAS* gene | • Thrombocytopenia frequent bleeding and bruising<br>• Bloody diarrhea<br>• Recurrent respiratory infections |
| Agammaglobulinemia | X-linked recessive | *Bruton tyrosine kinase* (*BTK*) gene | • Life-threatening viral/bacterial infection<br>• Atrophied tonsils<br>• No lymphadenopathy |
| Job's syndrome | Autosomal dominant | *STAT3* | • Recurrent skin and pulmonary bacterial infections<br>• Mucocutaneous candidiasis<br>• Facial asymmetry, prominent forehead, deep-set eyes, and broad nasal bridge<br>• Hyperextensibility of the joints<br>• Dental anomaly<br>• Aneurysms |
| Omenn syndrome | Autosomal recessive | *RAG-1* and *RAG-2* | • Life-threatening bacterial, viral and fungal infections<br>• Erythroderma<br>• Diarrhea<br>• Failure to thrive<br>• Hepatosplenomegaly<br>• Generalized lymphadenopathy |
| Leiner's disease | Autosomal dominant | *Dysfunctional complement protein 5* gene | • Seborrheic-like erythroderma<br>• Persistent gastrointestinal disturbance<br>• Wasting and weight loss<br>• Recurrent staphylococcal and candidal infections |
| Acrodermatitis enteropathica | Autosomal recessive | Zinc transporter gene *SLC39A4* | • Periorificial sharply-demarcated, dry, scaly erythematous plaques<br>• Brittle, dry, and lusterless hair<br>• Angular cheilitis<br>• Delayed wound healing<br>• Diarrhea<br>• Growth retardation |
| Phenylketonuria | Autosomal recessive | *Phenylalanine hydroxylase* (*PAH*) gene | • Musty odor in the breath, skin, or urine<br>• Lighter skin, hair, and eye color<br>• Microcephaly<br>• Delayed development<br>• Mental disorders, seizures |
| Hartnup disease | Autosomal recessive | *SLC6A19* is a gene | • Photosensitive pellagra-like skin rash<br>• Cerebellar ataxia<br>• Anxiety<br>• Depression<br>• Mild intellectual disability |
| Hurler syndrome | Autosomal recessive | *Alpha-L-iduronidase enzyme* gene | • Developmental delay<br>• Joint stiffness and contractures<br>• Short stature<br>• Ear, sinus, and pulmonary infections<br>• Cardiac and hepatic disease<br>• Coarse facies |

## CONCLUSION

The differential diagnosis of atopic dermatitis demands careful clinical evaluation to avoid misdiagnosis and inappropriate treatment. Overlapping features with psoriasiform, eczematous, infectious, and immunodeficiency-related conditions necessitate a structured, evidence-basedapproach incorporating history, morphology, and emerging diagnostic tools. As dermatology moves toward precision medicine, refining diagnostic algorithms through biomarkers and molecular profiling will enhance differentiation, leading to more tailored therapeutic strategies and improved patient outcomes.

## REFERENCES

1. Son JH, Chung BY, Kim HO, Park CW. Clinical Features of Atopic Dermatitis in Adults are Different according to Onset. J Korean Med Sci. 2017;32(8):1360-6.
2. Foti C, Bonamonte D, Cassano N, Vena GA, Angelini G. Photoallergic contact dermatitis. G Ital Dermatol Venereol. 2009;144(5):515-25.
3. Ilkit M, Durdu M, Karakaş M. Cutaneous id reactions: a comprehensive review of clinical manifestations, epidemiology, etiology, and management. Crit Rev Microbiol. 2012;38(3):191-202.
4. Dogra N, Shah S, Dogra D. Lichen scrofulosorum: an important marker of occult tuberculosis. Indian J Dermatol. 2008;53(2):91-2.
5. Synakiewicz J, Polańska A, Bowszyc-Dmochowska M, Żaba RW, Adamski Z, Reich A, et al. Generalized lichen nitidus: a case report and review of the literature. Postepy Dermatol Alergol. 2016;33(6):488-90.
6. Lee HS, Chun YS, Hann SK. Nevus depigmentosus: clinical features and histopathologic characteristics in 67 patients. J Am Acad Dermatol. 1999;40(1):21-6.
7. Wollina U. Pompholyx: a review of clinical features, differential diagnosis, and management. Am J Clin Dermatol. 2010;11(5):305-14.

CHAPTER 2.4

# Biologics in Atopic Dermatitis

*Disha Chakraborty, Abhishek De*

## INTRODUCTION

Atopic dermatitis is a recurrent inflammatory dermatosis with a genetic basis. Its etiology is multifactorial with a complex pathophysiology. The signs and symptoms, as well as the age at which they first appear, vary greatly in their clinical expression. Severe itching and dry skin are its hallmarks, which indicate a deterioration in the function of the barrier and immune system dysfunction. Type 2 helper T cell (Th2) malfunction is the predominant cause, while Th17, Th22, and Th1 pathways may also be at play.[1]

## ADVANTAGES OF USING BIOLOGIC TREATMENT OF ATOPIC DERMATITIS

- Biologic targets specific cytokines such as IL-4, interleukin 13 (IL-13), and IL-31 which are specific to the pathogenesis of atopic dermatitis (AD). The more targeted and selective approach compared to conventional systemic drugs, reduces the risk of systemic adverse effects.
- Clinical research suggests that biologics are more effective in reducing key signs and symptoms of AD including pruritus, rashes, barrier dysfunction, and also in improving quality of life.
- Biologics are more tailored for a longer-term safe and effective therapy option.
- Biologics reduce the need for long-term application of topical steroids, thereby lowering the risk of steroid-related side effects.
- Biologics also may reduce the chance of atopic march and other complications of AD.[1,2]

## WHEN TO USE BIOLOGICS IN AD?

Recent AAD guidelines for the management of AD suggest biologics like dupilumab should be used for moderate-to-severe AD, especially in patients in whom conventional topical and systemic therapies are of limited benefit.

The biologics that are approved for AD by various United States Food and Drug Administration (US FDA) are dupilumab, tralokinumab, and nemolizumab.

### Dupilumab[3-5]

Trade name: Dupixent®.

#### *Global Approval*

- Dupilumab was approved as the first targeted biologic treatment for AD.
- On March 28, 2017, dupilumab was approved in the United States for the treatment of individuals with moderate-to-severe AD.
- After receiving FDA approval, dupilumab was further approved by regulatory agencies worldwide, including the European Medicines Agency (EMA) and other national regulatory authorities.
- The treatment is now more widely available worldwide as a result of its universal acceptability.
- Non-FDA-approved indications—allergic contact dermatitis, hand dermatitis, chronic spontaneous urticaria, prurigo nodularis, and alopecia areata. It works effectively in all Th2-mediated inflammatory diseases.
- Dupilumab is currently being tested for bullous pemphigoid, eosinophilic esophagitis, and chronic obstructive pulmonary disease (COPD).

### *Approval in India*

It was approved on July 11, 2023, as the first biologic medication for the treatment of moderate-to-severe AD in adults whose disease is not adequately controlled with topical prescription therapies or when those therapies are not advised.

### *Mechanism of Action*

- It is an immunoglobulin G4 (IgG4) monoclonal antibody that is fully humanized and targets the alpha component of the IL-4 receptor.
- Type I and type II are the two types of IL-4 receptors. The IL-4R and the common chain (C) form a heterodimer in type I, whereas the IL-4R and the IL-13 alpha chain (IL-13R1) form a heterodimer in type II.
- The Th2 pathway's downstream signaling of IL-4 and IL-13, two crucial cytokines involved in B cell activation, dendritic cell differentiation, and IgE class switching, is suppressed by dupilumab.
- It also lowers the recruitment of eosinophils.

### *Adverse Effects*

- It is more tolerated and safer than most systemic medicines.
- The most common side effects include ocular and injection-site reactions, such as soreness and bruising.
- Common eye side effects include conjunctivitis, keratitis, pruritus, dry eyes, and blepharitis.
- The most common opportunistic infection with dupilumab is herpes simplex virus.
- Recent dupilumab facial redness (DFR) reports include erythema, scaling, papules, itching, rash, burning, and neck and face discomfort.

### *Administration*

- Dupilumab injection single-dose pre-filled syringes **(Fig. 1)** contain 300 mg/2 mL and 200 mg/1.14 mL. Sterile, preservative-free medicine.
- To prevent light damage, it is refrigerated in its original carton between 36° and 46°F (2° and 8°C).
- Dupilumab is injected subcutaneously into the thigh or abdomen, except the two inches around the navel.
- Adults should start with 600 mg dupilumab (two 300 mg injections at different places) and then 300 mg every 15 days. For therapeutic results, it should be continued for 16 weeks.

### *Doses in the Pediatric Age Group*

The doses in the pediatric age group are summarized in **Table 1**.

### *Use in Pregnancy and Lactation*

- Dupilumab for severe AD during pregnancy has not been found to harm mothers or fetuses.
- Dupilumab could weaken neonatal immunity, requiring further study. Nursing research on dupilumab is lacking.
- Although dupilumab is unlikely to pass into breast milk due to its large molecular weight, limited research warns against using it in breastfeeding moms.
- With topical prescription therapies ineffective or inappropriate, the FDA approved dupilumab in June 2022 for children aged 6 months to 5 years with moderate-to-severe AD.

## Selective Interleukin 13 Blockers

Developing drugs that specifically target IL-13 has the potential to optimize treatment effectiveness while minimizing adverse effects, as IL-13 plays a crucial role in the

**TABLE 1: Doses of dupilumab in the pediatric age group.**

| Body weight | Initial dose | Subsequent doses |
|---|---|---|
| 15 to <30 kg | 600 mg (two 300 mg injections) | 300 mg Q4W |
| 30 to <60 kg | 400 mg (two 200 mg injections) | 200 mg Q2W |
| 60 kg or more | 600 mg (two 300 mg injections) | 300 mg Q2W |

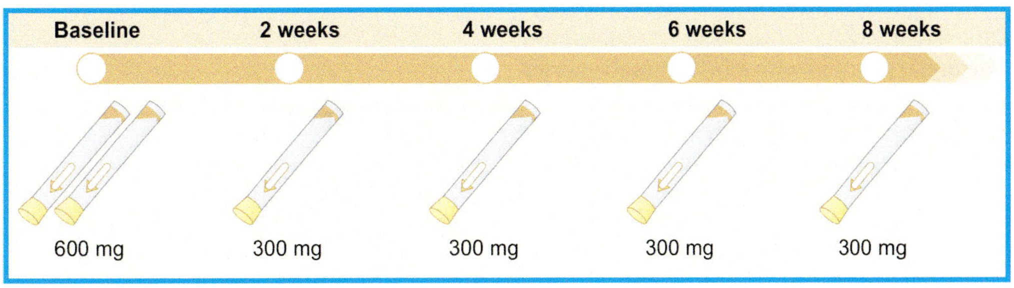


**FIG. 1:** Dosing schedule of dupilumab.

pathophysiology of (AD). Consequently, the emergence of novel targeted therapeutic approaches has been facilitated, as shown by the selective IL-13 inhibitors lebrikizumab and tralokinumab.

## Tralokinumab

### *Approval*

The US FDA (2021) and the European Union approved it for moderate-to-severe AD.

### *Mechanism of Action*

Competitively inhibits the binding of IL-13 to two receptors, IL-13Rα1 and IL-13Rα2.

### *Dose*

- *Initial dose*: 600 mg (four 150 mg subcutaneous injections) followed by 300 mg (two 150 mg injections) every other week.
- *Injection*: 150 mg/mL solution in a single-dose prefilled syringe with a needle guard.

### *Adverse Effects*

Upper respiratory tract infections, conjunctivitis, injection site responses, eosinophilia (incidence < 1%).[6]

## Lebrikizumab

It is not FDA-approved.

### *Mechanism of Action*

- A humanized IgG4 monoclonal antibody binds to soluble IL-13 with high affinity.
- It hinders IL4R/IL13Rα1 heterodimerization, hence, inhibiting downstream signaling.
- Lebrikizumab, unlike tralokinumab, allows IL-13 to continue to bind to the IL-13Rα2 decoy receptor, maintaining the hypothesized endogenous regulation mechanism.

### *Dose*

- The first treatment with lebrikizumab was for asthma.
- Lebrikizumab is injected subcutaneously at doses of either 250 mg/500 mg Q2W for up to 14 weeks, (phase III trials). The first treatment with lebrikizumab was for asthma.
- Lebrikizumab is injected subcutaneously at doses of either 250 mg/500 mg Q2W for up to 14 weeks (phase III trials).

### *Adverse Effects*

- In the phase II TREBLE trial, lebrikizumab-treated patients had the same number of adverse events (AE) as placebo, also, dropout rates, and infections.
- Average AE lasted 1–3 days and was mild to moderate.[7]
- Conjunctivitis occurred in 15 lebrikizumab (9.6%) and four placebo (7.5%) participants. Lebrikizumab-treated patients had infrequent and small herpetic infections and peripheral eosinophilia (3.8 and 3.2%).

## Nemolizumab

The proinflammatory cytokine IL-31 is implicated in the itch-scratch cycle that causes the skin barrier to be disrupted in AD by overexpressing IL-31 receptors on sensory nerves.

### *Approval*

- In Japan, patients 13 years of age and older with severe AD were first approved to receive nemolizumab (Mitchga) in 2022.
- Galderma received a Breakthrough Therapy status from the US FDA in 2019 to evaluate the drug's potential to reduce pruritus brought on by prurigo nodularis.

### *Mechanism of Action*

Nemolizumab is a humanized IgG2 monoclonal antibody that acts by blocking the IL31 receptor (IL31R).

### *Dose and Administration*

Nemolizumab is injected subcutaneously. It is licensed for use in Japan to treat AD at a dose of 60 mg administered subcutaneously once every 4 weeks.

### *Adverse Effects*

- The most common adverse events (AEs) linked to nemolizumab included upper respiratory tract infections, nasopharyngitis, and worsened AD.
- Furthermore, a dose-dependent increase in asthma-related occurrences was observed in patients having a history of asthma.[8]

# FUTURE TRENDS

**Table 2** summarizes newer updates in the treatment of AD with different biologicals.

**TABLE 2: Updates on different biologicals in atopic dermatitis.**

| Drug | Mechanism | Findings from clinical trials |
|---|---|---|
| Tezepelumab | • Tezepelumab is a fully human IgGλ2 (lambda chain) mAb binding TSLP<br>• TSLP stimulates dendritic cells to produce type 2 cytokines such as IL-4, IL-5, IL-13, and TNF | • Patients were randomized to receive either 280 mg of tezepelumab subcutaneous (SC) or a placebo q2w with concurrent TCS in a phase IIa trial<br>• At week 12 the primary endpoint, EASI-50 versus placebo, failed to attain statistical significance. Other secondary objectives, such as the EASI-75, EASI-90, SCORAD, and NRS scores at week 12, did not show significant improvements in tezepelumab-treated individuals compared to placebo[9] |
| ISB 830 (previously known as GBR 830) | • Humanized IgG1 anti-OX40 monoclonal antibody ISB 830<br>• OX40L from antigen-presenting cells boosts effector T-cell responses | ISB 830 was investigated for safety and efficacy in moderate-to-severe AD adults with insufficient topical treatment in a phase IIa trial. The results were favorable. Nasopharyngitis (8.7%) was the only treatment-related AE. The medication is in phase IIb for atopic dermatitis[10] |
| MOR106 | Mouse and human IgG1 anti-IL-17C mAb | • In a phase 1 trial, it demonstrated promising outcomes. At week 4, 83% of AD patients receiving MOR106 achieved the EASI-50, compared to 20% in the placebo group, and improvements persisted in the treatment group for the course of the subsequent 10 weeks<br>• But two phase 2 trials (NCT03568071 and NCT03864627) were stopped early because they did not show promising results in terms of their primary endpoints[11] |
| Omalizumab and ligelizumab | Recombinant anti-IgE monoclonal antibody | • In an AD systematic review and meta-analysis, fewer than 50% of patients treated with omalizumab showed significant clinical improvement (SCORAD-50, EASI-75, or IGA 0 or 2-point reduction)<br>• A 2013 phase 2 trial of ligelizumab (QGE031), a monoclonal antibody with stronger IgE affinity than omalizumab, was completed without findings, suggesting a lack of effectiveness in AD (NCT01552629)[12] |
| Fezakinumab | Human IgGλ2 (lambda chain) anti-IL-22 mAb | Currently not under trial[13] |

(AD: atopic dermatitis; IgE: immunoglobulin E; TNF: tumor necrosis factor; TSLP: thymic stromal lymphopoietin )

## CONCLUSION

In summary, the utilization of biological medicines has significantly transformed the approach to treating AD, presenting a promising prospect for patients with moderate to severe conditions that have proven unresponsive to traditional therapeutic interventions. Clinical trials and real-world research have provided substantial evidence regarding the effectiveness and safety characteristics of biologics, with a particular emphasis on dupilumab. Despite the persistent issues of cost and long-term safety monitoring, it is evident that biologic therapy offers significant benefits in terms of enhancing disease severity, increasing the quality of life, and alleviating the burden associated with AD. An ongoing investigation into novel biologic medicines and an improved comprehension of their mechanisms of action will augment our capacity to deliver efficacious and individualized treatment for individuals afflicted with AD.

## REFERENCES

1. Rajagopalan M, De A, Godse K, Krupa Shankar DS, Zawar V, Sharma N, et al. Guidelines on Management of Atopic Dermatitis in India: An Evidence-based Review and an Expert Consensus. Indian J Dermatol. 2019;64(3):166-81.
2. Dutta A, De A, Das S, Banerjee S, Kar C, Dhar S. A Cross-sectional Evaluation of the Usefulness of the Minor Features of Hanifin and Rajka Diagnostic Criteria for the Diagnosis of Atopic Dermatitis in the Pediatric Population. Indian J Dermatol. 2021;66(6):583-90.
3. Dhar S, De A, Srinivas SM. Real-World Effectiveness and Safety of Dupilumab for the Treatment of Moderate-to-Severe Atopic Dermatitis in Indian Patients: A Multi-Centric Retrospective Study. Indian J Dermatol. 2021;66(3):297-301.
4. Sanofi. (2016). Sanofi and Regeneron announce a marketing authorization application for Dupixent® (dupilumab) accepted for review by the EMA. [Online] Available from https://newsroom.regeneron.com/news-releases/news-release-details/regeneron-and-sanofi-announce-marketing-authorization [Last accessed January, 2025].
5. Wang FP, Tang XJ, Wei CQ, Xu LR, Mao H, Luo FM. Dupilumab treatment in moderate-to-severe atopic dermatitis: A systematic review and meta-analysis. J Dermatol Sci. 2018;90(2):190-8.
6. Tollenaere MAX, Molck C, Henderson I, Pollack S, Addis P, Petersen HH, et al. Tralokinumab Effectively Disrupts the IL-13/IL-13Rα1/IL-4Rα Signaling Complex but not the IL-13/IL-13Rα2 Complex. JID Innov. 2023;3(5):100214.
7. Bernardo D, Bieber T, Torres T. Lebrikizumab for the Treatment of Moderate-to-Severe Atopic Dermatitis. Am J Clin Dermatol. 2023;(5):753-64.
8. Kabashima K, Matsumura T, Komazaki H, Kawashima M; Nemolizumab JP01 and JP02 Study Group. Nemolizumab plus topical agents in patients with atopic dermatitis (AD) and moderate-to-severe pruritus provide improvement in pruritus and signs of AD for up to 68 weeks: results from two phase III, long-term studies. Br J Dermatol. 2022;186(4):642-51.
9. Simpson EL, Parnes JR, She D, Crouch S, Rees W, Mo M, et al. Tezepelumab, an anti-thymic stromal lymphopoietin monoclonal antibody, in the treatment of moderate-to-severe atopic dermatitis: A randomized phase 2a clinical trial. J Am Acad Dermatol. 2019;80(4):1013-21.
10. Rajagopalan M, Chitkara AJ, Dalwai S, De A, Gulati R, Mukherjee S, et al. Burden of Disease, Unmet Needs in the Diagnosis and Management of Atopic Dermatitis: An Indian Expert Consensus. Clin Cosmet Investig Dermatol. 2021;14:1755-65.
11. MorphoSys AG. (2019). MOR106 Clinical Development in Atopic Dermatitis Stopped for futility. [Online] Available from https://www.morphosys.com/media-investors/media-center/morphosys-ag-mor106-clinical-development-in-atopic-dermatitis-stopped [Last accessed January, 2025].
12. Chan S, Cornelius V, Cro S, Harper JI, Lack G. Treatment Effect of Omalizumab on Severe Pediatric Atopic Dermatitis: The ADAPT Randomized Clinical Trial. JAMA pediatrics. 2019;174(1):29-37.
13. Guttman-Yassky E, Brunner PM, Neumann AU, Khattri S, Pavel AB, Malik K, et al. Efficacy and safety of fezakinumab (an IL-22 monoclonal antibody) in adults with moderate-to-severe atopic dermatitis inadequately controlled by conventional treatments: A randomized, double-blind, phase 2a trial. J Am Acad Dermatol. 2018;78(5):872-81.e6.

2.5

CHAPTER

# Small Molecule in Atopic Dermatitis

***SK Shahriar Ahmed, Disha Chakraborty, Abhishek De***

## INTRODUCTION

Small molecules are nonbiologic pharmaceuticals that inhibit inflammatory cytokines by altering signaling pathways in immune cells. For moderate-to-severe atopic dermatitis (AD), several oral small molecules with various modes of action are suggested. Th2-associated interleukin (IL)-4, -13, -31, Th22-associated IL-22, and Th1-associated interferon (IFN)-γ are linked to the pathogenesis of AD.[1] It also causes downstream activation of the Janus kinase (JAK) and signal transducer and activator of the transcription (STAT) pathway. Phosphodiesterase-4 (PDE-4), which controls the generation of cytokines, has also been found in immunological and inflammatory cells, including T cells, B cells, monocytes, macrophages, neutrophils, and so on. This finding raises the possibility that PDE-4 is involved in regulating AD-associated inflammation. With their ability to selectively target AD immunological pathways, small molecules may be more successful than conventional systemic medicines for treating AD with fewer side effects and an easier-to-follow treatment plan.[2]

## JANUS KINASE INHIBITOR IN ATOPIC DERMATITIS

The JAK/STAT system regulates several immunological activities, including Th2 cytokines such as IL-4, IL-5, IL-13, IL-31, and thymic stromal lymphopoietin, which are responsible for the pathogenic mechanisms of AD. It is important to remember that JAK/STAT also affects the epidermal barrier functions. JAK/STAT-dependent IL-4 and IL-13 signaling contributes to the deregulation of keratinocyte function in AD, which results in the downregulation of elements of the skin barrier such as loricrin, involucrin, and filaggrin, etc. Not to mention, one of the main symptoms of AD is pruritus, which is caused by peripheral nerve activity that is regulated by JAK/STAT.[3]

While only seven JAK inhibitors are currently used in the treatment of AD, namely abrocitinib, baricitinib, gusacitinib, upadacitinib, tofacitinib, delgocitinib, and ruxolitinib. Abrocitinib and upadacitinib are the only Food and Drug Administration (FDA)-approved (in the year 2022) JAK inhibitors for the treatment of AD.

### Topical Janus Kinase Inhibitors

- In a study by Bissonnette et al., tofacitinib 2% ointment BID has significantly reduced (81.7%) the baseline eczema area and severity index (%EASI) at week 4 in comparison to vehicle (29.9%).
- Whereas ruxolitinib 1.5% cream BID versus vehicle achieved the primary endpoint of %EASI (71.6% vs. 15.5%). Delgocitinib 0.5% ointment has shown efficacy in reducing baseline modified EASI by 57.1% versus tacrolimus 0.1% (62%) versus placebo (12.2%).
- Brepocitinib (BREPO), a JAK1/tyrosine kinase 2 (Tyk2) inhibitor, is under investigation for topical and oral therapy, including AD.[4]

### Systemic Janus Kinase Inhibitors

- Tofacitinib is a first generation of JAK1 and JAK3 inhibitor implicated in the Th1 and Th2 signaling pathways. 66.6% reduction in the severity scoring of AD index (SCORAD) and 69.9% reduction in pruritus and sleep loss score was noticed with tofacitinib 5 mg BD in a study conducted by Levy et al. Side effects include weight gain, gastrointestinal perforations, deep vein thrombosis, pulmonary embolism, upper respiratory tract infection, diarrhea, nausea, etc.[5]

- Baricitinib (BARI), a first-generation oral JAK1/2 selective inhibitor, was FDA-approved in June 2018 at 2 mg QD for adult moderate-to-severe rheumatoid arthritis. A significant number of patients achieved EASI-50 using baricitinib 2 mg (57%) and 4 mg (61%) compared to placebo (37%) as described by Guttman-Yassky et al. Common laboratory changes included increased blood creatine phosphokinase (CPK) (grade 1) and elevated lipids, and minimal changes in hematologic, hepatic, and renal parameters.[6]
- Upadacitinib is a JAK1-selective inhibitor that was first FDA-approved in August 2019 for treatment of adult patients with moderate-to-severe rheumatoid arthritis (15 mg QD). Achieving primary endpoint (EASI-75) across different doses of upadacitinib was 74 versus 62 versus 39 versus 23% with 30 mg versus 15 mg versus 7.5 mg versus placebo. Common adverse events (AEs) included upper respiratory tract infection (URTI), acne, headache, increased blood CPK, nasopharyngitis, and nausea.[7]
- Abrocitinib is an oral, selective JAK-1 inhibitor recently approved (January, 2022) for the treatment of moderate-to-severe AD in adults. In a study by Bieber et al. by week 12, Investigator's Global Assessment (IGA) and EASI-75 responses were observed in 48.4 and 70.3% of patients in the 200 mg abrocitinib group, 36.6 and 58.7% in the 100 mg abrocitinib group, 36.5 and 58.1% in the dupilumab group, and 14.0 and 27.1% in the placebo group, respectively. The most common AEs are AD, URTI, headache, nausea, and diarrhea.[8]

## PHOSPHODIESTERASE-4 INHIBITOR IN ATOPIC DERMATITIS

- Leukocytes from AD patients with PDE-4 inhibitor show increased activity of PDE, an enzyme that catalyzes the conversion of cyclic adenosine monophosphate (cAMP) to AMP, resulting in leukocyte hyperactivity and inflammation, in comparison to controls. PDE-4 is one of the main forms of the 11 distinct human PDE isoenzymes that are expressed in leukocytes. Intracellular cAMP builds up when the PDE-4 signaling pathway is disrupted, which activates effector molecules and protein kinase A (PKA). Proinflammatory cytokines, neutrophil degranulation, chemotaxis, and endothelial cell adhesion are also inhibited.
- Treatment for mild-to-moderate AD with topical PDE inhibitors (PDEi) is effective. Apremilast is an oral PDE-4i that inhibits inflammatory pathways, enhances the synthesis of the anti-inflammatory cytokine IL-10, and suppresses the production of tumor necrosis factor (TNF), IL-12, IL-2, IFN-γ, IL-5, IL-8, leukotriene B4 (LTB4), and adhesion molecule CD18/CD11b (Mac-1). Crisaborole ointment is approved for mild to moderate AD, whereas apremilast is only approved for psoriasis.[9]
- In a study "Phase 2 trial" by Simpson et al., apremilast 40 mg twice daily showed a significant improvement of EASI versus placebo (–31.6% vs. –11%, $p < 0.04$) at week 12. There is no real-world data available regarding the efficacy of apremilast in AD. There are multiple side effects which have been reported with apremilast such as depression, nausea, vomiting, headache, cough, diarrhea, decreased appetite, joint pain, and allergic reaction.[10]
- In a vehicle-controlled phase III trial, more patients achieved Investigator's Static Global Assessment (ISGA) of 0 or 1 at day 29 in crisaborole 2% ointment-treated group versus placebo (48.5% vs. 29.7%, $p < 0.001$). Two randomized, double-blind, and vehicle-controlled phase 3 studies with 759 and 763 participants demonstrated that crisaborole improves pruritus compared with vehicle (56.6% vs. 39.5%; $p < 0.001$) as early as day 2 of therapy (34.3% vs. 27.3%; $p = 0.013$). Crisaborole ointment is very safe and can be used in >3 months age group. Local irritation and stinging sensation is the most common side effects. It could be a very good steroid-sparing topical agent which could be used for a longer duration.[11,12]

## HISTAMINE H4 RECEPTOR ANTAGONIST

It has also been individuals with AD which exhibits higher levels of H4R receptor expression on CD4+ T cells in comparison to healthy individuals. Th2 elevation of IL-31, a cytokine linked to AD severity, is the outcome of H4R stimulation. Furthermore, there is a favorable correlation between H4R activation and the rate of keratinocyte growth. H4R antagonist therapy reduces the size of lesions, and itching, attracts inflammatory cells, and produces inflammatory cytokines in several animal models of dermatitis. Most of the molecules are in phase 2 trial.[13]

## CRTH2 RECEPTOR ANTAGONISTS

The chemoattractant receptor-homologous molecule expressed on Th2 cells (CRTH2, sometimes referred to as prostaglandin D2 receptor/DP2) expressed on Th2 cells is a novel target for AD. Prostaglandin D2 (PGD2) has both pro- and anti-inflammatory properties. PGD2 attaches to DP1, which reduces inflammation and preserves epidermal barrier function; however, when it attaches to CRTH2, which induces leukocyte chemotaxis, inflammation is increased. Three oral small molecule CRTH2 receptor antagonists are now being investigated for AD: timapiprant (OC000459), fevipiprant (QAW039), and BBI-5000.[14]

## CONCLUSION

Small molecules have revolutionized the treatment landscape of atopic dermatitis, offering targeted, orally administered options that bridge the gap between conventional immunosuppressants and biologics. The emergence of JAK inhibitors, PDE-4 inhibitors, and other pathway-specific agents has expanded therapeutic choices, addressing both systemic inflammation and skin barrier dysfunction. Their rapid onset, broad immunomodulatory effects, and flexible dosing make them invaluable, particularly for patients who are non-responsive or intolerant to biologics. However, long-term safety, risk mitigation, and patient selection criteria remain key considerations. As research continues to refine efficacy, durability, and safety profiles, small molecules are poised to play an increasingly central role in the precision management of atopic dermatitis.

## REFERENCES

1. Gadina M, Gazaniga N, Vian L, Furumoto Y. Small molecules to the rescue: Inhibition of cytokine signaling in immune-mediated diseases. J Autoimmun. 2017;85:20-31.
2. Yoo J, Kim D, Park J, Kim YK, Park Choo HY, Woo HA. Novel Small Molecule Inhibitors Targeting the IL-6/STAT3 Pathway or IL-1β. Molecules. 2022;27(9):2696.
3. Raychaudhuri SP, Shah RJ, Banerjee S, Raychaudhuri SK. JAK-STAT Signaling and Beyond in the Pathogenesis of Spondyloarthritis and Their Clinical Significance. Curr Rheumatol Rep. 2024;26(6):204-13.
4. Alves C, Penedones A, Mendes D, Batel Marques F. Topical Janus kinase inhibitors in atopic dermatitis: a safety network meta-analysis. Int J Clin Pharm. 2023;45(4):830-8.
5. Berbert Ferreira S, Berbert Ferreira R, Scheinberg MA. Atopic dermatitis: Tofacitinib, an option for refractory disease. Clin Case Rep. 2020;8(12):3244-7.
6. Hagino T, Saeki H, Fujimoto E, Kanda N. Efficacy and safety of baricitinib treatment for moderate to severe atopic dermatitis in real-world practice in Japan. J Dermatol. 2023;50(7):869-79.
7. Silverberg JI, Gooderham MJ, Paller AS, Deleuran M, Bunick CG, Gold LFS, et al. Early and Sustained Improvements in Symptoms and Quality of Life with Upadacitinib in Adults and Adolescents with Moderate-to-Severe Atopic Dermatitis: 52-Week Results from Two Phase III Randomized Clinical Trials (Measure Up 1 and Measure Up 2). Am J Clin Dermatol. 2024;25(3):485-96.
8. Iznardo H, Roé E, Serra-Baldrich E, Puig L. Efficacy and Safety of JAK1 Inhibitor Abrocitinib in Atopic Dermatitis. Pharmaceutics. 2023;15(2):385.
9. De A, Chakraborty D, Grisilda BN, Chaudhuri S, Godse K, Dhar S. Efficacy and safety of crisaborole ointment in pediatric atopic dermatitis: A 4-week open-label study. Indian J Skin Allergy. 2024;3(1):60.
10. Simpson EL, Imafuku S, Poulin Y, Ungar B, Zhou L, Malik K, et al. A Phase 2 Randomized Trial of Apremilast in Patients with Atopic Dermatitis. J Invest Dermatol. 2019;139(5):1063-72.
11. Eichenfield LF, Gower RG, Xu J, Alam MS, Su JC, Myers DE, et al. Once-Daily Crisaborole Ointment, 2%, as a Long-Term Maintenance Treatment in Patients Aged ≥ 3 Months with Mild-to-Moderate Atopic Dermatitis: A 52-Week Clinical Study. Am J Clin Dermatol. 2023;24(4):623-35.
12. Paller AS, Tom WL, Lebwohl MG, Blumenthal RL, Boguniewicz M, Call RS, et al. Efficacy and safety of crisaborole ointment, a novel, nonsteroidal phosphodiesterase 4 (PDE4) inhibitor for the topical treatment of atopic dermatitis (AD) in children and adults. J Am Acad Dermatol. 2016;75(3):494-503.e6.
13. Schaper-Gerhardt K, Rossbach K, Nikolouli E, Werfel T, Gutzmer R, Mommert S. The role of the histamine H4 receptor in atopic dermatitis and psoriasis. Br J Pharmacol. 2020;177(3):490-502.
14. He R, Oyoshi MK, Wang JY, Hodge MR, Jin H, Geha RS. The prostaglandin $D_2$ receptor CRTH2 is important for allergic skin inflammation after epicutaneous antigen challenge. J Allergy Clin Immunol. 2010;126(4):784-90.

CHAPTER 2.6

# Management of Atopic Dermatitis in Adults

*Abhishek De, Disha Chakraborty*

## INTRODUCTION

The management of atopic dermatitis (AD) involves a multifaceted approach that includes identifying and avoiding triggers, maintaining proper skin care, and using appropriate medications. However, the management strategies can vary based on the severity of the condition and individual patient factors. This chapter aims to provide a comprehensive overview of the management of AD in adults, focusing primarily on evidence-based recommendations presented in tabular format. We will summarize key aspects of AD management, including controlling factors responsible for exacerbation, general care recommendations, topical and systemic treatment options, and other therapies such as phototherapy and emerging biologic therapies.

## GENERAL CARE IN THE MANAGEMENT OF ATOPIC DERMATITIS

General care is essential for managing AD. A consistent skincare routine with moderate, fragrance-free products and frequent moisturization will moisturize the skin and reduce skin flare-ups. Identifying and avoiding triggers such as stress is crucial. To optimize the management and quality of life, regular follow-up appointments with a healthcare professional are necessary to monitor the condition and adjust the treatment plan. Management also requires patient's education and psychological therapies in addition to medicinal interventions. Patient's education helps AD patients to comprehend, manage, and follow treatment. Thus, a comprehensive AD care strategy should involve patient's education and psychological well-being. Patient's education and psychological support are crucial to AD care in adults, and this section discusses how to incorporate these into professional practice **(Tables 1 and 2A and B)**.[1,2]

**TABLE 1: The role of patient's education and psychological counseling in the management of atopic dermatitis.**

| Aspect | Importance | Strategies |
|---|---|---|
| Patient's education | Crucial in improving treatment adherence and outcomes | • Provide detailed information on the condition, triggers, and treatment options<br>• Demonstrate proper skincare techniques |
| Psychological factors | Can significantly impact disease severity and quality of life | • Address stress and anxiety through counseling or relaxation techniques<br>• Encourage support from family and peers |
| Cognitive behavioral therapy (CBT) | Effective in reducing itch intensity and improving coping mechanisms | • Refer patients to CBT specialists for tailored therapy<br>• Incorporate CBT principles into routine dermatology visits |
| Stress management | Essential in preventing exacerbations and improving overall well-being | • Teach stress-reduction techniques such as mindfulness or yoga<br>• Encourage regular physical activity |
| Support groups | Provide emotional support and practical advice | • Connect patients with local or online support groups<br>• Discuss experiences and coping strategies with peers |

**TABLE 2A: The recommendations regarding the predisposing factors in the management of atopic dermatitis (AD).**

| Predisposing factors | Recommendations |
|---|---|
| Food allergens | • Empirical food restriction is *not* recommended. Common food allergens identified for triggering AD include milk and milk products, peanuts, eggs, soy, wheat, seafood, and shellfish<br>• However, food should be restricted based on clinical experience and food diagnosis procedures<br>• A specific food-free diet should only be considered when an allergy to the specific food trigger is identified based on proper procedures, including a food diary and allergy test by a specialist |
| Clothing | • Loose-fitting smooth cotton cloths are ideal for AD<br>• Avoid irritating fabrics and fibers such as wool, acrylic, and nylon<br>• Cotton is recommended as the best fabric for AD patients |
| Sweating | Occupational or recreational exposure to high temperature and humidity should be avoided as sweating can exacerbate AD |
| Environmental triggers | Allergens such as mites, house dust, pollens, and organic solvents such as formaldehyde and toluene should be avoided to reduce AD symptoms |

**TABLE 2B: The recommendations regarding the general care strategies in the management of atopic dermatitis (AD).**

| General care | Recommendations |
|---|---|
| Bathing and cleansing | • Once daily bathing with lukewarm water for 5–10 minutes is helpful to wash away perspiration, dirt, debris, and allergens from the skin surface<br>• Use low pH, hypoallergenic, nonirritant, and fragrance-free nonsoap cleansers (Syndet) for cleansing |
| Perfumes, personal hygiene products, and cosmetics | Avoid their use as they can irritate the skin and exacerbate AD symptoms |
| Vaccination | Continue the standard national vaccine program except during acute exacerbation; postpone vaccination until the skin condition has stabilized |

## TOPICAL TREATMENT IN THE MANAGEMENT OF ATOPIC DERMATITIS

The utilization of topical therapies is fundamental in the treatment of AD, as they offer focused alleviation for symptoms and aid in the restoration of the skin barrier. A variety of therapeutic products are included in this category, such as emollients, corticosteroids, calcineurin inhibitors, and phosphodiesterase-4 (PDE-4) inhibitors. Each category of topical drug possesses distinct mechanisms of action and indications; yet, they are frequently employed in conjunction to attain the most favorable results. The following table enumerates the significance of topical therapies in the treatment of AD, emphasizing their effectiveness, safety considerations, and practical suggestions for their implementation in clinical settings **(Table 3)**.[3]

## CONVENTIONAL SYSTEMIC MANAGEMENT

The implementation of systemic management is of utmost importance in the holistic care of AD, especially in instances where topical medications prove inadequate in symptom control or when the condition is severe. In this part, an examination is conducted on different systemic therapy modalities for AD, encompassing oral drugs and biologic therapies. These therapies aim to specifically address the fundamental immunological dysregulation and inflammation linked to AD. However, only cyclosporin is a molecule that has found its place in the management algorithm of AD in various national and international guidelines. Other conventional immunomodulators often lack robust data.

A comprehension of advantages, drawbacks, and factors to be taken into account regarding systemic therapy is useful for dermatologists and healthcare professionals to treat AD and enhance the overall well-being of patients.[4,5] **Table 4** summarizes the conventional treatment options for the treatment of AD.

## BIOLOGIC AND SMALL MOLECULE IMMUNOMODULATOR

Biologics and small molecules, which provide targeted therapy for specific disease processes in the pathophysiology of the illness, have completely revolutionized the systemic management of AD. They are especially impor-

**TABLE 3: Topical treatment in the management of atopic dermatitis (AD).**

| Topical treatment | Recommendations |
|---|---|
| Moisturizers | Regular use of moisturizer at least twice a day on moist skin has long-term steroid-sparing effects and reduces the frequency of acute episodes |
| Topical corticosteroids (TCS) | • They are the most commonly used, FDA-approved treatment for mild-to-severe AD<br>• Choose an effective and safe TCS considering patient's age, disease severity, and application areas. Apply twice daily for the treatment of AD; use the fingertip unit method to measure the quantity to be applied<br>• Long-term use of low- to mid-potency TCS is reasonably safe, but superpotent TCSs are not preferred<br>• For more sensitive areas like the face or flexures or genitalia only a mild topical steroid for a short duration time is recommended |
| Topical calcineurin inhibitors (TCIs) | Consider for treatment of AD flares. Tacrolimus 0.1% ointment and pimecrolimus 1% cream are approved for use in AD. TCIs are safe and effective, with common side effects being skin burning and irritation |
| Wet wrap therapy | Considered for moderate-to-severe AD without risk of infection to quickly reduce AD severity |
| Topical PDE-4 inhibitor | • Crisaborole 2% ointment, FDA-approved for mild-to-moderate AD, showed a small but significant improvement in dermatitis in multiple studies also demonstrated efficacy in reducing pruritus. The safety profile of crisaborole was favorable, with a small percentage of patients experiencing application-related adverse events<br>• Recent AAD guidelines strongly recommend its use based on high-certainty evidence |
| Topical JAK-inhibitor | • Topical ruxolitinib 1.5% cream was FDA-approved for short-term and noncontinuous chronic treatment of mild-to-moderate AD<br>• It demonstrated efficacy in improving IGA scores and reducing itch compared to vehicles. Adverse events were rare and similar to a vehicle, with application site burning, pain, and pruritus occurring at similar or lower rates<br>• The recommendation for topical JAK inhibitors is based on moderate certainty evidence, pending long-term safety data |
| Antimicrobials | • Antimicrobials are sometimes necessary to treat infected lesions of AD, such as impetigo<br>• However, the use of topical antibiotic and steroid-antibiotic combination for uninfected AD is limited and should be avoided<br>• Various antimicrobials were studied, but the evidence is limited by small sample sizes and short treatment durations |
| Others | • Studies on topical doxepin, used for 1 week, led to a reduction in pruritus compared to the control group. However, withdrawal due to adverse events was higher in the experimental group<br>• Reported side effects included drowsiness, which occurs due to systemic absorption, and allergic contact dermatitis<br>• Coal tar preparations can help to reduce itching, inflammation, and scaling. They are often used in combination with other therapies for AD<br>• Topical vitamin D analogs such as calcitriol and calcipotriene can help to regulate immune responses and reduce inflammation in AD<br>• Topical antipruritics such as menthol, camphor, and pramoxine can help to relieve itching associated with AD but has the risk of developing contact sensitization. |

(AAD: American Academy of Dermatology; AD: atopic dermatitis; FDA: Food and Drug Administration; IGA: Investigator's Global Assessment; JAK: Janus kinase; PDE-4: phosphodiesterase-4)

**TABLE 4: Conventional systemic management.**

| Systemic treatment | Recommendation |
|---|---|
| Oral antihistamines | Use to control pruritus, but their role is limited. Hydroxyzine, cetirizine, and other antihistamines can have a steroid-sparing effect by producing sedation and pruritus relief |
| Systemic antibiotic | Avoid indiscriminate use. Short courses for widespread infection with clinical evidence of localized infection |
| Systemic corticosteroids | • Use with caution, particularly in selected scenarios to control acute flares<br>• Start with an initial dose of 0.5 mg prednisolone/kilogram of the body weight/day and then followed by a slow taper |

*Continued*

*Continued*

| Systemic treatment | Recommendation |
|---|---|
| Cyclosporine | • Approved in Europe for short-term treatment of severe atopic dermatitis (AD)<br>• Consider as first choice among systemic immunomodulators for moderate-to-severe unresponsive cases<br>• Used in adults and also pediatric age group 2–16 years<br>• It is the most commonly used and well-tolerated systemic agent for severe AD in 2–16 years in the USA and Canada<br>• Administer twice a day at a daily dose of 3–5 mg/kg/day with regular strict monitoring to avoid side effects<br>• Median duration of treatment is 4.6 months<br>• If hypertension develops, dose reduction or discontinuation is advised after patient's evaluation<br>• Patients need to be monitored for nonmelanoma skin cancer<br>• Monitoring serum electrolytes, renal function test, and serum lipid levels is necessary |
| Methotrexate | • It is a systemic immunosuppressive drug used off-label to treat severe AD that does not respond to traditional treatments<br>• Consider as a second-line choice after cyclosporine<br>• It functions by preventing the synthesis of DNA, RNA, and proteins via the enzyme dihydrofolate reductase. This inhibition leads to a reduction in skin inflammation<br>• *Dosage:* 10–25 mg of methotrexate given orally or by subcutaneous injection once a week is the usual dosage for treating AD. With routine monitoring of blood counts and liver function tests, the dose may be changed by the patient's response and tolerance<br>• Research indicates that methotrexate can lessen the severity of AD and enhance a patient's quality of life in certain cases. It is frequently taken into consideration when more systemic treatments have not worked or are inappropriate. However, each person will react differently to methotrexate, and it could take a few weeks to months before symptoms noticeably improve<br>• Several side effects, including liver toxicity, bone marrow suppression, gastrointestinal side effects, and an elevated risk of infections, are possible with methotrexate. To identify and control these adverse effects regular monitoring is crucial |
| Azathioprine | • Azathioprine is an immunosuppressive medication effective in managing severe AD by modulating the immune response. It is frequently employed as a systemic second-line therapy in cases where traditional treatments have not worked or are intolerable. Its dose is between 2 and 2.5 mg/kg daily<br>• It is very effective in severe AD and is a cheaper choice for patients who cannot afford cyclosporine<br>• The use of azathioprine necessitates strict monitoring due to possible adverse effects, which include bone marrow suppression, liver toxicity, and an increased risk of infections. However, it can reduce inflammation and improve symptoms of AD |
| Mycophenolate mofetil | • Also, an immunosuppressive medication<br>• It is anti-inflammatory in AD by preventing T- and B-cell proliferation<br>• It is often considered when other systemic treatments have not been effective or are not suitable<br>• Its dose is between 2 and 3 g divided twice daily<br>• Though generally well-tolerated, adverse effects may include increased risk of infections, bone marrow suppression, and gastrointestinal distress<br>• Throughout treatment, it is advised to regularly assess liver function and blood levels |
| Systemic PDE-4 inhibitor, apremilast | • Apremilast is a phosphodiesterase-4 (PDE-4) inhibitor that modulates inflammatory responses by inhibiting the production of proinflammatory cytokines and increasing the anti-inflammatory cytokines<br>• It is available in 10, 20, and 30 mg doses. It is started with a 10 mg once daily dose and gradually titrated up to 30 mg twice daily dose as the patient is gradually able to tolerate<br>• It has shown some promise in treating AD, despite being largely utilized in the treatment of psoriasis and psoriatic arthritis. Its effectiveness in lessening the severity of AD and enhancing the quality of life for people with moderate-to-severe AD has been shown in clinical trials<br>• The most frequent side effect of apremilast is diarrhea, which is often easily tolerated. Others are headaches, nausea, and weight loss<br>• It has to be used with caution in patients with a creatinine clearance of <30 mL/min |

(DNA: deoxyribonucleic acid; RNA: ribonucleic acid)

tant for individuals with moderate to severe disease not responding to traditional treatments. By targeting the inflammatory pathway they have demonstrated exceptional success in reducing the symptoms of AD and enhancing quality of life. The significance of small molecules and biologics in the systemic treatment of AD is examined in this section, with particular attention paid to their mechanisms of action, clinical efficacy, safety profiles, and implications for use in clinical practice.[5,6] Summary of biologics, JAK inhibitors, and other therapies used in the treatment of AD is provided in **Table 5**.

**TABLE 5: The biologics, Janus kinase (JAK) inhibitors, and other therapies in the management of atopic dermatitis (AD).**

| Therapy | FDA approval and age group | Mechanism of action | Dose (adult) | Evidence |
|---|---|---|---|---|
| Dupilumab | • Yes (2017) for adults and children >6 years<br>• Approved in India for adult patients of AD | • Fully humanized IgG-4 monoclonal antibody<br>• Suppresses the downstream signaling of IL-4 and IL-13, cytokines of the Th2-pathway involved in B-cell activation, dendritic cell (DC) differentiation, and IgE class switching | 600 mg dosage of dupilumab (two 300 mg injections, given at separate locations), followed by 300 mg once every 15 days | Efficacy established in large RCTs. Excellent safety record with few major safety concerns after >5 years in clinical practice |
| Tralokinumab | Yes (2021) | Completely humanized IgG-4 monoclonal antibody that precisely targets IL-13, for the treatment of moderate-to-severe AD | An initial dose of 600 mg (four 150 mg subcutaneous injections) followed by 300 mg (two 150 mg injections) given every other week. Patients <100 kg who get clear or nearly clear skin after 16 weeks of treatment may be given a dose of 300 mg every 4 weeks | Significant improvement in signs/symptoms of AD and QOL in multiple clinical trials. No major safety concerns were identified |
| Nemolizumab | No. In Japan, it has been approved | A humanized IgG-2 monoclonal antibody that acts by blocking the IL-31 receptor (IL-31R) | Subcutaneously administered. at a dose of a 60-mg subcutaneous injection to be given at intervals of 4 weeks | In a 16-week phase 3 trial, Japanese AD patients with moderate-to-severe pruritus and poor response to topical medicines and antihistamines were randomized to SC nemolizumab (60 mg) or placebo q4w with topical medications. Results were favorable in the nemolizumab group |
| Upadacitinib | Yes (2022) for adults and children of 12 years and older for moderate-to-severe refractory AD | Inhibits intracellular cytoplasmic enzymes JAK. They are a group of four tyrosine kinases (JAK 1, 2, 3, and tyrosine kinase) associated with immune-mediated inflammatory processes | For <65 years—15 mg once daily and can be increased to 30 mg once daily. For >65 years—15 mg once daily. | Demonstrated very high efficacy in reducing signs/symptoms of AD and improving QOL. Rapid onset of action. High certainty evidence |

*Continued*

*Continued*

| Therapy | FDA approval and age group | Mechanism of action | Dose (adult) | Evidence |
|---|---|---|---|---|
| Abrocitinib | • Yes (2021) for adults with moderate-to-severe AD<br>• Approved in India for adult patients of AD | Oral JAK-1 inhibitor | Starting and maintenance dose of 100 mg once daily. It can be increased to 200 mg once a day | Demonstrated very high efficacy in reducing signs/symptoms of AD and improving QOL. Rapid onset of action. High certainty evidence |
| Baricitinib | Off-label | Oral JAK-1 and JAK-2 inhibitor | 2 mg once daily up to 4 mg/day | Effective for AD but less efficacious than upadacitinib and abrocitinib. Network meta-analysis suggests lower efficacy |

(FDA: Food and Drug Administration; Ig: immunoglobulin; IL: interleukin; QOL: quality of life; RCT: randomized controlled trial; SC: subcutaneously)

## CONCLUSION

Finally, treating adult AD requires a customized approach. Regular skin care, lifestyle adjustments, and patient's education are essential. Topical corticosteroids and calcineurin inhibitors are first line for mild-to-moderate cases, whereas phototherapy and biologics are for moderate-to-severe cases. In **Flowchart 1**, we have provided a flowchart for the stepwise approach in treating AD in adults according to the disease severity. Based on evidence-based recommendations and shared decision-making, these treatments can enhance AD outcomes and quality of life. More research is needed to improve adult AD treatment **(Flowchart 1)**.

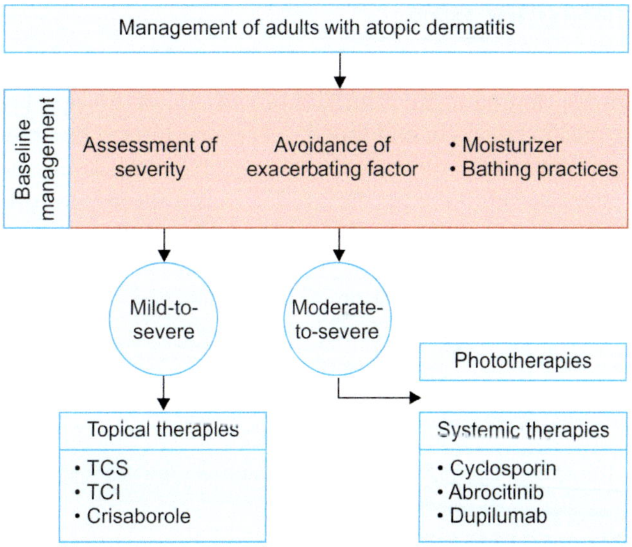


**FLOWCHART 1:** Recommended management algorithm for treatment of adult patients with atopic dermatitis (AD).
(TCI: topical calcineurin inhibitor; TCS: topical corticosteroids)

## REFERENCES

1. Rajagopalan M, Chitkara AJ, Dalwai S, De A, Gulati R, Mukherjee S, et al. Burden of Disease, Unmet Needs in the Diagnosis and Management of Atopic Dermatitis: An Indian Expert Consensus. Clin Cosmet Investig Dermatol. 2021;14:1755-65.
2. Rajagopalan M, De A, Godse K, Krupa Shankar DS, Zawar V, Sharma N, et al. Guidelines on Management of Atopic Dermatitis in India: An Evidence-based Review and an Expert Consensus. Indian J Dermatol. 2019;64(3):166-81.
3. Sideris N, Paschou E, Bakirtzi K, Kiritsi D, Papadimitriou I, Tsentemeidou A, et al. New and upcoming topical treatments for atopic dermatitis: a review of the literature. J Clin Med. 2022;11(17):4974.
4. Dhar S, De A, Saha A, Chitnis KR, Mane A, Dhoot D, et al. Intermittent or Sequential Topical Tacrolimus in Atopic Dermatitis: Systematic Review and Meta-analysis. Cureus. 2023;15(12):e50640.
5. Dhar S, De A, Srinivas SM. Real-World Effectiveness and Safety of Dupilumab for the Treatment of Moderate to Severe Atopic Dermatitis in Indian Patients: A Multi Centric Retrospective Study. Indian J Dermatol. 2021;66(3):297-301.
6. Dhar S, Datta S, De A. Use of Janus kinase inhibitors in atopic dermatitis—an update. Indian J Dermatol Venereol Leprol. 2023:1-8.

2.7

CHAPTER

# Management of Atopic Dermatitis in Children

***Deepika Halder, Disha Chakraborty***

## INTRODUCTION

Atopic dermatitis (AD) is a chronic inflammatory disorder that can affect individuals of all age groups but typically begins in childhood. It is characterized by itchy, eczematous skin lesions that are recurrent in nature and often associated with elevated serum immunoglobulin E (IgE) levels. The development of AD is influenced by several factors:

- Genetic predisposition
- Immune dysregulation
- Skin barrier dysfunction
- Environmental triggers

Diagnosis is primarily clinical and may be supported by established diagnostic criteria.

## MANAGEMENT

As per Indian ethnic, socioeconomic, resource-based, and demographic characteristics, Skin Allergy Research Society of India has updated its evidence-based consensus statement for the management of AD.[1]

Management usually depends upon the severity of the disease.

### Skin Care Management

#### *Daily Bathing and Moisturization*

The treatment of AD focuses on controlling inflammation, addressing triggers, relieving pruritus, and managing xerosis, a key feature of the condition. Topical moisturizers are fundamental, preventing dehydration, softening skin, and reducing the need for pharmacological treatments. They are first-line therapy for mild AD and an essential component in moderate-to-severe cases, helping to alleviate inflammation, xerosis, and pruritus while minimizing reliance on corticosteroids and antibiotics.

Daily bathing with warm water complements moisturization by hydrating the skin and removing allergens and irritants. Crucially, applying moisturizers immediately after bathing enhances hydration and therapeutic efficacy, as bathing without moisturization can worsen symptoms. The main takeaways from this are the following:

- *Bathing*: A single daily bath with lukewarm water (~27–30°C) for 5–10 minutes during daytime is recommended.
- *Cleansers*: Use hypoallergenic, fragrance-free, non-soap gentle cleansers (Syndets) with a neutral or low pH. Avoid scrubbing or rubbing the skin; gently pat dry with a soft towel.
- *Moisturization*: Apply moisturizers within three minutes of bathing while the skin is still damp to lock in moisture.
- *Effective moisturization techniques*: Moisturize at least twice daily to maintain hydration.
- *Personal skincare and cosmetics*: Avoid hygiene and cosmetic products containing fragrances, formaldehyde, lanolin, nickel, neomycin, or preservatives such as parabens.[2]

### Pharmacological Management

#### *First Line Therapy*

##### Moisturizers

**Moisturizers in AD:** Moisturizers are a cornerstone of therapy for AD, offering long-term steroid-sparing effects and reducing the frequency of acute flares.

*Mechanism of action*

- *Prevention of transepidermal water loss (TEWL)*: Forms a barrier to reduce water evaporation.
- *Maintenance of skin integrity*: Supports the structural health of the skin.
- *Restoration of lipids*: Replenishes essential skin lipids, attracting water to maintain the skin barrier.

*Types of moisturizers*

- *Occlusives*:
  - Prevent TEWL by mimicking the intracellular lipid bilayer, free fatty acids, and cholesterol.
  - Common ingredients: Beeswax, paraffin, and petrolatum.
- *Humectants*:
  - Water-attracting substances that mimic the natural moisturizing factor (NMF) of the stratum corneum.
  - Draw water from deeper epidermal and dermal layers to the skin surface.
  - Common ingredients: Alpha hydroxy acids, hyaluronic acid, glycerin, urea.
- *Emollients*:
  - Fill gaps between desquamating corneocytes and mimic natural skin lipids.
  - *Common ingredients*: Linoleic acid, linolenic acid, stearic acid, and oleic acid.

*Key ingredients to consider*

- *Anti-inflammatory properties:*
  - *Aloe vera in olive oil cream*: Proven to be as effective as 0.1% betamethasone cream.
  - *Virgin coconut oil*: Helps control acute flares effectively.

*Clinical recommendations*

- Moisturizers are essential for all AD patients, regardless of severity (mild, moderate, or severe).
- Continuous use during remission helps maintain skin integrity and prevents recurrences.[2]

## Wet Wrap and Bleach Therapy

Wet-wrap therapy, combined with topical treatments, is a proven approach for managing AD flare-ups. This method involves applying topical agents to the skin, followed by a layer of wet tubular bandage and an outer dry bandage, enhancing the efficacy of moisturizers by smoothing the skin and minimizing water loss. Bleach baths have also been explored as a treatment option, inspired by observations of improvements in eczematous lesions after exposure to chlorinated swimming pools.

Huang et al. demonstrated the effectiveness of bleach baths, combined with intranasal mupirocin, in reducing *Staphylococcus aureus* colonization and preventing secondary infections. This therapy typically involves soaking in a solution of diluted bleach (1/4 cup in 35–40 L of water) for 5–10 minutes. However, conflicting evidence exists, with some studies finding bleach baths ineffective for AD management.

In addition to bleach, antiseptic agents such as triclosan, potassium permanganate, and chlorhexidine gluconate are utilized for managing infected skin and as a preventive measure in AD. While these agents help reduce bacterial load on the skin, their efficacy on inflamed AD lesions varies across studies. Notably, combination therapies involving antibiotics and antiseptic agents have shown greater success in treating clinically infected AD skin.[3]

## Topical Anti-inflammatory Treatment Options

Anti-inflammatory therapy using topical calcineurin inhibitors (TCIs) such as tacrolimus and pimecrolimus, alongside topical corticosteroids (TCS), is considered highly effective for managing acute flares of AD. These treatments work by reducing the excessive inflammatory response in the skin during flare-ups. Both TCS and TCIs function by suppressing T lymphocyte activity and inhibiting the release of proinflammatory cytokines from immune cells. As a result, these agents effectively control inflammation, alleviate pruritus, and manage skin eruptions.

### Topical Corticosteroids

- *Role in management*: TCS is essential for managing acute flares of AD and is used alongside moisturizers. Randomized controlled trials (RCTs) have demonstrated the safety and efficacy of repeated courses of low- to midpotency TCS for up to 5 years in children and one year in adults.
- *Proactive approach*: To prevent flares in stabilized AD, a proactive regimen of low- to midpotency TCS applied twice weekly is effective in both adults and children.
- *Selection criteria*: The choice of TCS depends on factors, such as:
  - Patient's age
  - Affected body areas
  - Severity of xerosis
  - Patient preference
  - Cost of the medication
- *Safety considerations*:
  - Low to midpotency TCS are generally safe for long-term use.
  - High-potency TCS, however, may cause local side effects, including:
    - Striae rubrae+
    - Skin atrophy
    - Telangiectasia
    - Burning, erythema, and acneiform eruptions

 - Rarely, hypothalamic-pituitary-adrenal (HPA) axis suppression may occur, especially in children due to their higher body surface area-to-mass ratio, leading to increased systemic absorption.
- *Application guidelines*: While no universal standard exists, one commonly recommended method is using one adult fingertip unit (~0.5 g) for an area equivalent to two adult palms.

### Topical Calcineurin Inhibitors

- *Introduction and approval*: TCIs, such as pimecrolimus 1% cream and tacrolimus (0.03% and 0.1% ointment), have been approved since 2002 for their anti-inflammatory effects in AD.
- *Safety profile*:
  - TCIs are safe for long-term use, up to 12 months.
  - The most common side effect is a transient burning sensation, which resolves within one week in 80% of patients.
- *Concerns about malignancy risk*:
  - There is no convincing evidence supporting the boxed warning about an increased risk of malignancy.
  - A slight increase in the likelihood of viral infections has been reported.

By effectively combining TCS and TCIs with moisturizers, a personalized approach to AD management can minimize flares and maintain long-term skin health.[2]

## Phosphodiesterase-4 Inhibitors

Crisaborole, a phosphodiesterase 4 (PDE-4) inhibitor, received Food and Drug Administration (FDA) approval in 2016 for the topical treatment of mild-to-moderate AD in children aged 3 months and older. By targeting PDE-4, crisaborole reduces the production of inflammatory cytokines involved in AD pathogenesis.

Phase 3 trials demonstrated significant improvement in both skin symptoms and pruritus severity. Adverse effects were mostly mild, with stinging or burning at the application site being the most common. The drug maintains a favorable safety profile within the first year of use, though long-term data are still limited.[4]

## Systemic Therapies

Here is an overview of the various systemic therapies for the management of pediatric AD **(Table 1)**.

### Phototherapy

Phototherapy, particularly narrowband ultraviolet B (NBUVB), is an effective adjunct for managing severe, refractory pediatric AD, with sessions typically administered two to three times weekly. NBUVB suppresses Th2-mediated inflammation and has shown efficacy, with 40% of children achieving significant improvement after ten or more treatments and experiencing prolonged remission. However, adverse effects such as skin burning, erythema, pruritus, herpes simplex reactivation, and a potential long-term risk of skin cancer, particularly with psoralen (PUVA), warrant caution, especially in children. Challenges in scheduling, ensuring protection and limited long-term safety data often discourage its use in infants and young children, though studies support its safety in older pediatric patients.[5,6]

## Biologics and Emerging Therapies

The emergence of targeted biologic therapies has revolutionized dermatology, with dupilumab being the only FDA-approved treatment for pediatric AD in patients aged six months and older. By inhibiting the interleukin 4 IL-4 and IL-13 signaling pathways, dupilumab effectively suppresses the Th2-driven inflammation central to AD pathophysiology. Beyond dupilumab, new biologics are advancing through clinical trials. Lebrikizumab, an IL-13 inhibitor, demonstrated promising outcomes in the phase 2b trial for adults with moderate-to-severe AD, and phase 3 trials for adolescents are nearing completion.

- *Dupilumab*: It is an FDA-approved IL4 receptor alpha antagonist for moderate-to-severe AD.
  - *Results from key clinical trials*: Three 16-week Phase III trials—LIBERTY AD PRESCHOOL, PEDS, and ADOL—evaluated dupilumab's efficacy and safety in pediatric AD. PRESCHOOL and PEDS focused on infants and children using dupilumab with TCS, while ADOL examined its use as monotherapy in adolescents. All studies utilized weight- and age-adjusted doses. At week 16, dupilumab significantly improved key endpoints, including Investigator Global Assessment (IGA) 0/1, Eczema Area and Severity Index (EASI)-75, EASI-50, and EASI-90, compared to placebo, demonstrating its effectiveness in reducing symptoms and improving quality of life. Combination therapy with TCS was found to be more effective than monotherapy. Notably, the PRESCHOOL trial suggested that early intervention may alter the atopic march, though further studies are needed to confirm this.

Real-world studies supported these findings, showing sustained improvements in EASI, numeric rating scale (NRS), and Children Dermatology Life Quality Index (CDLQI) scores across age groups. Younger children (2–6 years) experienced faster initial responses than older groups, potentially due to weight-based dosing differences. Long-term studies, including a 52-week

**TABLE 1: Various systemic therapies for the management of pediatric atopic dermatitis.**

| Agent | Mechanism of action | Route of administration and dose | Efficacy | Recommended monitoring | Side effects |
|---|---|---|---|---|---|
| Cyclosporine A (CsA)[5] | Calcineurin inhibitor | *Oral*: 3–5 mg/kg/day | Multiple trials, including a systematic review, have highlighted the effectiveness of CsA in improving severe AD symptoms in children and adults. It is considered a first-line systemic treatment, generally recommended for up to 1 year of use | Blood pressure, complete blood count (CBC), comprehensive metabolic panel (CMP) with liver function tests (LFTs), creatinine, and optionally lipid panel | Nausea, headache, tingling sensations, high blood pressure, increased hair growth, gum overgrowth, kidney toxicity, and potential cancer risks |
| Azathioprine (AZA)[5] | Purine analog and antimetabolite | *Oral*: 2.5–3.5 mg/kg/day in patients with normal levels of thiopurine methyltransferase | Several case studies and clinical trials indicate that AZA provides modest improvements in AD symptoms. Although effective, it is typically regarded as less potent than CsA, making it a second-line option | CBC, CMP with LFTs, thiopurine methyltransferase enzyme analysis, and pregnancy testing if applicable | Digestive disturbances, liver toxicity, blood abnormalities, bone marrow suppression, potential teratogenic effects, and long-term cancer risk |
| Methotrexate (MTX)[5] | Folate antagonist | *Oral, intramuscular, subcutaneous*: 0.2–0.7 mg/kg/week for children | Retrospective data from 55 pediatric cases suggest that 76% of severe AD patients show improvement with MTX, primarily reducing affected skin areas and reliance on topical corticosteroids. Its efficacy is thought to parallel that of AZA | CBC, CMP with LFTs and creatinine, viral hepatitis screening, and pregnancy testing if required | Digestive issues, liver toxicity, oral ulcers, blood count abnormalities, bone marrow suppression, lung fibrosis, and potential effects on pregnancy |
| Mycophenolate mofetil (MMF)[5] | Inhibitor of inosine monophosphate dehydrogenase | *Oral*: 40–50 mg/kg daily | A comparative trial with CsA demonstrated similar efficacy between the two for maintenance therapy. MMF shows a slower onset but more sustained response post-treatment withdrawal. It is often used after remission is induced with CsA | CBC, CMP with LFTs, pregnancy testing when applicable, and tuberculosis screening if needed | Digestive discomfort, fatigue, headaches, abnormal blood counts, bone marrow suppression, risks of birth defects, and potential long-term cancer risks |
| Corticosteroids[5] | Multifaceted anti-inflammatory and immunosuppressive action | Oral, intramuscular | Limited evidence from two trials and one case series supports the short-term use of agents such as bedomethasone, flunisolide, and methylprednisolone. These agents are noted for their rapid symptom control and moderate efficacy in AD management | Routine monitoring is generally unnecessary for short-term use | Growth suppression, weight gain, high blood pressure, adrenal gland suppression, weakened bones, eye conditions like cataracts/glaucoma, diabetes, and mood changes |

multicenter analysis and a 24-week single-center trial, confirmed continued efficacy with no serious adverse events reported, aside from mild injection site reactions and conjunctivitis. These results highlight dupilumab's safety, efficacy, and potential to enhance quality of life in pediatric AD while emphasizing the need for further research on optimal dosing and long-term safety in infants.

- *Side effects*: Dupilumab has consistently demonstrated a strong safety profile in treating pediatric AD, with adverse reaction rates comparable to placebo and no need for organ toxicity monitoring. A clinical trial involving patients with severe comorbidities, such as malignancies, immunodeficiencies, and organ transplants, confirmed similar adverse event rates between dupilumab-treated and control groups. Common side effects included injection site reactions, conjunctivitis, and mild, reversible conditions, such as eczema of the head and neck, rosacea, and dry eye. Proactive management of these reactions often prevents treatment discontinuation.

In the PRESCHOOL and PEDS trials, adverse events were more frequent in placebo groups, while ADOL showed similar rates across treatment arms. Dupilumab q2w dosing had slightly higher adverse event rates than q4w dosing, but discontinuation due to serious effects was rare, and no deaths were reported. Dupilumab reduced skin infection rates by half compared to placebo, reflecting improved skin integrity, although conjunctivitis was more frequent in dupilumab groups. Interestingly, a drug-disease interaction was suggested by studies showing higher conjunctivitis rates in AD patients but not in asthma patients treated with dupilumab. These findings confirm dupilumab's safety and efficacy, with outcomes in children paralleling those observed in adults.[6]

### *Other Biologics*

Doses of dupilumab are summarized in **Table 2**.

Other biologics include tralokinumab, an IL-13 inhibitor already approved for adults with moderate-to-severe AD, showing encouraging results in a completed phase 3 trial for adolescents. Additionally, nemolizumab, a selective IL-31 inhibitor targeting Th2 inflammation and itch signaling, is under investigation, with multiple phase 3 trials exploring its efficacy in both pediatric and adult AD.

#### Janus Kinase (JAK) Inhibitors

JAK inhibitors represent a promising treatment for pediatric AD, available in both oral and topical formulations. Topical ruxolitinib, FDA-approved as a 1.5% cream, is indicated for mild-to-moderate AD in immunocompetent patients aged 12 years and older with <20% body surface area affected. In two phase 3 trials, ruxolitinib showed significant efficacy, with rapid itch relief, likely due to its effects on JAK signaling in sensory nerves. It is well-tolerated with minimal application-related discomfort, though it carries the same boxed warning as oral JAK inhibitors despite limited systemic absorption.

**TABLE 2: Dosing regimens for phase III clinical trials.[6]**

| Dosing | Age | Weight | Dosage |
|---|---|---|---|
| Preschool | 6 months to 5 years | • ≥15 kg to <30 kg<br>• ≥5 kg to <15 kg | • 300 mg + TCS q4w<br>• 200 mg + TCS q4w |
| Pediatric age | 6–11 years | • ≥15 kg to <30 kg<br>• ≥30 kg<br>• All body weight | • 100 mg + TCS q2w<br>• 200 mg + TCS q2w<br>• 300 mg + TCS q4w |
| Adolescent | 12–17 years | • <60 kg<br>• ≥60 kg<br>• All body weight | • 200 mg q2w<br>• 300 mg q2w<br>• 300 mg q4w |

(TCS: topical corticosteroids; q4w: every 4 weeks; q2w: every 2 weeks)

Oral JAK inhibitors have also gained traction. Upadacitinib, approved in 2022 for patients aged 12 and older with refractory moderate-to-severe AD, demonstrated over 90% improvement in Eczema Area and Severity Index (EASI) scores in phase 3 trials. It also surpassed dupilumab in skin clearance and itch relief in adult head-to-head trials.

Abrocitinib, currently approved for adults, has shown favorable results in adolescents during trials, particularly for itch improvement, though approval for younger populations is pending.

Adverse effects of oral JAK inhibitors include nausea, acne, nasopharyngitis, headache, and increased susceptibility to infections, such as herpes zoster. Other risks involve elevated creatine phosphokinase levels, thrombosis, malignancies, and cardiovascular events, necessitating a boxed warning. For safety monitoring, laboratory evaluations are recommended at baseline, 1 month after starting treatment, and every 3 months thereafter.[7]

### *Adjunctive Therapies*

#### Antihistamines

- *Role in managing pruritus*: Antihistamines are recommended for managing itching but their role is limited.

- *Sedating versus nonsedating*: Sedating antihistamines can be used for short-term, under supervision, especially in children under the age of 2 years where sleep is disturbed due to severe pruritus.[2] Hydroxyzine and cetirizine (also shows steroid-sparing effect) can control both pruritus and disturbed sleep.

#### Antibiotics and Antimicrobials

- *Management of secondary infections*: Depending upon the clinical evaluation short course of oral antibiotics can be considered in generalized infection.
- *Topical versus oral antibiotics*: Topical antibiotics should be considered in localized infection.
- *Preventing antibiotic resistance*: There is no role of preventive antibiotic therapy. Long-term use of topical or systemic antibiotics should be avoided to prevent bacterial resistance and sensitization.[8]

#### Probiotics

The connection between gut health and skin barrier function has gained attention in recent studies. The gut microbiome is believed to regulate the immune system, and its disruption, or dysbiosis, may reduce immune tolerance and increase susceptibility to skin conditions, such as acne, psoriasis, and AD. Probiotics, particularly *Lactobacillus* species, have been explored as potential adjunctive treatments for pediatric AD. A randomized controlled trial reported a significant reduction in SCORAD (SCORing Atopic Dermatitis) scores among children with moderate-to-severe AD following twice-daily supplementation with *Lactobacillus fermentum*. Additionally, a systematic review suggested that topical probiotics may also reduce AD severity. However, challenges regarding optimal dosing, formulation, efficacy, and safety have hindered their routine clinical application.[9]

### *Lifestyle and Environmental Modifications*

#### Identifying and Avoiding Triggers

- *Common environmental triggers*: Allergens such as mites, house dust, pollens, and organic solvents such as formaldehyde and toluene can aggravate AD symptoms.
- *Food allergens and dietary modifications*: Foods that may trigger AD are milk, milk-related products, soy protein, shellfish, and peanuts. There is no recommendation for empirical food exclusion and large panel-based allergy testing. A specific food-free diet can be considered after proper testing by an allergy specialist and maintaining a food diary.
- Keeping an eczema diary.

## CLOTHING AND FABRICS

- *Choosing appropriate fabrics*: Loose-fitting cotton clothes are recommended for AD patients. Woolen, acrylic, nylon, or any other irritating fabrics should be avoided. Silver coated and silk are the best fabrics for AD patients but in terms of the Indian context they are costly.
- *Laundry practices*: Detergents and fabric softeners that contain dyes, and perfumes may be left on the fabric after washing and drying. It can irritate sensitive skin. The use of hypoallergic and fragrance-free liquid products is safe.
- *Importance of breathable, nonirritating materials*: As sweating can exacerbate AD, breathable and nonirritating materials could help, and washing away sweat by bathing can improve symptoms.

## HOME ENVIRONMENTS

- Managing indoor air quality
- Using humidifiers
- Reducing dust mites and pet dander

## Psychological Support and Education

- *Parental and caregiver education*:
  - Teaching proper skincare routines
  - Educating about the chronic nature of the disease
  - Strategies for managing acute flareups
- *Support groups and resources*:
  - Connecting with other families
  - Accessing educational materials
  - Role of healthcare providers in support
- *Regular follow-up*:
  - Importance of regular checkups
  - Adjusting treatment plans
  - Monitoring growth and development
  - Recognizing signs of infection
  - Addressing treatment side effects
  - Managing comorbid conditions (e.g., allergies and asthma)[10]

## FUTURE DIRECTIONS IN ATOPIC DERMATITIS MANAGEMENT

- *Research and emerging therapies*:
  - Advances in understanding the pathophysiology of AD.
  - New and emerging treatment options.
  - Potential role of gene therapy and personalized medicine.

- *Improving quality of life*:
  - Innovations in skincare products
  - Dietary supplements (vitamin D and essential fatty acids) and probiotics supplements have some protective role and reduce the severity of AD.
  - Role of mental health support

## CONCLUSION

Owing to the chronicity and relapsing nature of the disease, management depends on the severity, mental status, socioeconomic status, and affordability of the patient. Individualized treatment plans should be provided to every atopic patient.

## REFERENCES

1. Rajagopalan M, De A, Godse K, Shankar KDS, Zawar V, Sharma N, et al. Guidelines on Management of Atopic Dermatitis in India: An Evidence-based Review and an Expert Consensus. Indian J Dermatol. 2019;64(3):166-81.
2. Bieber T. Atopic dermatitis. Ann Dermatol. 2010;22(2):125-37.
3. Nicol NH, Boguniewicz M. Wet wrap therapy in moderate to severe atopic dermatitis. Immunol Allergy Clin North Am. 2017;37(1):123-39.
4. Chakraborty D, De A, Khan A, Dhar S, Raychaudhuri SP. Comparative evaluation of the efficacy and safety of crisaborole ointment (2%) versus tacrolimus ointment (0.1%) for the topical treatment of atopic dermatitis: an open-labeled single-blinded randomized controlled trial. Int J Dermatol. 2024.
5. Johnson H, Yu J. Current and emerging therapies in pediatric atopic dermatitis. Dermatol Ther (Heidelb). 2022;12(12):2691-703.
6. Harb H, Chatila TA. Mechanisms of dupilumab. Clin Exp Allergy. 2020;50(1):5-14.
7. Bieber T, Simpson EL, Silverberg JI, Thaçi D, Paul C, Pink AE, et al. Abrocitinib versus placebo or dupilumab for atopic dermatitis. N Engl J Med. 2021;384(12):1101-12.
8. Munday J, Bloomfield R, Goldman M, Robey H, Kitowska G, Gwiezdziski Z, et al. Chlorpheniramine is no more effective than placebo in relieving the symptoms of childhood atopic dermatitis with a nocturnal itching and scratching component. Dermatology. 2002;205(1):40-5.
9. Mahmud MR, Akter S, Tamanna SK,Mazumder L, Esti IZ, Banerjee S, et al. Impact of gut microbiome on skin health: gut-skin axis observed through the lenses of therapeutics and skin diseases. Gut Microbes. 2022;14(1):2096995.
10. Solomon I, Ilie MA, Draghici C, Voiculescu VM, Căruntu C, Boda D, et al. The impact of lifestyle factors on evolution of atopic dermatitis: An alternative approach. Exp Ther Med. 2019;17(2):1078-84.

CHAPTER 2.8

# Atopic Dermatitis in Pregnancy

*Arnab Dutta, Disha Chakraborty*

## INTRODUCTION

Skin changes in pregnancy can be either physiological either due to the influence of maternal hormones, or there may be changes in preexisting skin diseases or the development of new pregnancy-specific dermatoses.[1] Atopic eruption in pregnancy (AEP) may occur as de novo or as a recurrence or exacerbation of known or preexisting AD.

## SYNONYMS

- Early onset prurigo of pregnancy
- Prurigo of pregnancy
- Prurigo gestationis
- Pruritic folliculitis of pregnancy
- Eczema of pregnancy

## EPIDEMIOLOGY

Atopic dermatitis (AD) is the most common skin disease during gestation which makes up to about 50% of all pregnancy dermatoses. The term *atopic eruption of pregnancy* was coined in 2006 by the authors of a large retrospective study that supported a clinical overlap among patients with gestational AD. 75% of cases occur before the third trimester of pregnancy. The eruption is seen more commonly in primigravida with singleton pregnancy. AD in pregnancy has a strong tendency to recur in subsequent pregnancies.

## PATHOPHYSIOLOGY

Pregnancy is characterized by a lack of strong maternal cell-mediated immune function and T-helper 1 (Th1) cytokine production (e.g., IL-12 and interferon-gamma) with a dominant humoral immune response and T-helper 2 (Th2) cytokine production (e.g., IL-4 and IL-10).[2] Exacerbation of AD in pregnancy may be due to the Th2 shift. Patients may have an atopic background with raised total serum immunoglobulin E (IgE) levels.

## CLINICAL FEATURES

Two-thirds present with widespread eczematous changes (so-called E-type AEP) often affecting typical atopic sites such as the face, neck, and flexural surfaces of the limbs, whereas one-third of patients have papular lesions (P-type AEP).

## MORPHOLOGICAL PATTERNS

Refer to **Table 1**.

## PROGNOSIS

Maternal prognosis is good even in severe cases as skin lesions usually respond quickly to therapy. Recurrence in subsequent pregnancies is common. Fetal prognosis is unaffected, but the infant may be at risk of developing atopic skin changes later.

## DIFFERENTIAL DIAGNOSIS (TABLE 2)

Atopic eruption in pregnancy must be differentiated from other pregnancy-specific dermatoses which is summarized in **Table 2**.

## MANAGEMENT (BOX 1)

Topical therapies to improve itching and relieve dryness, such as urea and 1–2% menthol, are initial treatment recommendations. Adequate skin hydration is critical

**TABLE 1: Two types of morphological patterns are currently described.**

| Entity | Onset | Clinical features | Diagnosis | Prognosis |
|---|---|---|---|---|
| Prurigo of pregnancy | Occurs in all trimesters | • History of atopy[3]<br>• Multiple itchy, excoriated papules over the abdomen and extensor surface of limbs | • *Histopathology (HPE)*: Parakeratosis, and acanthosis, with perivascular lymphocytic infiltrate around upper dermal vessels<br>• Immunofluorescence—negative | • Lesions persist throughout pregnancy<br>• Itching settles after delivery<br>• Mother and fetus are unaffected<br>• May recur in subsequent pregnancies |
| Pruritic folliculitis | Occurs in the second and third trimester of pregnancy | • May be mistaken for acne or folliculitis<br>• Multiple follicular papules or pustules occurring typically on the shoulders, upper back, arms, chest, and abdomen | • *Histopathology (HPE)*: Nonspecific folliculitis with upper dermal infiltrate<br>• Immunofluorescence—negative | • Lesions usually resolve spontaneously a few weeks after delivery<br>• No association with fetal or maternal morbidity[4] |

**TABLE 2: Differentiation of atopic eruption in pregnancy from other pregnancy-specific dermatoses.**

| Dermatoses | Age of onset | Risk factors | Clinical features | Prognosis | Investigations |
|---|---|---|---|---|---|
| Polymorphic eruption of pregnancy | Affects primigravidae in the last few weeks of pregnancy or immediately postpartum (15%) | • Maternal obesity<br>• Primigravida<br>• Multiple pregnancies | • Starts on the abdomen, often within the striae distensae<br>• Severely pruritic urticarial papules that coalesce into plaques, spreading to the buttocks and proximal thighs. Umbilical sparing is a characteristic finding | Maternal and fetal prognosis is unimpaired and there is no cutaneous involvement of the newborn. Lesions are self-limiting and the disease does not recur | • HP—epidermal and upper dermal edema, with a perivascular infiltrate of lymphocytes and histiocytes. There may be a striking number of eosinophils (as there may be in pemphigoid gestationis)<br>• DIF—negative<br>• IIF—negative |
| Pemphigoid gestationis (PG) | Late pregnancy or the immediate postpartum period | • Trophoblastic tumors (choriocarcinoma and hydatidiform mole)<br>• HLA DR3 and DR4 | • Intense pruritus that occasionally may precede skin lesions<br>• Erythematous urticarial papules and plaques typically develop on the abdomen, characteristically involving the periumbilical region<br>• Lesions progress to tense blisters which resemble those of bullous pemphigoid<br>• Facial and mucous membranes are usually spared | • Pemphigoid gestationis can recur in subsequent pregnancies and with the use of oral contraceptive therapy. When PG recurs, it often presents at an earlier gestation and with increased severity<br>• Fetal increase in prematurity and small-for-date babies. About 10% of newborns may develop mild skin lesions (neonatal PG) which resolve spontaneously within days to weeks | • HPE—the prebullous stage is characterized by edema of the upper and middle dermis accompanied by a predominantly perivascular inflammatory infiltrate, composed of lymphocytes, histiocytes, and a variable number of eosinophils. bullous stage-subepidermal blistering that, ultrastructurally, is located at the lamina lucida of the dermoepidermal junction<br>• DIF—linear C3 deposition along the dermoepidermal junction in 100% of cases and additional IgG deposition in 30% of cases<br>• *IIF*: IgG + in 30–100% cases |

*Continued*

*Continued*

| Dermatoses | Age of onset | Risk factors | Clinical features | Prognosis | Investigations |
|---|---|---|---|---|---|
| Intrahepatic cholestasis of pregnancy (ICP) | Second or third trimester | ICP recurs during subsequent pregnancies in an estimated 45–70% of patients | Patients are classically present during the third trimester with moderate-to-severe pruritus, which may be either localized to the palms and soles or generalized. Pruritus begins during the first and second trimesters in 10% and 25% of cases, respectively. Intense pruritus is often associated with secondary excoriations | • Maternal—after delivery, pruritus disappears spontaneously within days to weeks but may recur with subsequent pregnancies and oral contraception<br>• Fetal—increased risk of prematurity, fetal distress, and stillbirth[5] | ALP and serum bile acids raised |

**BOX 1 Recommendations for the use of phototherapy.**

*First line*:
- Topical emollients
- Topical corticosteroids
- *Oral antihistamines*: loratadine and cetirizine

*Second line*: Narrow-band ultraviolet B (UVB) phototherapy

*Third line*:
- Prednisolone
- Azathioprine

as fundamental therapy. Antihistamines such as chlorpheniramine, loratadine, and cetirizine may also be used which are considered safe in pregnancy. Topical medium to high-potency steroids are considered safe in pregnancy. Oral corticosteroids may be needed in nonresponders to topical therapy when initial treatment is not successful. Prednisone or prednisolone at a maximum dose of 0.5 mg/kg/day for 2–3 weeks may be necessary to control symptoms. Broad and narrowband ultraviolet B (UVB) and ultraviolet A (UVA)-1 light therapy have also been utilized. Cyclosporin A and azathioprine (off-label use) may be used in pregnancy when benefits to the mother are deemed to outweigh any potential risk to the fetus. Methotrexate and mycophenolate mofetil, Janus kinase inhibitors, baricitinib, upadacitinib, and abrocitinib are also contraindicated for use in pregnancy.

## CONCLUSION

Managing atopic dermatitis in pregnancy requires a delicate balance between disease control and fetal safety, necessitating individualized, risk-stratified approaches. Physiological changes during pregnancy can alter disease trajectory, with some patients experiencing exacerbation while others see improvement. Topical therapies remain first-line, while systemic options must be carefully selected to minimize fetal risk. Emerging evidence on the safety of biologics and small molecules offers new possibilities, yet long-term data remain limited. A multidisciplinary approach, incorporating dermatology and obstetric expertise, is essential for optimizing maternal and fetal outcomes while ensuring adequate disease control and patient well-being.

## REFERENCES

1. Balakirski G, Novak N. Atopic dermatitis and pregnancy. J Allergy Clin Immunol. 2022;149(4):1185-94.
2. Wilder RL. Hormones, pregnancy, and autoimmune disease. Ann N Y Acad Sci. 1998;840:45-50.
3. Vaughan Jones SA, Black MM. Pregnancy dermatoses. J Am Acad Dermatol. 1999;40(2 Pt 1):233-41.
4. Zoberman E, Farmer ER. Pruritic folliculitis of pregnancy. Arch Dermatol. 1981;117(1):20-2.
5. Lammert f, Marschall HU, Glantz A, Matern S. Intrahepatic cholestasis of pregnancy: molecular pathogenesis, diagnosis and management. J Hepatol. 2000;33(6):1012-21.

SECTION

# 3

# Contact Dermatitis

***Section Editor:*** Sathish Pai B

***Assistant Editor:*** Lisa Jennifer Dsouza

3.1

CHAPTER

# Irritant Contact Dermatitis

*Delvin Poulose, Shrutakirthi D Shenoi*

## INTRODUCTION

Irritant contact dermatitis (ICD) is a localized, inflammatory skin response to a wide range of chemical or physical agents. ICD results from the direct cytotoxic effect of irritants and is not immune-mediated and does not require prior sensitization. ICD is a multifactorial disorder influenced by the physical and chemical properties of the irritating substance, host-related susceptibility factors, and environmental factors.

The clinical manifestations of ICD can be similar to those of other acute or chronic eczematous dermatitides, including atopic dermatitis and allergic contact dermatitis. ICD, allergic contact dermatitis, and atopic dermatitis may coexist in the same patient.

## PREVALENCE

Irritant contact dermatitis is the most common type of contact dermatitis. ICD represents approximately 80% of occupational contact dermatitis and is considered the most frequent cause of hand eczema.[1] In the general population, the estimated prevalence of hand eczema ranges from 0.4 to 4%. Females are more frequently affected than males, particularly between the ages of 20–59 years.[1,2] Because many patients with hand eczema do not seek medical care, the true prevalence of hand eczema may be higher.[2] In a study of over 68,000 patients referred for patch testing, approximately 13% were diagnosed with ICD, with nearly one-half of the cases related to occupation.[3]

## RISK FACTORS

The development of ICD is influenced by host-related and environmental factors.

### Host Related

- *Age*: The reactivity of skin to irritants is highest in infants and it decreases with age.[4]
- *Sex*: The prevalence of ICD in general, and of hand dermatitis in particular, is greater in females than in males. However, the higher risk in females is probably due to increased domestic and occupational exposure to detergents.[1]

#### *Body Site*

The response to irritants varies among different sites due to differences in the thickness of the stratum corneum and barrier function. The face, dorsum of the hands, and finger webs are more prone to irritation from chemical substances than the palms, soles, or back.[5]

#### *Atopy*

People with atopic dermatitis are more sensitive to irritants due to a persistently compromised barrier function. Sixty-four percent of respondents with ICD in a population-based study of patients with occupational skin disease reported having a personal or family history of atopic dermatitis or exhibiting typical and/or mild indications of the condition.[6]

#### *Environmental*

The skin's reaction to irritants is influenced by environmental conditions, including temperature, air movement, humidity, and occlusion. The function of the epidermal barrier appears to be compromised by high temperatures and airflow, which also facilitates the penetration of irritants such as sodium lauryl sulphate, a surfactant found in many detergents.[7]

## PATHOGENESIS

The development of ICD is attributed to a number of mechanisms, some of which are not fully understood:

- Loss of lipids and disruption of the epidermal barrier
- Damage to the membranes of keratinocyte cells
- Cytotoxic effect on keratinocytes
- Keratinocytes secrete proinflammatory cytokines
- Activation of innate immunity
- *Acute ICD*: The acute disruption of the epidermal barrier caused by surfactants (e.g., sodium lauryl sulphate) in experimental animal and human models causes preformed cytokines, such as interleukin (IL) 1-alpha, IL-1-beta, IL-6, and tumor necrosis factor (TNF)-alpha, to be released from keratinocytes.[8] The release of proinflammatory chemokines (such as CCL20, CCL21, and CXCL8), which draw mononuclear and polymorphonuclear cells to the site of damage, is primarily signaled by IL-1-alpha and TNF-alpha.
- *Chronic ICD*: Even though the pathogenesis is not completely understood, prolonged exposure to mild irritants or damp conditions suppresses the inflammatory response while promoting the growth and differentiation of cells. Compared to nonirritated skin, chronically irritated skin had greater levels of IL-1RA and lower levels of TNF-alpha and IL-1-alpha.[9]

## MECHANISM OF ACTION OF IRRITANTS

It is possible for various substances to work in concert to cause dermatitis. While detergents remove both lipids and hygroscopic (water-holding) compounds (such as the breakdown products of filaggrin), solvents only remove the lipids from the stratum corneum. There is an additive effect when solvents and detergents are exposed together.[10]

### Chemical Irritants

#### *Water and Wet Work*

Water erodes skin by acting as a cytotoxic agent since it is hypotonic. Prolonged exposure to water on intact skin results in stratum corneum enlargement, disruption of intercellular lipids, increased skin permeability, and increased susceptibility to irritants.[11]

#### *Detergents and Surfactants*

Detergents used for domestic and industrial cleaning remove lipids and hygroscopic substances in the stratum corneum, denature proteins, and damage the cell membranes.

- *Solvents*: Solvents remove lipids and hygroscopic substances and damage cell membranes.
- *Oxidizing agents*: Oxidizing agents, such as sodium hypochlorite (bleach) or benzoyl peroxide, are cytotoxic agents.
- *Acids*: Strong acids (e.g., sulfuric acid) cause protein coagulation and cell necrosis.
- *Alkalis*: Alkaline solutions disrupt the cross-links in keratin, dissolve molecules that retain water, saponify surface lipids, and induce cell expansion.

### Physical Irritants

Chronic microtrauma or friction damages the stratum corneum, impairs the skin barrier, and induces the release of preformed cytokines from keratinocytes.

## CLINICAL MANIFESTATIONS

Irritant contact dermatitis can present with a variety of clinical symptoms, including erythema and moderate skin dryness, as well as acute or chronic eczematous dermatitis and even skin necrosis.

### Acute Irritant Contact Dermatitis

Acute ICD often results from a single exposure to an irritant or caustic chemical. Clinical features include erythema, edema, vesicles, bullae, and oozing **(Fig. 1)**. The reaction usually just affects the area of touch and is accompanied by a scorching, stinging, or painful feeling.

### Chronic Irritant Contact Dermatitis

Repetitive exposure to mild irritants or low concentrations of severe irritants causes chronic ICD. Erythema, scaling, lichenification, hyperkeratosis, and fissuring are clinical features of chronic ICD **(Fig. 2)**. While itching

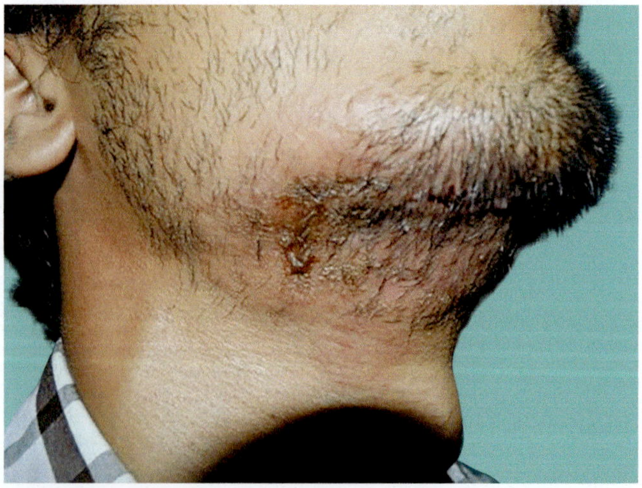

**FIG. 1:** Acute irritant contact dermatitis secondary to antiseptics showing erythema, vesicles, crusting and mild oozing.

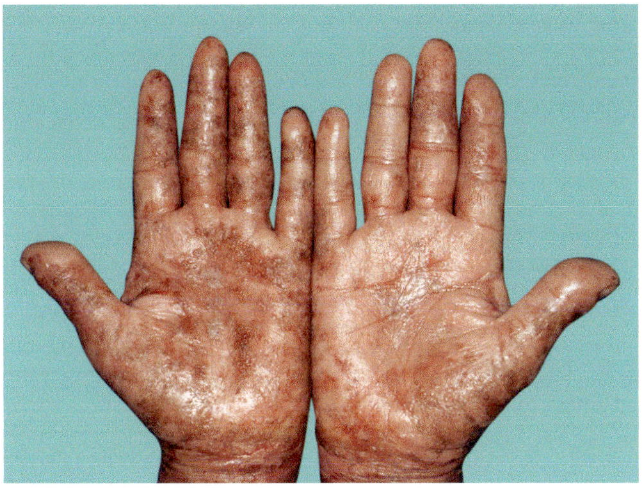

**FIG. 2:** Chronic irritant contact dermatitis of hands showing erythema, scaling and hyperkeratosis.

might occur, it is frequently a less obvious sign than burning and pain.

## DIAGNOSIS

The clinical observation of localized dermatitis in a patient with a history of exposure to chemical or physical irritants serves as the basis for the diagnosis of ICD. To make the right diagnosis, a thorough skin examination and precise history collection are essential.

### Skin Examination

A complete skin examination should be performed to evaluate the extent of the skin involvement and concomitant skin disorders. The morphology, localization, and temporal course of dermatitis often suggest the diagnosis of ICD. In most cases, the affected sites are exposed areas, such as the dorsum of hands, face, and neck.

### History

- Daily activities, including occupation, home exposure, and hobbies
- Types of substance or machinery used at the workplace
- Workplace environment (temperature, humidity, and dust)
- Use of protective gloves or gear
- Wet work (including the use of occlusive gloves)
- Hand washing habits
- Use of cleansers skin-protecting creams and cosmetic products

#### *Patch Testing*

In many cases, patch testing is required to rule out allergic contact dermatitis. Typically, a common set of allergens is utilized for preliminary screening. Depending on the patient's history of exposure, testing for additional series or particular allergens connected to the workplace can be necessary.

#### *Skin Biopsy*

It is not routinely performed, but it is useful to differentiate ICD from psoriasis or other types of inflammatory dermatoses.

#### *Histopathology*

Acute ICD is characterized by mild spongiosis, intra-epidermal vesicles or bullae, and necrosis of keratinocytes. A perivascular mononuclear cell infiltrate may be seen. Electron microscopy shows a condensed cytoplasm containing aggregated keratin filaments, lipid vacuoles, membrane-bound vesicles, disrupted cell membranes, and pyknotic nuclei with condensed chromatin.

- Chronic ICD is characterized by hyperkeratosis, parakeratosis, hypergranulosis, and acanthosis.

## DIFFERENTIAL DIAGNOSIS

- *Allergic contact dermatitis*: A positive patch test to the relevant exposure is generally diagnostic of allergic contact dermatitis, along with relevant history of longstanding eczema.
- *Atopic dermatitis*: A history of atopic dermatitis and/or involvement of flexural areas suggest the diagnosis of atopic dermatitis.
- *Psoriasis*: Nonpustular palmoplantar psoriasis may be extremely difficult to differentiate from hyperkeratotic, chronic ICD, and biopsy may not differentiate the two.
- *Fungal infection*: Tinea manuum or pedis are typically unilateral or asymmetrical. Potassium hydroxide (KOH) examination of scales can clarify the diagnosis.

## MANAGEMENT

- Identification and avoidance of the offending irritant(s).
- Treatment of skin inflammation.
- Restoration of the epidermal barrier function.
- Prevention of further exposure.

### Avoidance

Avoidance of offending irritants and adoption of protective measures are critical in the management of ICD. For hand dermatitis, general measures include **(Flowchart 1)**.

- Using vinyl gloves with cotton lining if wet work cannot be avoided.

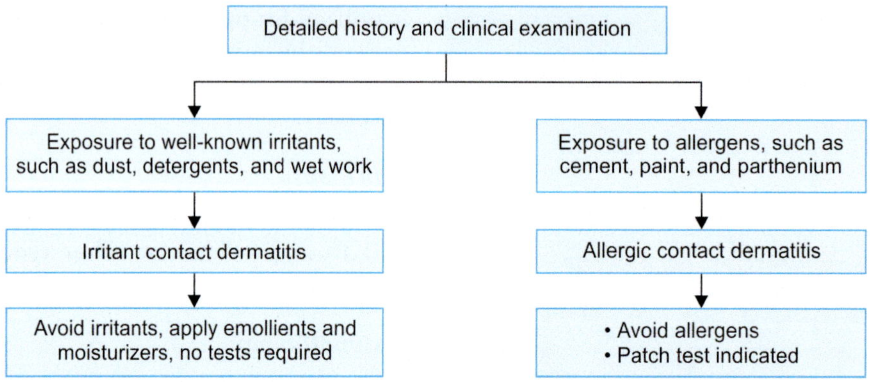


**FLOWCHART 1:** Approach to a case of suspected irritant contact dermatitis (ICD).

- Using lukewarm water and small amounts of mild, fragrance-free, and soap-free skin cleansers for hand washing.
- Using moisturizers and barrier creams frequently, particularly with work-associated exposure to irritants and after-hand hygiene.

## Active Treatment

### *Emollients and Moisturizers*

Emollients and moisturizers are beneficial in all patients with ICD. They soften the stratum corneum, reduce the transepidermal water loss (TEWL), and attract water to the stratum corneum. Emollients and moisturizers are used to decrease irritation and improve or restore the skin barrier function in ICD.

### *Topical Corticosteroids*

Topical corticosteroids in combination with emollients are frequently used in clinical practice for the treatment of ICD. Preparations of different potencies are selected based on the severity and location of dermatitis, as described below. In general, ointments are preferred to creams.

**Flowchart 1** summarizes the approach to a case of suspected ICD.

## Prevention

Gloves and barrier creams combined with adequate skin care are widely recommended as the most important measures of personal protection in occupations at increased risk of ICD. Depending on the nature of the irritant exposure, the use of personal protective equipment (e.g., suits, face masks, and goggles) may be beneficial. Worker education programs are also effective at preventing occupational ICD.

### *Education*

Numerous studies outline the importance of appropriate education on primary prevention of occupational dermatitis, including ICD, for workers involved in health care, hairdressing, wet work, food preparation, cleaning, and manufacturing. Educational training may occur in vocational schools or on-the-job training sessions and includes information on hand hygiene, proper use of personal protective equipment, and application of moisturizers or barrier creams.

# CONCLUSION

Irritant contact dermatitis (ICD) is a common and prevalent skin condition caused by exposure to various irritants, with hand eczema being a primary manifestation. Diagnosis involves a thorough clinical assessment and testing to distinguish ICD from other dermatitis types. Effective management focuses on irritant avoidance, skin protection, and appropriate use of emollients and corticosteroids.

# REFERENCES

1. Thyssen JP, Johansen JD, Linneberg A, Menné T. The epidemiology of hand eczema in the general population--prevalence and main findings. Contact Dermatitis. 2010;62(2):75.
2. Crane MM, Webb DJ, Watson E, Cunliffe T, English J. Hand eczema and steroid-refractory chronic hand eczema in general practice: prevalence and initial treatment. Br J Dermatol. 2017;176(4):955.
3. Loman L, Uter W, Armario-Hita JC, Ayala F, Balato A, Ballmer-Weber BK, et al. European Surveillance System on Contact Allergies (ESSCA): Characteristics of patients patch tested and diagnosed with irritant contact dermatitis. Contact Dermatitis. 2021;85(2):186.
4. Jakasa I, de Jongh CM, Verberk MM, Bos JD, Kezić S. Percutaneous penetration of sodium lauryl sulphate is increased in uninvolved

skin of patients with atopic dermatitis compared with control subjects. Br J Dermatol. 2006;155(1):104.

5. Rougier A, Dupuis D, Lotte C, Roguet R, Wester RC, Maibach HI. Regional variation in percutaneous absorption in man: measurement by the stripping method. Arch Dermatol Res. 1986;278(6):465-9.
6. Berardesca E, Vignoli GP, Distante F, Brizzi P, Rabbiosi G. Effects of water temperature on surfactant-induced skin irritation. Contact Dermatitis. 1995;32(2):83-7.
7. Ohlenschlaeger J, Friberg J, Ramsing D, Agner T. Temperature dependency of skin susceptibility to water and detergents. Acta Derm Venereol. 1996;76(4):274-6.
8. Spiekstra SW, Toebak MJ, Sampat-Sardjoepersad S, van Beek PJ, Boorsma DM, Stoof TJ, et al. Induction of cytokine (interleukin-1 alpha and tumor necrosis factor-alpha) and chemokine (CCL20, CCL27, and CXCL8) alarm signals after allergen and irritant exposure. Exp Dermatol. 2005;14(2):109-16.
9. Visscher MO, Said D, Wickett R. Stratum corneum cytokines, structural proteins, and transepidermal water loss: effect of hand hygiene. Skin Res Technol. 2010;16(2):229-36.
10. Wigger-Alberti W, Krebs A, Elsner P. Experimental irritant contact dermatitis due to cumulative epicutaneous exposure to sodium lauryl sulphate and toluene: single and concurrent application. Br J Dermatol. 2000;143(3):551-6.
11. Warner RR, Boissy YL, Lilly NA, Spears MJ, McKillop K, Marshall JL, et al. Water disrupts stratum corneum lipid lamellae: damage is similar to surfactants. J Invest Dermatol. 1999;113(6):960-6.

CHAPTER 3.2

# Allergic Contact Dermatitis

*Zoya A, Shrutakirthi D Shenoi*

## INTRODUCTION

Many adverse events can occur as a consequence of contact with various irritants, allergens, or other extrinsic factors, such as UV radiation and microbes. Contact dermatitis (CD) is an inflammatory condition caused by irritant or toxic effects of the chemicals or contact allergens that can induce an immune response predominantly of T-cell type. Two forms of CD include irritant contact dermatitis (ICD) and allergic contact dermatitis (ACD), although the former is more frequent than the latter, the prevalence of ACD is 15–25% of CD cases.[1] The cutaneous responses of ACD and ICD are governed by the chemical concentration, frequency and duration of exposure, host susceptibility, and integrity of the skin barrier. CD represents one of the most common occupational skin diseases in many countries causing a significant impact on healthcare and industrial productivity.

Allergic contact dermatitis is a type 4 delayed hypersensitivity reaction triggered when the skin comes in contact with a hapten/molecule (size < 500 Da) to which the individual has not previously been sensitized.[2] For instance, molecules such as in jewelry, plants, personal care products, preservatives, fragrances, hair dyes, photoallergens as well as chemicals at work can cause allergic reactions. ACD can affect all age and gender groups although it is found to be more common in females.[3] Clinical presentation can be more confined to the contact site or diffuse at times. Patch test is the gold standard diagnostic test that aids in the identification of potential allergens and diagnosis of ACD. The main principle of treatment is patient counseling regarding avoidance of the triggering factor or allergen.

## PATHOPHYSIOLOGY

Allergic contact dermatitis is a cell-mediated hypersensitivity reaction with two distinct phases. The afferent phase is a sensitization phase that occurs when a foreign substance penetrates through the skin and induces the formation of antigen complexes. On subsequent reexposure of the antigen, there is activation of hapten-specific T-cells which induce acute inflammatory response within 2 days called as efferent or elicitation phase.

There are a series of fundamental events that occur following contact with an allergen. The first step includes percutaneous penetration of the allergen via the stratum corneum followed by activation of innate immune mechanisms within the skin which stimulates the release of pro-inflammatory cytokines, such as interleukin (IL)-1, tumor necrosis factor-alpha (TNF-α), IL-8, IL-18, and granulocyte-macrophage colony-stimulating factor (GM-CSF). These activate the dendritic and Langerhans cells which present antigenic peptides to the naïve T-cells via MHC molecules. As a result, naïve CD4+ and CD8+T cells are primed, activated, and cloned to form specific subsets of effector T-cells (Th1, Th2, Th17, and Treg cells) which migrate from the lymph node to the skin and trigger cytokine-induced proliferative localized inflammatory response.[4]

## CLINICAL FEATURES

Allergic contact dermatitis presents with itchy lesions on the exposed or covered areas of the body. A detailed history regarding the onset, site of initial lesion, duration, and progression of the lesions, patient's occupation, household activities, or any hobbies pertaining to the exposure of a particular allergen are obtained along with cutaneous examination. The classical appearance of ACD in the acute stage is often as a pruritic eczematous eruption with papules, edema, and vesiculation at the site of contact **(Figs. 1 to 3)**. On frequent chronic exposure, lichenification or scaly plaques are observed. Apart from the acute stage, there are two other stages of progression of ACD. In the second stage due to lymphatic spread, locally disseminated erythematous or erythema-multiforme-like lesions are found at the primary site. In the third stage, hematogenous dissemination of antigen results in "idic reaction" and "systemic contact dermatitis."[5] Airborne CD and photoallergic CD represent other types of ACD.

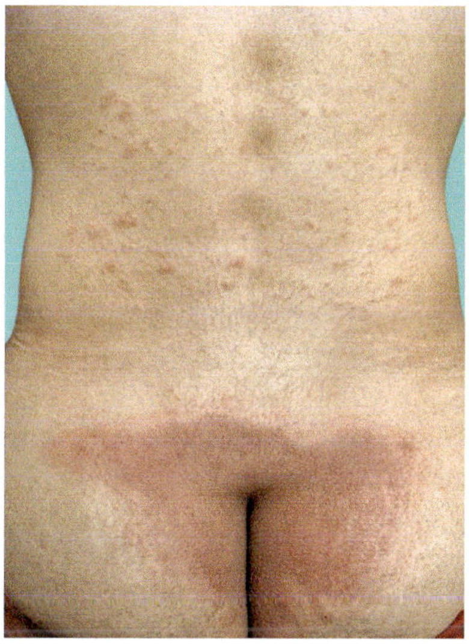

**FIG. 1:** Allergic contact dermatitis (ACD) with idic reaction to lignocaine ointment.

Other rare forms reported include nummular, bullous, pigmented, purpuric, lichenoid, lymphomatoid, pustular, and granulomatous ACD.

## DIFFERENTIAL DIAGNOSIS

The differential diagnosis of ACD includes other exogenous and endogenous forms of eczema such as ICD, atopic dermatitis, stasis dermatitis, and hand and foot dermatitis. Other conditions such as urticaria, drug reactions, tinea corporis, psoriasis and rarely other causes of erythroderma are to be ruled out.

## INVESTIGATIONS

### Histopathology

The histopathological findings are nonspecific. For a definitive diagnosis, clinical correlation and patch testing are needed. In the acute stage of ACD, there is a variable degree of spongiosis, vesiculation, and mixed dermal inflammatory infiltrate of lymphocytes, eosinophils, and histiocytes. In the chronic stage, there is hyperkeratosis, marked acanthosis with minimal epidermal edema.

### Patch Test

Patch test is a standardized diagnostic method that is to be performed in all suspected cases of CD. Patients on immunosuppressants, corticosteroids, or with active dermatitis should not be tested. Indian standard series of 20 allergens **(Table 1)** as recommended by the Contact and Occupational Dermatoses Forum of India is the screening test. Subsequently, additional batteries such as cosmetic, fragrance, and footwear series may be used.

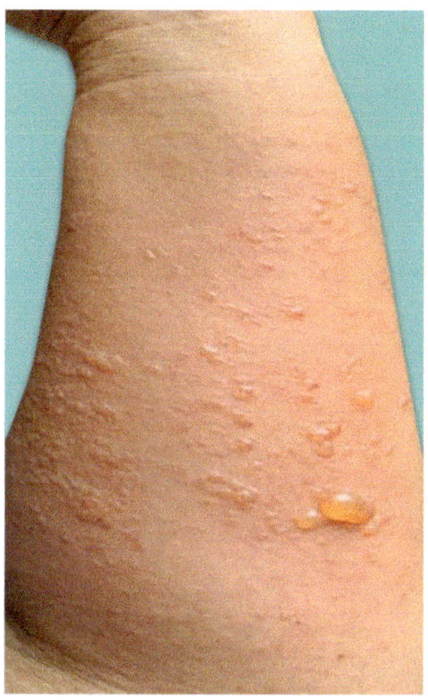

**FIG. 2:** Acute allergic contact dermatitis (ACD) to plant.

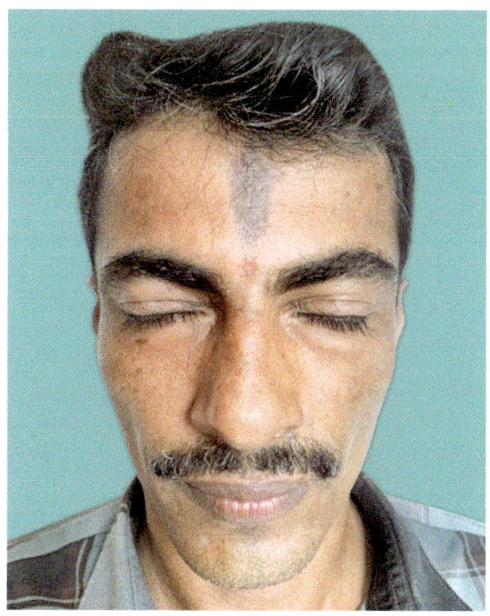

**FIG. 3:** Allergic contact dermatitis (ACD) to sandalwood paste.

The allergens are applied over the non-hairy areas of the upper back and results are read after 48 and 72 hours respectively. Interpretation of the results is done using the International Grading System (macular erythema—?, palpable erythema—1+, vesicular reaction—2+, bullous/ulcerative reaction—3+). In a study of 582 patients, 177 patients showed positive patch test results, nickel sulphate (49%) being the most common allergen followed by potassium dichromate (28%), cobalt (26%), p-Phenylenediamine (23%), neomycin (16%), and fragrance mix (15%).[6]

**TABLE 1: Allergens in Indian standard battery series.**

| Allergens | Sources |
|---|---|
| Lanolin | Cosmetics and topical agents |
| Peru balsam | Cosmetics and perfumes |
| Formaldehyde | Fabrics, paints, disinfectants, and cleaners |
| Mercaptobenzothiazole | Rubber |
| Potassium dichromate | Cement, shoes, metals |
| Nickel sulphate | Jewelers, metals, and coins |
| Cobalt sulphate | Cement, paint, and metals |
| Colophony | Ink, paper, glue, and dental materials |
| Epoxy resins | Adhesive |
| Parabens mix | Preservative |
| Paraphenylenediamine | Hair dyes and leather shoes |
| Parthenium | Plant |
| Neomycin | Antibiotic |
| Benzocaine | Local anesthetic |
| Chlorocresol | Lubricant and cosmetics |
| Fragrance mix | Perfumes and cosmetics |
| Thiuram mix | Rubber |
| Nitrofurazon | Topical bactericide |
| Black rubber mix | Rubber |

In cases when a patch test cannot be performed, a repeat open application test (ROAT) can be performed. The product to be tested is applied over the antecubital fossa of the forearm over an area of 5 cm$^2$ twice daily for a week. The test is reported positive when frank dermatitis is observed at the site of application.

**Flowchart 1** provides an algorithm for the approach to a patient with allergic CD.

## MANAGEMENT

Once the offending agent has been identified, the primary aim of the management is to counsel and educate the patient about the allergen and their sources in order to avoid further exposure. There are instances wherein cross reactions to other allergens can occur, hence patient is to be warned about the same. Patients should be instructed to read the labels of the products before use.

Moderate to high-potency topical corticosteroids along with emollients are the first line of treatment for ACD. Symptomatic treatment with antihistamines soaks in cases of oozing lesions, and antibiotics when there is evidence of secondary bacterial infection are advised. Tapering doses of systemic corticosteroids are indicated in acute, severe, and extensive forms of eczema **(Table 1)**.

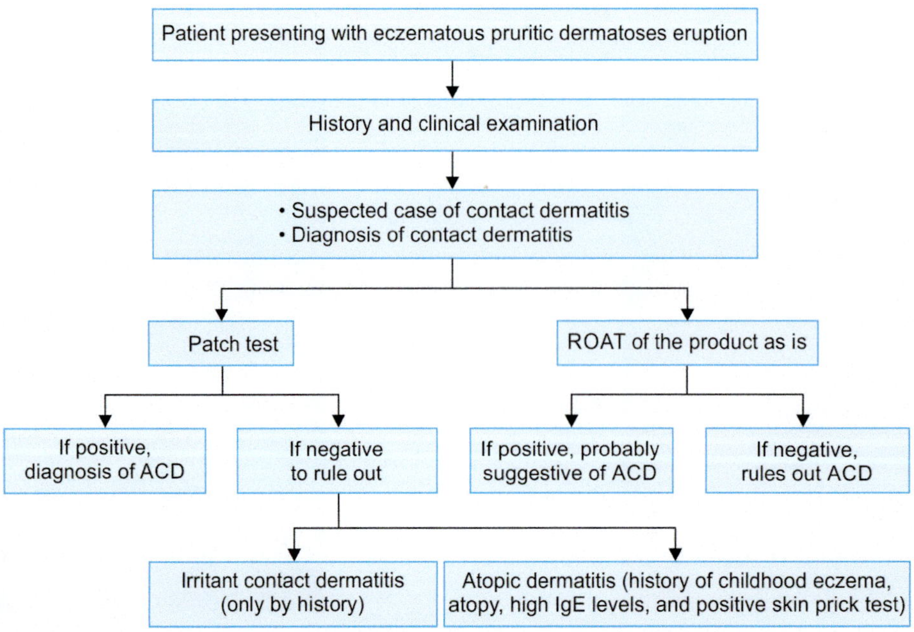


**FLOWCHART 1:** Approach to a case of ACD.

(ACD: allergic contact dermatitis; IgE: immunoglobulin E; ROAT: repeat open application test)

## CONCLUSION

Allergic contact dermatitis (ACD) is a skin condition caused by an immune response to specific allergens, typically diagnosed through patch testing. The primary treatment involves avoiding triggers, using topical corticosteroids, and emollients. In more severe cases, systemic corticosteroids and antibiotics may be required to manage the condition effectively.

## REFERENCES

1. Novak-Bilić G, Vučić M, Japundžić I, Meštrović-Štefekov J, Stanić-Duktaj S, Lugović-Mihić L. Irritant and allergic contact dermatitis - skin lesion characteristics. Acta Clin Croat. 2018; 57(4):713-20.
2. Divkovic M, Pease CK, Gerberick GF, Basketter DA. Hapten-protein binding: from theory to practical application in the in vitro prediction of skin sensitization. Contact Dermatitis. 2005;53(4):189-200.
3. Murphy PB, Atwater AR, Mueller M. Allergic Contact Dermatitis. In: Treasure Island (FL): StatPearls Publishing; 2025.
4. Kaplan DH, Igyártó BZ, Gaspari AA. Early immune events in the induction of allergic contact dermatitis. Nat Rev Immunol. 2012;12(2):114-24.
5. Lachapelle J-M. Allergic contact dermatitis: clinical aspects. Rev Environ Health 2014;29(3)185-94.
6. Hassan I, Akhtar S, Zeerak S, Rasool F, Rather P, Bhat Y, et al. Clinicoepidemiological and patch test profile of patients attending the contact dermatitis clinic of a tertiary care hospital in North India: A 7-year retrospective study. Indian Dermatol Online J. 2019;10(6):669-75.

# 3.3

CHAPTER

# Airborne Contact Dermatitis

*Meghashree G, Shrutakirthi D Shenoi*

## INTRODUCTION

Airborne contact dermatitis (ABCD) is an inflammatory reaction caused by exposure to particles suspended in the air.[1] Contact dermatitis is considered as airborne based on the history of the patient, existence of dust or airborne allergens and volatile causative agents, the morphology and distribution of the lesions, and the results of epicutaneous tests.[2]

## EPIDEMIOLOGY

The prevalence of ABCD is difficult to estimate primarily, because it is difficult and cumbersome to prove an ABCD, especially of irritant type, and secondly the term airborne has been used less often in literature. Epidemiologically, ABCD can be classified into occupational and nonoccupational ABCD, the former being more common than the latter.[1]

## IMMUNOLOGY AND PATHOGENESIS

Airborne contact dermatitis can be classified as either airborne allergic contact dermatitis (ABACD) or airborne irritant contact dermatitis (ABICD), based on its etiology and the mechanism of inflammation.

Allergic contact dermatitis (ACD) is a type IV (delayed) hypersensitivity reaction and is characterized by an immune response to a specific antigen. Skin lesions resulting from allergen exposure may extend outside the initial sites of exposure, including the covered areas.

Irritant contact dermatitis is a nonallergic inflammatory response to a physical or chemical irritant, resulting in skin lesions confined to the area of initial exposure.[3]

A study on cytokine profile of patients with *Parthenium* dermatitis showed increased levels of proinflammatory cytokines like interleukin (IL)-6, IL-8, IL-17 and tumor necrosis factor alpha (TNF-α), and decreased levels of anti-inflammatory cytokines like IL-4 and IL-10.[4] Polymorphism of TNF-α (TNF-308 A allele) was associated with polysensitization.[5]

## ETIOLOGY

Based on the causative agents, ABCD can be categorized as of: (1) Plant origin and (2) nonplant origin.[3]

### Plant-related Airborne Contact Dermatitis

Two major families of plants that are responsible for ABCD are the Compositae family and the Anacardiaceae family. Plants of the Compositae family include ragweed, goldenrod, sunflowers, and chrysanthemums. The flowers, leaves, stems, and pollens of these plants are coated with sesquiterpene lactones, which are the primary substances responsible for producing an allergic reaction upon exposure. Airborne exposure can occur through direct contact with sesquiterpene lactones (SLs) coating the pollen or through the release of these chemicals into the air through incineration.[3]

In India, *Parthenium* dermatitis, caused by *Parthenium hysterophorus*, is an important cause of ABCD. *Parthenium* belongs to Compositae family. Parthenin present in

*Parthenium* belongs to the pseudoguaianolide class of SLs, which induces allergic reaction. The other components, namely thiophenes, monoterpenes, and acetylenes, are known to cause phytophotodermatitis. *Parthenium* allergens contaminate herbal ingredients, which are used in culinary, cosmetic, and medicinal products.[1]

The other group of plants commonly responsible for ABCD reactions belong to the genus *Toxicodendron* of the Anacardiaceae family. These plants include poison ivy, poison oak, and poison sumac and produce sap, which contains the highly allergenic oil urushiol.[3]

### Nonplant-related Airborne Contact Dermatitis

The airborne contactants can also be classified on the basis of their physical state as:

- Volatile airborne contactants such as acids, alkalis, ammonia, and pesticides
- Droplets such as insecticides, perfumes, and hair sprays
- Powders which include aluminum, anhydrous calcium silicate, and metallic oxides
- Particles such as tree-sawing particles, wool, and plastics

Many agents have been reported in literature to cause ABCD. Those causing ABACD include dust particles from wood, cement (potassium dichromate), and metals including nickel, silver, mercury, gold, and arsenic salts, pharmaceutical agents such as azathioprine, budesonide, famotidine, lansoprazole and methotrexate, pesticide additives, rubber latex, and even particles from cigarettes. The development of ABCD in response to medications can occur during the manufacturing process, during the compounding process at the pharmacy or after distribution to healthcare professionals and patients.

Agents implicated in causing ABICD include phosphates, metal dusts, carbon fiber and fiberglass, epoxy resin, isothiazolinones, animal dander, ammonia, anhydrous calcium sulfate, cleaning products, and formaldehyde.[1]

## CLINICAL FEATURES

Clinically, airborne dermatitis can be classified into five different types:[6]

1. Airborne irritant contact dermatitis
2. Airborne allergic contact dermatitis

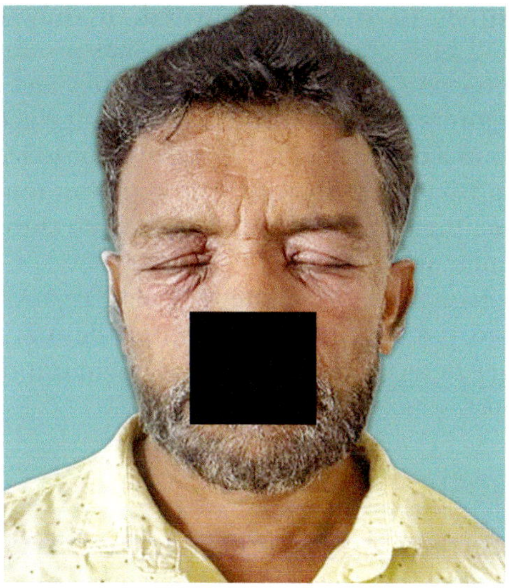

**FIG. 1:** A case of airborne contact dermatitis.

3. Airborne phototoxic reactions
4. Airborne photoallergic reactions
5. Airborne contact urticaria

Rare presentations include acneiform lesions, lichenoid eruptions, fixed drug eruptions, exfoliative dermatitis, telangiectases, paresthesias, purpura, erythema multiforme-like eruption, pellagra-like dermatitis, and lymphomatoid contact dermatitis (CD).

The most common sites for ABCD are the parts of the body that are exposed to the air such as face, neck, upper aspect of the chest, "V" region of the neck, hands, wrists, underarms, and sometimes, lower legs in women **(Fig. 1)**.

Other areas distinctly involved in ABCD include the upper eyelids, posterior ears, and nasolabial folds and submandibular region, which are the shadowed areas of the face that are spared in photodermatitis.[1,7]

The upper eyelids are commonly affected in ABCD for two reasons: (1) Airborne materials are easily deposited on the upper eyelid, while the eye is closed and are then trapped and occluded when the eye is opened, and (2) the skin of the eyelids is particularly thin, which allows chemicals to penetrate easily.[8]

Some agents cause more than one type of reaction. *P. hysterophorus* can produce allergic CD, photocontact dermatitis, and a lichenoid eruption. Similarly, formaldehyde and phosphorus sesquisulfide can lead to an airborne irritant or allergic CD and contact urticaria.[1]

Sawdust from teak, redwood, mahogany, and rosewood may contain sensitizers that produce a dry dermatitis, particularly on the face, penis, and scrotum in carpenters and woodworkers. Cement dust usually presents as a dry, lichenified dermatitis due to its alkaline and hygroscopic properties. The eruption tends to be dry rather than oozy in cases of ACD to the chromium or cobalt content in cement.[1]

A personal history of atopy is also associated with increased risk for ABCD, as in atopic dermatitis there is barrier defect which allows easy penetration of the allergens.[3]

## DIAGNOSIS

Diagnosing ABCD and determining the causative agent can be quite difficult and cumbersome, especially in ABICD. Diagnosis depends on history, the timeline of the disease, history of atopy and occupational exposures as well as the physical examination.

Allergic contact dermatitis can be confirmed by patch testing and photopatch test. There are no specific tests for irritant contact dermatitis as the diagnosis is based mainly on history of exposure to known irritants and the clinical findings.

In case of occupational ABCD, the patient can collect a small amount of dust from open areas in the workplace and bring it to the physician, who can then mix the dust with a tiny amount of petrolatum and use this mixture in a patch test. This method, although not standardized, can provide important evidence to either support or argue against the diagnosis of occupational ABCD. Alternatively, the sampling of air in the suspected environment and analysis of the concentrations of specific allergens or irritants can also be pursued, but is rarely helpful.[1,3]

Other tests include epicutaneous procedures such as open test, repeated open application tests, and use tests. In cases of airborne contact urticaria, prick tests are warranted.[7]

## TREATMENT

In cases of ABCD due to *Parthenium*, one should avoid going outdoors on days when pollens are present in high concentrations in air, especially in summers and in the months from September to November. Air conditioning decreases indoor pollen counts. Simple routine measures like taking a bath after coming indoors, wearing fresh clothes, and eliminating weeds and grasses near the house can be beneficial. Use of a barrier cream on the exposed areas after every wash is important to slow down penetration of antigen into the skin. Other measures which can be used are photoprotection, sunscreens, change of job, change of residence, antihistamines, drying agents in cases of weeping eruptions such as aluminum sulfate and calcium acetate, and emollients for lichenified areas.[1,9]

For localized dermatitis, topical steroids are the mainstay of therapy. They decrease the number of human leukocyte antigen (HLA) DR+ Langerhans cells (LCs) and inhibit the production and function of IL-1, IL-2, and interferon gamma (IFN-γ). Systemic steroids decrease T-cell proliferation and are indicated when there is involvement of more than 25% body surface area.[1]

Psoralens and ultraviolet A (PUVA) decreases HLA DR+ LC, whereas UVB induces epidermal hyperplasia and prostaglandin E.[1]

Immunosuppressives are indicated for severe, recalcitrant photosensitive dermatitis. The most commonly used immunosuppressive agent is azathioprine at the dose of 1–2.5 mg/day. It blocks DNA replication by incorporating 6-thioguanine into DNA and prevents lymphocytic proliferation after antigenic stimulation and also reduces the number and antigen-presenting capacity of LC.[10]

Other drugs include betamethasone 1–2 mg/day during exacerbations and methotrexate 15 mg/week.[1]

Hyposensitization refers to introduction of an antigen into the body by a route different from the natural one, to induce such a change in the immune system that the body does not develop clinical manifestations when the antigen is introduced into the body through normal route. In a study which evaluated the effect of oral hyposensitization as an alternative therapeutic modality in *Parthenium* dermatitis, there was a gradual improvement in 70% of patients and exacerbation in 30% during the course of the study.[11]

Although the diagnosis of ABCD is generally straightforward, the challenge lies in differentiating ABICD from ABACD. A knowledge of irritants and allergens at work and home with appropriate testing becomes crucial in management.

**Flowchart 1** depicts the approach to a case of ABCD.

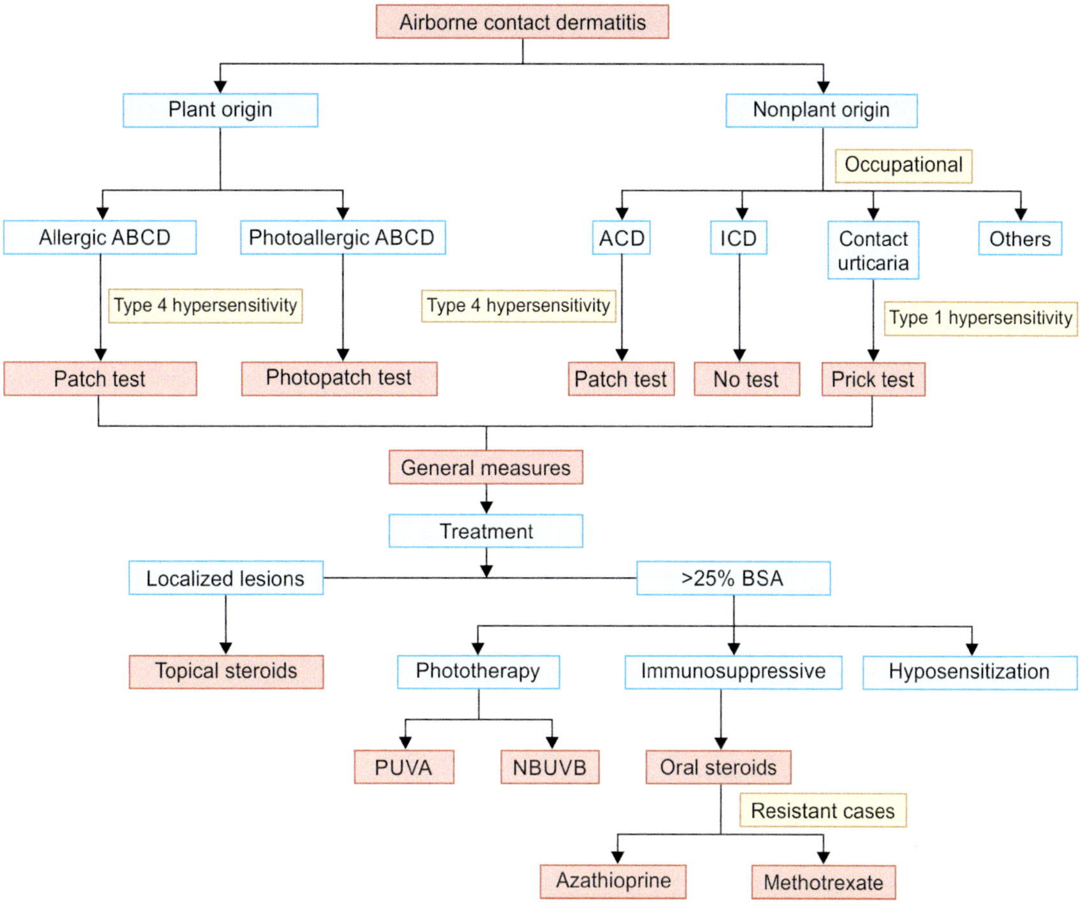


**FLOWCHART 1:** Approach to a case of ABCD.

(ABCD: airborne contact dermatitis; ACD: allergic contact dermatitis; BSA: body surface area; ICD: irritant contact dermatitis; NBUVA: narrowband ultraviolet A; PUVA: psoralens and ultraviolet A)

## CONCLUSION

Airborne contact dermatitis (ABCD) is a challenging condition caused by exposure to airborne irritants or allergens. Diagnosis requires careful history-taking, clinical examination, and appropriate testing. Treatment focuses on avoiding triggers, managing symptoms with medications, and in severe cases, using immunosuppressive therapies.

## REFERENCES

1. Handa S, De D, Mahajan R. Airborne contact dermatitis – current perspectives in etiopathogenesis and management. Indian J Dermatol. 2011;56:700-6.
2. Santos R, Goossens AR. An update on airborne contact dermatitis: 2001–2006. Contact Dermatitis. 2007;57:353-60.
3. Schloemer JA, Zirwas MJ, Burkhart CG. Airborne contact dermatitis: common causes in the USA. Int J Dermatol. 2015;54:271-4.
4. Akhtar N, Verma KK, Sharma A. Study of pro- and anti-inflammatory cytokine profile in the patients with parthenium dermatitis. Contact Dermatitis. 2010;63:203-8.
5. Westphal GA, Schnuch A, Moessner R, Koenig IR, Kränke B, Hallier E, et al. Cytokine gene polymorphisms in allergic contact dermatitis. Contact Dermatitis. 2003;48:93-8.
6. Dooms-Goosens A, Deleu H. Airborne contact dermatitis: An update. Contact Dermatitis. 1991;25:211-7.
7. Bonamonte D, Romita P, Filoni A, Angelini G, Foti C. Airborne contact dermatitis. Open Dermatol J. 2020;14:31-7.
8. Habif TP. Contact dermatitis and patch testing. In: Habif TP (Ed). Clinical Dermatology: A Color Guide to Diagnosis and Therapy, 5th edition. St Louis, MO: Mosby (Elsevier); 2009. pp. 130-53.
9. Nicholson PJ, Llewellyn D, English JS. On behalf of the Guidelines Development Group. Evidence-based guidelines for the prevention, identification and management of occupational contact dermatitis and urticaria. Contact Dermatitis. 2010;63:177-86.
10. Patel AA, Swerlick RA, McCall CO. Azathioprine in dermatology: The past, the present, and the future. J Am Acad Dermatol. 2006;55:369-89.
11. Handa S, Sahoo B, Sharma VK. Oral hyposensitisation in patients with contact dermatitis from Parthenium hysterophorus. Contact Dermatitis. 2001;44:279-82.

3.4

CHAPTER

# Eyelid Dermatitis

*Gatha M Upadya*

## INTRODUCTION

Eyelid dermatitis, which is also called periocular or periorbital dermatitis, presents with erythematous, scaly lesions on upper or lower eyelid, especially periorbital area. Patients may experience itching, burning, stinging, and the lids are red and scaly. The lids may get swollen with recurrent dermatitis. Eye lids may get thickened and lichenified. The lid margin also may get affected then it is called blepharitis.[1]

## EPIDEMIOLOGY

It is usually seen in adults and teens and less common in children. Eyelid dermatitis is seen very commonly in clinical practice. Main causes are allergic contact dermatitis, irritant contact dermatitis, and atopic dermatitis (AD).[2] When it is due to allergic contact dermatitis, females out member males. Various causes of allergic contact dermatitis are metals, shellac, preservatives, topical antibiotics, fragrances, and surfactants.[1] Airborne contact dermatitis is caused by exposure to antigens or irritant particles suspended in the air. These include plant antigens, rubber, glues, industrial dust pesticides, etc. Protein contact dermatitis is an immunoglobulin E (IgE)-mediated allergic contact dermatitis due to sensitization to plants or animal protein including foods, pollen, and animal hair. Irritant contact dermatitis which exacerbates eyelid dermatitis include soaps, shampoos, and fragrances.

Eyelid dermatitis may occur in patients with a history of childhood atopy[2] or asthma or seasonal allergy. Some of the irritants play a major role in the development of eyelid dermatitis in these patients. Eyelid dermatitis can also be triggered by various conditions such as seborrheic dermatitis, AD, ocular rosacea, dermatomyositis, and psoriasis.[1] Seborrheic dermatitis can affect eyelids, leading to yellow greasy flakes, red itchy skin affecting the eyelids margins and creases. People with AD have a defective skin barrier, hence are more prone to develop inflammation and itching leading to marked lichenification of the skin of the eyelids and dermatitis. Dennie–Morgan lines are prominent symmetrical folds below the lower eye lids. Eyelids are commonly involved on AD, and the second most common cause of eyelid dermatitis is AD seen in 10% of patients analyzed with eyelid dermatitis **(Flowchart 1)**.[3,4]

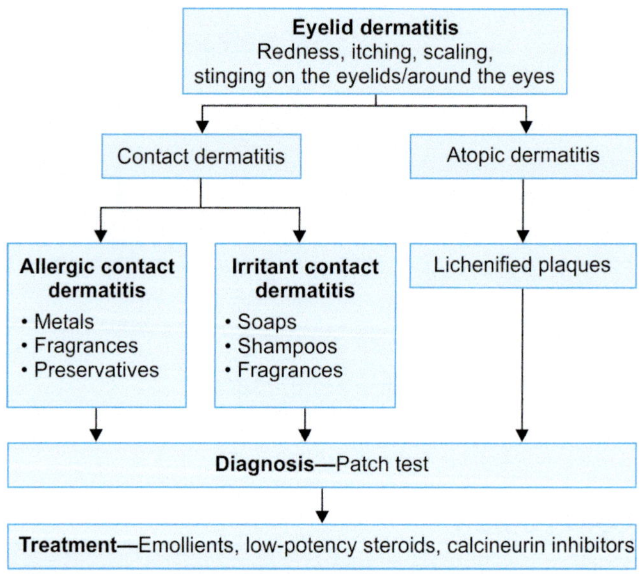


**FLOWCHART 1:** Management of eyelid dermatitis.

## CLINICAL FEATURES

Generally, these patients present as erythematous scaly, itchy rash on the upper and lower eyelids **(Figs. 1A and B)**.

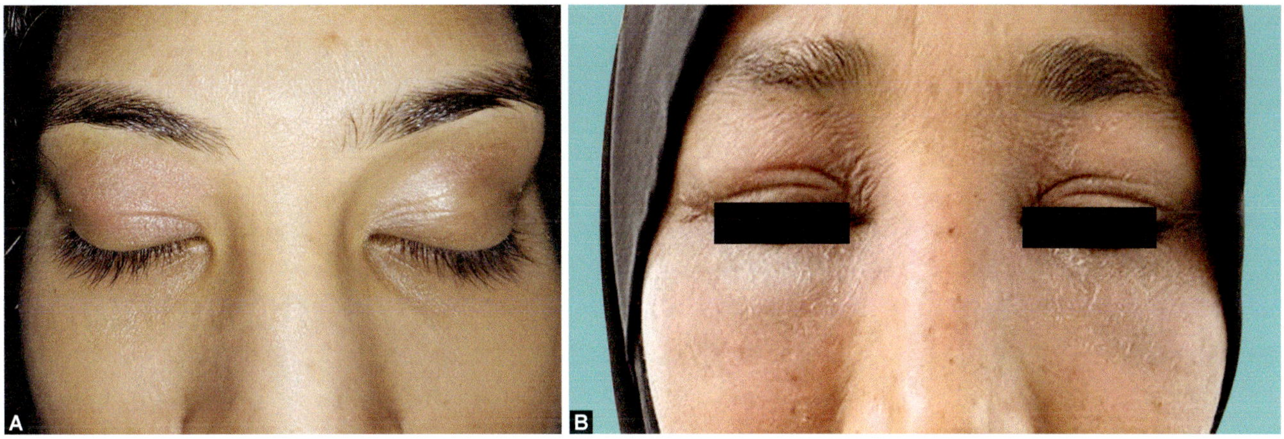


**FIGS. 1A AND B:** Eyelid dermatitis.

Some of them may be burning, and swelling of the lids may be unilateral or bilateral. Lids may become dry and cracked. Course may be chronic in patients with atopic etiology. There may be seasonal variation depending on the etiology. Occupational eyelid dermatitis may worsen in workplace exposure and improve with time off work.

## DIAGNOSIS

Mostly disease is diagnosed clinically bases on the history, symptoms, and appearance of the lesions. Anyone with eyelid dermatitis whose course is prolonged for more than 8 weeks, should be considered for patch test. If patch test is negative, then the other causes should be considered for. Atopic eyelid dermatitis is suspected in childhood onset AD with history of asthma and seasonal allergies. This is often associated with flexural involvement.

Any patient with ongoing eyelid dermatitis beyond 4–8 weeks should be considered for patch testing to find out if there are any contact sensitization. Frequent contact sensitizers would be nickel sulfate, fragrance mix, balsam of Peru, and paraphenylene diamine.[4] If the patch test is negative or not relevant to the current dermatitis then diagnosis of irritant contact dermatitis should be considered.

## MANAGEMENT

Management depends upon the avoidance of allergens and irritants for patients with contact dermatitis and usage of topical corticosteroids and calcineurin inhibitors.[1] Skin care is very important and bland emollients can be directly applied onto the eyelids. Usage of perfume and aerosol hair sprays should be avoided.

Low-potency corticosteroids are the first line of therapy. They can be safely used for short term (up to 2 weeks). If the patients require therapy for more than 4 weeks, they can be switched over to topical calcineurin inhibitors **(Flowchart 1)**. Long-term use of topical corticosteroids on the eyelids can lead to complications such as atrophy and periorbital dermatitis.[1] Hence, topical calcineurin inhibitors can be applied twice daily for 2–4 weeks or until the improvement is noted and then may be tapered.

## CONCLUSION

Eyelid contact dermatitis is an inflammatory reaction involving the eyelid skin that is caused by contact with a trigger substance. It may be due to contact dermatitis or atopic dermatitis. Presents with erythematous scaly itchy rashes on eyelids along with swelling. The dermatitis is treated with emollient, low potency steroids or calcineurin inhibitors.

## REFERENCES

1. Reeder MJ. (2024). Eyelid dermatitis (eczema). [online] Available from https://www.uptodate.com/contents/eyelid-dermatitis [Last accessed January, 2025].
2. Graves JE, Brodell RT. Erythematous scaling eyelids: patient history, exposure to allergens and irritants are keys to diagnosis. Postgrad Med. 2005;117:43-5.
3. Wolf R, Orion E, Tüzün Y. Periorbital (eyelid) dermatides. Clin Dermatol. 2014;32(1):131-40.
4. Guin JD. Eyelid dermatitis: Experience in 203 cases. J Am Acad Dermatol. 2002;47(5):755-65.

3.5

CHAPTER

# Hand Dermatitis

*Gatha M Upadya*

## INTRODUCTION

Hand dermatitis is a very common inflammatory disease, which involves both palmar and dorsal aspect of the hands due to various causes. It is distressing, because it has an impact on quality of life due to appearance and social functioning. The main complaints include redness, thickening of the skin, skin peeling, swelling, vesicles, cracks, etc.

It is common in young adult female and accounts for 20–35% of all forms of dermatitis, which may be seen in any age.[1] It is common in people with history of atopic dermatitis.[2] It is the most common occupational dermatosis seen among health workers, food handlers, housewives, and hairdressers. Strong risk factors include atopic dermatitis, allergic rhino conjunctivitis, and bronchial asthma. Dermatitis is aggravated by irritants such as fragrances, cleansers, raw fruits and vegetables, spices, plants, detergents, acids, alkalis, and friction. These can damage the stratum corneum removing lipids and impairing the barrier function of the skin. Further damage to the barrier function can happen because of water loss and inflammation.

## PATHOGENESIS[3]

This involves both genetic and environmental factors. There is a strong association between hand eczema and loss of function mutation in the filaggrin gene, which is important for the epidermal barrier. This results in water loss and easy penetration by allergens and irritants. Studies on occupational hand eczema show the association with handwashing practices and unprotected wet work. Hand dermatitis may be a manifestation of T-cell-mediated delayed hypersensitivity reaction. It may be a part of contact urticaria/protein contact dermatitis. Patients usually have a patch test, which is positive or increased immunoglobulin E (IgE) to certain food but negative for patch test. Usually, it starts as urticarial allergy over period of time this leads to chronic eczema.

## ETIOLOGY[4]

- *Exogenous*:
  - Chemical (soaps, detergents, and solvents)
  - Physical (friction and dryness)
  - Contact allergens (delayed hypersensitive reaction)
  - Ingested allergens (drugs)
  - Infection
- *Endogenous*:
  - Idiopathic (discoid and hyperkeratotic)
  - Immunological (atopic)
  - Psychosomatic (stress)
  - Dyshidrosis (sweat aggravated)

## CLINICAL MANIFESTATIONS

Hand dermatitis in its acute stage classically presents with erythema, oozing, swelling, and vesiculation. This can be shifted to chronic stage with lichenification and fissuring with a subacute stage in between. This can involve both the sides of the hands with itching and/or burning. In long-standing cases, there may be nail changes with loss of cuticle, nail fold swelling, and ridging in the nail plates.

## CLINICAL TYPES[4-6]

- Dyshidrotic eczema
- Chronic fissured hand dermatitis
- Hyperkeratotic palmar eczema
- Fingertip eczema
- Nummular eczema
- Interdigital eczema (apron dermatitis)
- Recurrent focal palmar peeling

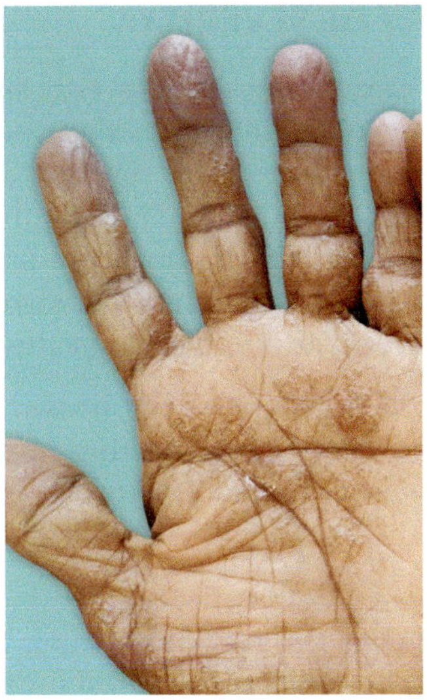

**FIG. 1:** Pompholyx.

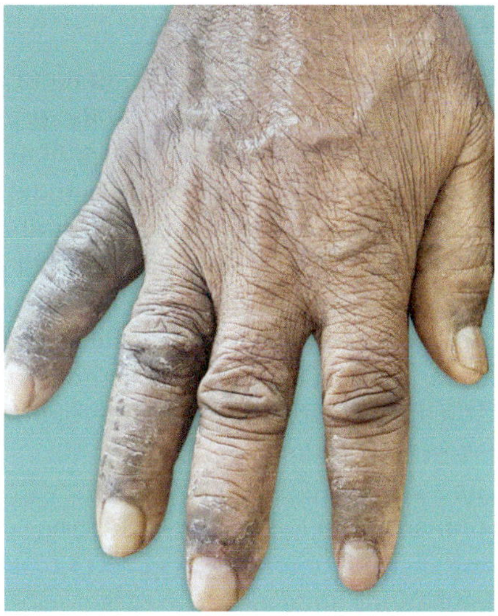

**FIG. 2:** Hyperkeratotic eczema.

Distribution of the lesions will be according to the etiology. Irritant contact dermatitis is mostly due to wet work and exposure to irritants. It affects the webspace's first, then to fingers, and finally to dorsum of the hands.

*Allergic contact dermatitis*: There are innumerable allergens, which may affect the hand like rubber, nickel, potassium dichromate, and para phenylenediamine. This may lead to periodic flare ups.

*Dyshidrotic eczema*: This usually presents with intensely itchy, sudden onset of the skin colored deep-seated vesicles on the palms and sides of the fingers. This can be exacerbated by sweating. Multiple relapses may lead to chronic hand dermatitis with lichenified, red, scaly plaques with fissuring. Also called as pompholyx **(Fig. 1)**.

*Hyperkeratotic palmar eczema*: It is a chronic non-inflammatory dermatitis, characterized by highly irritable, scaly, fissured hyperkeratotic plaques on the palms, which mimics palmar psoriasis and is less well circumscribed **(Fig. 2)**.

*Fingertip eczema*: It is limited to tips of single or several fingers. Skin is dry and cracked and can break down into painful fissures. It is a cumulative irritant dermatitis, which worsen in winter.

*Nummular eczema*: It tends to affect the dorsum of the hands with well-defined discoid plaques.

*Interdigital eczema*: It affects the finger webs, which resembles an apron. Common in women and may be endogenous in origin.

*Recurrent focal palmar peeling*: It is also called keratolysis exfoliative. During summer small superficial area of desquamation develops on sides or palmar aspect of the hands.

## DIAGNOSIS

Diagnosis depends on good history thorough examination and a patch testing. One has to consider:

- Acute relapsing, chronic course
- History of skin allergy
- Type of work or hobbies
- Frequency of exposure
- Type of personal protective equipment used by the healthcare workers
- Personal or family history of atopy

*Physical examination*: While assessing the patient one should examine the pattern of the lesion, extension of the lesion, whether nails are affected or not. Look for skin changes in other parts of the skin.

As the disease is multifactorial, finding out a cause is not easy, and needs thorough work up. The patients may require patch test and sometimes skin biopsy or scraping for fungus to rule out other causes, such as:

- *Psoriasis*: Symmetrical, well-defined, erythematous plaques with silvery scales
- *Tinea manuum*: Asymmetrical plagues with active, raised border
- *Palmoplantar pustulosis*: Recurrent crops of deep-seated sterile pustules in the palmar surface

## PATCH TEST[1]

Simple test done to identify the cause in hand dermatitis due to allergy **(Fig. 3)**. This is based on the principle that the skin of an allergic contact dermatitis patient is capable of reacting with the causative antigen. A standard quantity of the allergen applied on the aluminum chambers is stuck on the back of the patient. The allergen is left in contact with the skin for 48 hours and then removed to see any local inflammatory reaction. After removing the patches, the test reaction is read after half an hour and graded as negative to +++ based on the recommendation of international contact dermatitis research group **(Table 1)**.

Total and differential leukocyte count with evidence of eosinophilia, serum IgE level, skin biopsy, scraping for fungus, and radioallergosorbent (RAST) test are some other investigations done in case to case.

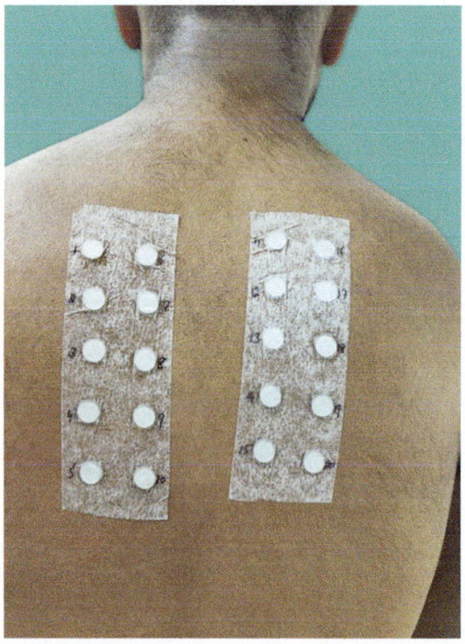

**FIG. 3:** Patch test.

**TABLE 1: Patch test—morphology and interpretation.**

| Symbol | Morphology | Interpretation |
|---|---|---|
| – | No reaction | Negative |
| ? | Erythema only no infiltration | Doubtful reaction |
| + | Erythema, infiltration, discrete papules | Weak positive reaction |
| ++ | Erythema, infiltration, papules, and vesicles | Strong positive reaction |
| +++ | Erythema, infiltration, and confluent vesicles | Extreme positive reaction |
| IR | Different type of reaction vesicles, blisters, and necrosis | Irritant reaction |

## ASSESSMENT OF SEVERITY[5]

It is very necessary to assess the severity and extent of the dermatitis. In regular clinical practice, several tools have been developed to assess the severity. They are Hand Eczema Severity Index, Physicians Global Assessment (PGA), and Dermatology Life Quality Index (DLQI).

Physicians Global Assessment tool is a relatively simple tool to assess the severity and extent of the involvement.

*Mild eczema*: It is the presence of two or more mild skin changes (erythema scaling, hyperkeratosis, lichenification, vesiculation, fissures, pruritus, and pain) involving less than 10% of the hand surface.

*Moderate eczema*: It is the presence of two or more mild to moderate skin changes (erythema scaling, hyperkeratosis, lichenification, vesiculation, fissures, pruritus, and pain) involving 10–30% of the hand surface.

*Severe eczema*: It is the presence of two or more moderate to severe skin changes (erythema scaling, hyperkeratosis, lichenification, vesiculation, fissures, pruritus, and pain) involving more than 30% of the hand surface.

## TREATMENT[2,7]

General principles include patient education regarding the avoidance of irritants/allergens, use of nonsoap cleansers, and use of protective gloves.

### Patient Education

Change in the behavior is an integral part of the management of hand dermatitis.

*Topical steroids*: This reduce the inflammation. Potent topical steroids can be used on the dorsum of the hands, and an ultrapotent topical steroid should be used in the palms. Cream formulation is best for vesicular dermatitis and ointment form for chronic dermatitis. They should be applied once or twice daily to the affected areas for several weeks, then discontinued after reducing the frequency gradually. Potent steroids under occlusion can be tried for short time if the standard applications have not been effective.

### Mild-to-moderate Disease

Liberal use of emollients and moisturizers are advised in patients with hand dermatitis. Moisturizers containing humectants will improve skin barrier function. Emollients such as petrolatum, dimethicone, and waxes soothe the dry, scaly skin, and prevent water loss by providing some occlusion.

First line of treatment for mild to moderate type of hand eczema would be topical steroids. Patient should be educated about the cause and need of avoidance of triggers, adoption of preventive methods, skin protection measures, and the importance of adherence to the treatment. Treatment is challenging to the patients as well as dermatologists. Counseling plays an important role in the management. Patient should be counseled about the triggering factors both in home and work environment. They should be advised to avoid common irritants and allergens such as solvents, detergents, alkalis, dust, and plants. Handwashing and drying should immediately be followed by the application of generous amount of hand cream and emollient. Repetitive handwashing should be discouraged. Overuse of soaps and cleansers may hamper the epidermal barrier function and delay healing.

Personal protection equipment such as gloves should be worn throughout cooking, gardening, and washing to minimize the exposure to the irritants. Barrier creams contain ceramides free fatty acids, and cholesterol should be used to minimize the entry of hazardous chemicals into the skin.

Steroids should be applied once or twice daily until there is stable improvement in the disease. Emollients are liberally used multiple times in a day. After remission, it can be maintained with mid potency topical steroid, slowly tapered over several months. In patients with recurrent relapse, topical calcineurin inhibitors may be an alternative and also a steroid-spacing agent.

## Phototherapy

Phototherapy using ultraviolet A (UVA) and UVB rays administered by a special hand/foot machine may be recommended. It may be delivered 2–3 times per week.

## Severe/Recalcitrant Dermatitis

Patients with severe, recalcitrant hand dermatitis, who do not respond to super potent corticosteroids, may require systemic treatment including oral steroids, immunosuppressives such as cyclosporin or methotrexate, or phototherapy.

## Systemic Therapy

Short-term oral corticosteroids is given for those who do not respond to super potent corticosteroids. Prednisolone 0.5–1 mg/day can be considered and tapered once the patient is stabilized.

*Alitretinoin* (9-cis-retinoic acid): It is an anti-inflammatory, immunomodulatory, antiproliferative drug with apoptotic effects. It is a strong drug, hence should be used with caution in female patients with childbearing age.

*Dupilumab*: An IL-4/IL-13 receptor antagonist is approved in the management of atopic dermatitis. It is effective in nonatopic chronic hand eczemas as well.

*Conventional immunosuppressives*: Like cyclosporine, methotrexate and azathioprine have been occasionally used in the management of recalcitrant diseases.

*How to look after your hands*:

- Use emollient soap substitute or leave an emollient to wash with. Apply emollient immediately.
- Never wash hands while wearing a ring. Soap can get collected under the ring and may cause irritation.
- While washing your hands, wear a cotton-lined rubber or polyvinyl chloride (PVC) gloves or 100% cotton gloves underneath. Better to use powder-free gloves.
- While drying the hands, particularly take care in between the fingers where skin is more prone to dryness or cracking.
- Do not peel vegetables with bare hands. They are irritants.
- If you have hand dermatitis, choose your career with utmost care, so that occupation will not aggravate the dermatitis.

Overall algorithm for hand management is shown in **Flowchart 1**.

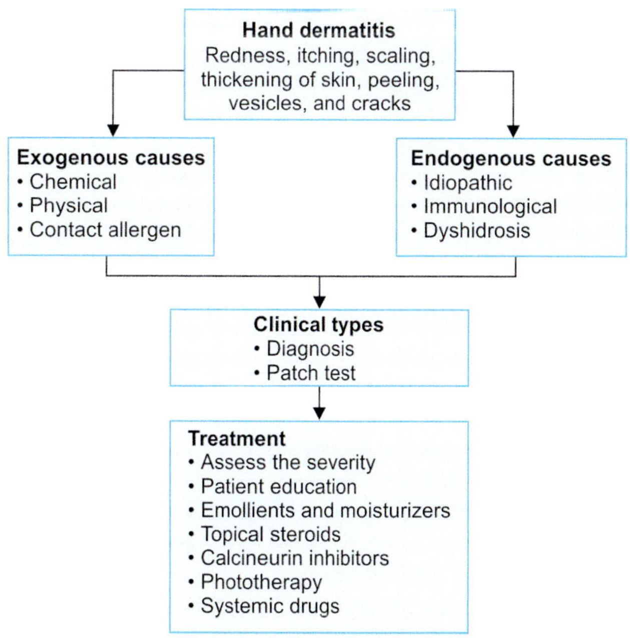


**FLOWCHART 1:** Management of hand dermatitis.

## CONCLUSION

Hand eczema is the commonest occupational skin disease affecting the hand. Mild forms are picked up only during occupational screening. There are some exogenous and endogenous causes. Important risk factors are wet work, atopy and contact allergy. There are many clinical types of hand dermatitis and the diagnosis depends upon a good history and clinical examination. However, patch test may pick up the cause. Preventive measures may play an important role in the therapy. Treatment includes assessment of the severity, patient education, phototherapy, topical and systemic drugs.

## REFERENCES

1. Agarwal US, Besarwal RK, Gupta R, Agarwal P, Napalia S. Hand eczema. Indian J Dermatol. 2014;59(3):213-24.
2. Coenraads PJ. Hand eczema. N Engl J Med. 2012;367:1829.
3. de Jongh CM, Khrenova L, Verberk MM, Calkoen F, van Dijk FJ, Voss H, et al. Loss-of-function polymorphisms in the filaggrin gene are associated with an increased susceptibility to chronic irritant contact dermatitis: a case-control study. Br J Dermatol. 2008;159(3):621-7.
4. DermNet NZ. (2024). Hand dermatitis. [online] Available from https://dermnetnz.org/topics/hand-dermatitis [Last accessed January, 2025].
5. Sheehan MP. (2024). Chronic Hand Eczema. [online] Available from https://www.uptodate.com/contents/chronic-hand-eczema [Last accessed January, 2025].
6. Lakshmi C, Srinivas CR. Hand Eczema: An update. Indian J Dermatol Venereol Leprol. 2012;78(5):569-82.
7. Thyssen JP, Schuttelaar MLA, Alfonso JH, Andersen KE, Angelova-Fischer I, Arents BWM, et al. Guidelines for diagnosis, prevention and treatment of hand eczema. Contact Dermatitis. 2022;86(5):357-78.

CHAPTER 3.6

# Perioral Dermatitis

*Raghavendra Rao, Nandana C*

## INTRODUCTION

In 1957, Frumess and Lewis described a recurrent dermatitis of the perioral area under the name "Light-sensitive seborrheic," that later came to be known as periorificial dermatitis, rosacea-like dermatitis, or perioral dermatitis (POD).[1]

It is an inflammatory and chronic disorder characterized by the presence of erythematous papules, papulovesicles, and pustules primarily distributed around the mouth.

## EPIDEMIOLOGY

Though the condition has been described in all racial and ethnic background, it is found to be more common in females between the ages of 16 and 45 years. A granulomatous form of periorificial dermatitis has been described in African-American population.

## ETIOPATHOGENESIS

Various factors that have been implicated in the causation of POD are shown in **Table 1**. It may be difficult to identify an underlying cause in a given patient. Physical factors such as ultraviolet (UV) rays, wind, and heat may cause worsening symptoms. Many studies indicate that patients with POD are usually atopic. Despite the evidence linking the onset of POD to the use of potent topical corticosteroid (TCS) usage, the mechanism by which TCS induces POD is unclear. It has been postulated that the TCS induces damage to the epidermal barrier function, thereby enhancing the penetration of allergens.[2] Recently, an increased incidence in POD following mask usage during COVID times has been observed.[3] It is postulated that the changes in local microbiome sebum secretion, skin temperature, hydration, and erythema under occlusion may be the contributing factors for this association. Few studies have indicated that there is increased transepidermal water loss in patients with POD, but this has very little or no significance in clinical or laboratory diagnosis of a patient.

**TABLE 1: Possible causes for perioral dermatitis (POD).[1]**

| | |
|---|---|
| Drugs | • Topical steroids<br>• Inhaled steroid sprays<br>• Oral contraceptives |
| Cosmetics | • Fluorinated toothpastes<br>• Skincare ointments and creams<br>• Lipstick |
| Physical factors | • Heat<br>• Wind<br>• Ultraviolet light |
| Microbiologic factors | • *Demodex folliculorum*<br>• *Candida albicans*<br>• *Fusiform spirilla* bacteria |
| Immunocompromised state | Children with leukemia |
| Miscellaneous factors | • Latex gloves<br>• Lip licking<br>• Hormonal fluctuations in women<br>• Malabsorption<br>• Emotional stress<br>• Increased mask usage[3] |

## CLINICAL MANIFESTATIONS

Skin lesions may appear as discrete or confluent erythematous papules, pustules, or vesicles concentrated predominantly over the perioral area. Vermillion border of the lip is characteristically spared with a border of normal skin that separates the lesional skin from the lip. Less often, there can be involvement of perinasal and periorbital areas. The lesions of POD may either be asymptomatic or associated with mild-to-moderate burning sensation or itching that usually resolves without scarring in a few months even without pharmacologic therapy. Although initial improvement may be noticed using TCS, its continued usage may cause exacerbation of the disease and can contribute to its chronicity.

### Variants of Perioral Dermatitis

*Granulomatous periorificial dermatitis* is a clinical variant of POD that is usually common in childhood and may present as multiple skin-colored to red-brown inflammatory papules in perioral, perinasal, or periocular areas.

*Lupus-like POD* is characterized by the presence of inflammatory papules that show yellowish discoloration on diascopy and heals with scarring.

## DIFFERENTIAL DIAGNOSIS

Perioral dermatitis is usually a straightforward clinical diagnosis, but the exclusion of some common and a few uncommon dermatological conditions is warranted. Various differential diagnoses are summarized in **Table 2**. Other possible but rare differentials include gram-negative folliculitis, eosinophilic folliculitis, cutaneous sarcoidosis, or syringomas.

**TABLE 2: Differential diagnoses of perioral dermatitis (POD).[1]**

| Differential diagnosis | Differentiating features |
|---|---|
| Seborrheic dermatitis | Examine perinasal and retroauricular areas, eyebrows and scalp for erythema, scaling |
| Rosacea | • Centrofacial distribution commonly<br>• Erythema, flushing after sun exposure<br>• Rhinophyma may be present or absent |
| Acne | • Comedones, scars, papulopustules, and nodules<br>• Adolescents age group mainly |
| Facial demodicosis | • Acute history more common<br>• Isolation of the organism |
| Impetigo | • Children<br>• Erosions, vesicles and honey-colored crusts |
| Allergic contact dermatitis | • Intense pruritus is the main symptom<br>• Prominent scaling in lesions |
| Irritant contact dermatitis | • History of contact with irritant substances<br>• Burning sensation more than pruritus<br>• Erythema, scaling, oozing, and edema common |
| Lupus miliaris disseminatus faciei | • Scarring common<br>• Eyelid involvement |
| Haber syndrome (familial rosacea-like dermatosis) | • Begins in childhood<br>• Intraepidermal epitheliomas<br>• Scars and keratotic plaques |

## DIAGNOSIS

It is based mainly on clinical ground. Few points that support the diagnosis include:

- Border of normal skin between the lesional skin and lip
- Burning or stinging sensation with features of eczematous dermatitis
- Recent history of TCS use and disease flares following withdrawal
- Absence of comedones

## HISTOPATHOLOGY

Skin biopsies are rarely necessary but helps to rule out other differential diagnosis when faced with diagnostic uncertainty. Biopsy specimens should ideally be taken from the chin and should include at least one papule. Histopathology of early lesions shows spongiotic reaction pattern with mild acanthosis, epidermal edema and parakeratosis, perifollicular and perivascular edema with lymphocytic infiltration, as well as occasional follicular abscesses. Later papular lesions may have diffuse hypertrophy of connective tissue and sebaceous gland hyperplasia. Caseating granulomas may be present in granulomatous POD.

## MANAGEMENT

- Strict discontinuation of topical steroids as well as all cosmetic products, soaps, or detergents being used on the face.

- Regular face wash with tap water; all kinds of soaps and cosmetic products should be discontinued.
- *"Null or Zero therapy"*: All topical medications including TCS which patient may be using should be discontinued, and patient should be reassured.
- Some experts advice switching over from potent TCS to low-potent TCS in the transition phase, which gradually should be weaned to prevent the rebound flare up. Frequency of application should be reduced prior to cessation of treatment.
- For initial treatment of mild POD, topical calcineurin inhibitors (TCIs) such as pimecrolimus or tacrolimus may be used.
- Topical antibiotics (erythromycin 2% gel twice daily or metronidazole 1% once daily) has been found to be effective.
- Topical antipruritic agents without corticosteroid agents, including pramoxine hydrochloride may be used to give symptomatic relief.
- *Oral therapies*: Patient who does not demonstrate improvement within 4–8 weeks of topical treatment may be advised oral therapies. This includes tetracycline group of drugs (tetracycline, doxycycline, and minocycline) or azithromycin.

## PREVENTION[4]

- Patients predisposed to POD, including those with history of atopy, may be advised to avoid TCS preparations.
- Gentle skin care practices include using mild cleansers for the face, and neutral or bland cosmetic agents without fragrance or potential irritants as and when necessary.
- Once stable remission is attained, the patients may be advised to slowly restart the skin care products that were being used one by one and closely monitor the effects of each product on skin.
- Any product that seems to induce recurrences may be discontinued.

## CONCLUSION

Perioral dermatitis is a chronic recurrent condition with variable causes and triggering factors. The early and correct identification of this relatively common condition, and differentiating from other similar differentials is monumental in a faster initiation of treatment, thus improving the quality of life of the patients suffering from the condition significantly.

## REFERENCES

1. Tempark T, Shwayder TA. Perioral dermatitis: a review of the condition with special attention to treatment options. Am J Clin Dermatol. 2014;15:101-13.
2. Dirschka T, Tronnier H, Fölster-Holst R. Epithelial barrier function and atopic diathesis in rosacea and perioral dermatitis. Br J Dermatol. 2004;150:1136-41.
3. Nahm WJ, Nagler AR, Milam EC. Association of perioral dermatitis with facial mask usage during the COVID-19 pandemic: A retrospective study. JAAD Int. 2023;10:86-7.
4. Ljubojević S, Lipozencić J, Turcić P. Perioral dermatitis. Acta Dermatovenerol Croat. 2008;16:96-100.

3.7

CHAPTER

# Face Dermatitis

*Raghavendra Rao, Priya Bhesaniya*

## INTRODUCTION

The face is one of the most exposed parts of the body, and therefore it is given great importance. It is constantly exposed to various agents either directly by application of products or indirectly via airborne and hand to face exposure. According to various studies, in the general population, the prevalence of face dermatitis is about 10%.[1] Apart from an underlying skin condition such as seborrheic dermatitis and atopic dermatitis, other common causes include cosmetics, fragrance, hair dye and preservatives present in skin care products that may cause allergic contact dermatitis.

## CLINICAL FEATURES

Taking a thorough history can give a clue to find out the cause. The first complaints are often dryness of the skin and itching. A detailed history regarding the usage of daily facial care products should be taken. Special emphasis should be given to find out if there is any change in the pattern of usage or switch to a new product prior to development of rash. However, patients may develop dermatitis to a product they have been using for years as hypersensitivity may develop to an allergen previously not sensitive to. Hence, history may be misleading in these cases.

## PATTERNS OF FACIAL CONTACT DERMATITIS[1]

- *Lateral facial dermatitis*: The sites involved in lateral facial dermatitis are pre-/postauricular region, mandibular region, and sides of the neck. Common causes causing dermatitis in these areas are shampoos, conditioners, and rinsing hair dye (as water flows down along these areas). Seborrheic (postauricular region) and atopic dermatitis (neck) can also involve these areas.
- *Central facial dermatitis*: In central facial dermatitis, forehead, nose, cheeks, and chin are affected. Allergens which are likely to causes central facial dermatitis include cosmetics, moisturizers, bindi application, kumkum application, topical medications as patients mostly apply these over the central part of the face compared to the lateral aspect of the face. History of application of pain-relieving balms should be sought.
- *Generalized facial dermatitis*: When the dermatitis involves entire face, airborne allergens such as *Parthenium*, powders of metallic salt, cement dust, and cosmetics that are applied throughout the face are the causative allergens. Occupational history is important as *Parthenium* exposure frequently occur among farmers; on the other hand, carpenters may be exposed to variety of wood dusts, which can also lead to the development of generalized facial dermatitis. Sparing of the skin creases, retroauricular region, submental region, and upper eyelids along with photoaggravation should arouse a strong suspicion of photodermatitis.
- *Unilateral facial dermatitis*: When dermatitis is localized, an ectopic source such as transfer of allergen from hands should be suspected as in the case of allergic dermatitis due to nail varnishes, soaps, and moisturizers applied to the hand. In addition to this, cosmetics, fragrances, or dyes used by the partner can cause connubial or consort contact dermatitis.

## KUMKUM/SINDOOR/TILAK DERMATITIS

In India, it is a common practice for married women to apply sindoor in the parting of their hair and for men to apply kumkum over the forehead or neck. So, if the patient develops dermatitis in these areas, history regarding its use should be taken. Kumkum has constituents like brilliant lake red R, Sudan I, fragrances, groundnut oil,

| TABLE 1: Causes of pigment contact dermatitis.[7] | |
|---|---|
| Cosmetics | Hair dye (PPD), lipstick, kumkum, and preservatives |
| Fragrance | Jasmine absolute, sandalwood oil, benzyl salicylate, etc. |
| Textiles | Azo dye |
| Others | Minoxidil, PTBPF (para tertiary butyl phenol formaldehyde), nickel sulfate |

(PPD: para-phenylenediamine)

tragacanth gum, para-phenylenediamine (PPD), and paraben among others, all of which can cause dermatitis. Sindoor contains allergens like mercury and the black paste lead sulfide. Pigment contact dermatitis (slate grey pigmentation) occurs more often than allergic contact dermatitis.[2] Furthermore, photoallergic reactions can be seen due to "*chandan*," which can be a component of kumkum. Hence, in such cases a photo-patch test should be done **(Table 1)**.

## *BINDI* DERMATITIS

*Bindi* is commonly applied over the glabella; para-tertiary butyl phenol (PTBP) whose concentration can be up to 80% in the glue is known to cause dermatitis as well as contact leukoderma.[3] Erythema and pruritus may be the first signs and symptoms following its application, which is subsequently followed by development of depigmentation. It may take months or years to develop.[4] Allergic contact dermatitis due to the epoxy resin can be another manifestation.

## DERMATITIS DUE TO BALMS

In Southeast Asia, it is very common to apply balms over the forehead or at other sites of pain. Many very commonly used balms may contains peppermint, clove oil, and ammonia solution, which can cause contact dermatitis.

## FACE MASK DERMATITIS

Wearing a face mask had become the "new normal" during the COVID pandemic. According to a study done by Niesert et al., most common symptoms were itching and erythema of skin following the use of masks.[5] These were more common in those who wore surgical masks compared to cloth mask. Common risk factors for dermatitis were increased temperature and moisture. They also observed aggravation of existing dermatosis including seborrheic dermatitis **(Table 1)**.

## PIGMENTED CONTACT DERMATITIS (RIEHL'S MELANOSIS)

It is a variant of noneczematous dermatitis in which patients present with greyish or greyish brown pigmentation over the face and neck.[6] In some, erythema and itching may also be present due to its inflammatory component. This occurs when there is repeated exposure to an allergen in small quantities due to T type IV cytolytic reaction. Hence, it leads to pigment incontinence rather than an eczematous reaction. The affected patients may remain asymptomatic for months to years. This is then followed by the development of greyish or brown pigmentation. The most common site involved is the preauricular region and sides of cheeks followed by the forehead, temples, chin, and neck.

## STATUS COSMETICUS

This refers to the nonspecific irritation, which can occur due to the application of cosmetics or soaps that may be free from common allergens. Despite having no significant findings on clinical examination, patients may complain of burning or stinging sensation and itching. Few patients may present with mild erythema over the nose and malar region, few follicular oriented papules, or slight periorbital edema. In these cases, the symptoms are disproportionate to the clinical picture. Few agents that can cause it include benzoic acid, sodium lauryl sulfate (SLS), lactic acid, and urea. "Anti-irritants" such as heavy mineral oils and polypropylene glycol can be used to neutralize the stinging.

## PATCH TESTING

- *Semi-open test*:[8] It is to assess the products, which have solvents and emulsifiers in them causing irritation (shampoos, dyes, varnishes etc.):
  - Using a cotton swab, product is applied onto a 2 × 2 cm area, and it is covered with an adhesive tape. The reading is taken at 48 and at 96 hours.
- *Repeated open application test (ROAT)*:[8] Commercial products are applied twice a day for 7 days to the anterior portion of the arm, antecubital fossa, or scapular region. The development of eczema between 2 and 4 days suggests that a sensitizer was present.

Management of facial dermatitis includes finding out the agent responsible for it by patch testing **(Flowchart 1)**. Avoiding contact with that agent is crucial to prevent further episodes. To alleviate the symptoms of the patient, topical mild to mid potency steroids, topical tacrolimus, and antihistamines can be prescribed.

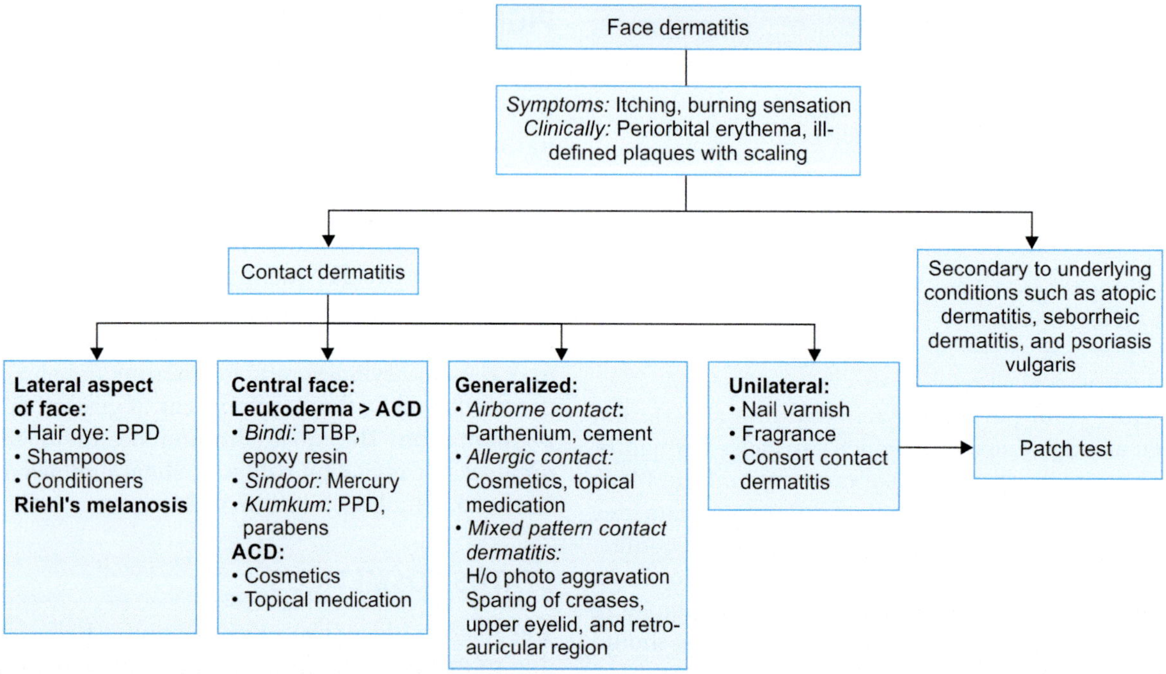


**FLOWCHART 1:** Approach to a patient with dermatitis of the face.

(ACD: allergic contact dermatitis; H/o: history of; PPD: para-phenylenediamine; PTBP: para-tertiary butyl phenol)

## CONCLUSION

Dermatitis affecting the face is commonly encountered in clinical practice especially with raise in usage of skin care products. It remains a challenge to arrive at the precise diagnosis. A thorough history, detailed clinical examination and patch testing with relevant series will help at the diagnosis in most cases. Avoidance of allergens along with mild topical steroid or topical calcineurin inhibitors often helps to give symptomatic relief.

## REFERENCES

1. Bruusgaard-Mouritsen MA, Garvey LH, Johansen JD. Facial contact dermatitis caused by cosmetic-relevant allergens. Contact Dermatitis. 2021;85(6):650-9.
2. Nath AK, Thappa DM. Kumkum-induced dermatitis: An analysis of 46 cases. Clin Exp Dermatol. 2007;32:385-7.
3. Bajaj AK, Gupta SC, Chatterjee AK. Contact depigmentation from free para-tertiary-butylphenol in bindi adhesive. Contact Dermatitis. 1990;22:99-102.
4. Gupta D, Thappa DM. Dermatoses due to Indian cultural practices. Indian J Dermatol. 2015;60(1):3-12.
5. Niesert AC, Oppel EM, Nellessen T, Frey S, Clanner-Engelshofen BM, Wollenberg, A et al. "Face mask dermatitis" due to compulsory facial masks during the SARS-CoV-2 pandemic: Data from 550 health care and non-health care workers in Germany. Eur J Dermatol. 2021;31(2):199-204.
6. Kim MS, Chung BY, Chang SE, Oh SH, Ryu HJ, Kim DH, et al. Pigmented contact dermatitis and hair dyes: A retrospective case-control multicentre study in Korea. J Eur Acad Dermatol Venereol. 2023;37(12):2543-9.
7. Shenoi SD, Rao R. Pigmented contact dermatitis. Indian J Dermatol Venereol Leprol. 2007;73:285-7.
8. Lazzarini R, Duarte I, Ferreira AL. Patch tests. An Bras Dermatol. 2013;88(6):879-88.

3.8

CHAPTER

# Noneczematous Contact Dermatitis

*Prabhakar Mallikarjuna Sangolli*

## INTRODUCTION

Contact dermatitis (CD) is a common entity with a classical eczematous rash at the site of contact. Besides the classic eczematous form, various noneczematous clinical variants can occur. Both allergic contact dermatitis (ACD) and irritant contact dermatitis (ICD) may show these noneczematous patterns.

## NONECZEMATOUS ALLERGIC CONTACT DERMATITIS

Noneczematous ACDs are discussed further.

### Erythema Multiforme-like Contact Dermatitis

The most common variant wherein the lesions resemble to that of target/urticarial lesions. They have been described as urticarial papules and plaque eruptions (UPPE) to distinguish them from the erythema multiforme.[1]

#### Causes

Plants and plant-related products: *Dalbergia nigra* (Brazilian rosewood), *Toxicodendron radicans* (poison ivy), *Machaerium scleroxylon* (pao ferro), *Eucalyptus saligna* (gum), tincture of capsicum, contact to natural rubber and airborne exposure to pyrethrum.[2,3]

Patients with such reactions should be analyzed for systemic involvement as previous reports have shown nephritis as an associated feature.[4]

#### Drugs and Chemicals

Ethylenediamine, sulfamide, econazole, promethazine, balsam of Peru, scopolamine, mafenide acetate, neomycin, vitamin E, budesonide, bufexamac, ketoprofen, triamcinolone acetonide, idoxuridine, phenylbutazone, brominated compounds, epoxy resin, formaldehyde, disperse blue 124, trichloroethylene, dinitrochlorobenzene and diphenylcyclopropenone.

#### Metals

Contact allergy to nickel and cobalt, 9-bromofluorene, and percutaneous/transrespiratory exposure to chemicals, such as formaldehyde/trichloroethylene.

#### Pathology

It has been postulated that an immune complex reaction and circulating antibodies, evoked by the causative allergen are responsible for UPPE.

#### Clinical Features

It arises usually as an eczematous lesion at the site of contact following which urticarial papules and plaques appear, in the same site and also at distant sites, in a few days. The urticarial eruptions persist longer than the primary eczematous lesions.

#### Diagnosis

A positive patch test reaction to the allergen can be elicited and is usually eczematous in nature.

#### Histopathology

Spongiosis, upper dermal edema, and perivascular lymphohistiocytic infiltrate can be seen. Occasionally vacuolar degeneration of basal cells is present. However, classical features of erythema multiforme such as epidermal dyskeratotic cells, and interface dermatitis are usually absent.

### Purpuric Contact Dermatitis

It is characterized by petechial and purpuric lesions, usually involving the lower limbs. The eruption evolves in several weeks even after the withdrawal of the offending agent and resolves leaving a pigmentation. Vasculitis, bleeding diathesis, and pigmented purpuric dermatosis are the main differential diagnoses.

### Causes

The following agents have been identified:
- *Rubber compounds*: N-isopropyl-N-phenyl-paraphenylenediamine (IPPD), and mercapto-benzothiazole are common causes. "PPPP syndrome" is defined as an ACD characterized by pruritus, petechiae, and purpura, caused by IPPD.
- *Textile compounds*: Optical whiteners, azoic dyes, Disperse Blue 85, formaldehyde resins, and paraphenylenediamine are common culprits. Petechial and itchy dermatitis occur in those areas that are in close contact with clothes.
- *Plants*: Agave americana L, Zea mays L, *Frullania*, and D-Limonene.
- *Others*: Vasculitic purpuric eruptions to balsam of Peru, ethylenediamine, benzoyl peroxide, and proflavine have also been reported. Fiberglass can cause pruritic follicular purpuric papules in exposed and unexposed sites.[5]

### Pathology

Purpuric CD can be either toxic or allergic in nature. A selective effect on endothelial cells either directly or secondary to lymphokines released in response to a lymphocytic reaction to the antigen at the perivascular site, has been proposed.

### Clinical Features

The lesions are usually limited to the site of exposure and resolve more rapidly once the cause is removed, in irritant form. The allergic form of purpuric CD generally is diffuse and has polymorphic manifestations.

### Diagnosis

Patch test gives a positive reaction to a causative allergen the majority of times. Blood workup and immunofluorescence can rule out other causes of vasculitis/purpura.

### Histopathology

Spongiosis, lymphocytic exocytosis in the epidermis, and leukocytoclastic vasculitis in the upper dermis are noted.

## Lichenoid Contact Dermatitis

The lesions resemble to that of classical lichen planus and can involve both skin and mucous membranes.

### Causes

Color developers, substances derived from para-phenylenediamine, are the most common cause of allergic contact with lichenoid eruption. Nickel, epoxy resins, aminoglycoside antibiotics, methacrylic acid esters for industrial use, chromates, cobalt, and palladium can cause similar lesions. Oral mucosae-involved forms are due to copper, zinc, and mercury contained in dental restorations.[6] Pigmented photocontact lichenoid dermatitis due to photosensitization by fragrances and plants such as parthenium is also known **(Figs. 1 and 2)**.

### Clinical Features

Lichenoid lesions occur either in association with eczematous lesions or per se in this type. The eruption

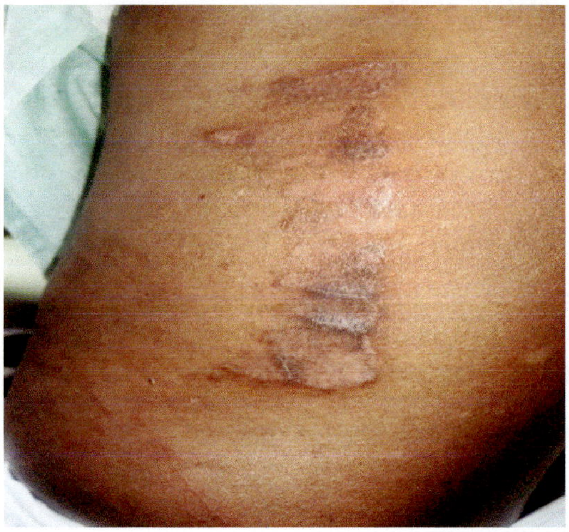

**FIG. 1:** Lichenoid rash secondary to capsicum plaster for pain.

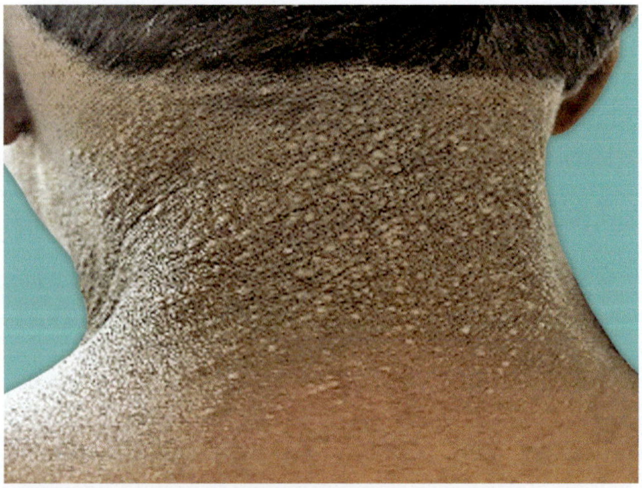

**FIG. 2:** Lichenoid contact dermatitis on the nape of the neck (patch test positive for parthenium).

mostly involves contact sites, later widely spreading with mucosal sparing (except in a few cases).

### Diagnosis

Positive reactions to patch tests are eczematous in nature but rarely might turn lichenoid.

## Lymphomatoid Contact Dermatitis

They clinically present with itchy papulonodular lesions resembling plaque parapsoriasis or an early-stage mycosis fungoides (MF).

### Causes

The following agents have been identified; para-phenylenediamine, para-tert-butylphenol resin, gold, ethylenediamine, nickel, cobalt, and kaolin are typically associated with this subtype of ACD.[7]

### Clinical Features

They can clinically present with infiltrative patches/papulonodular lesions at the contact site associated with an intense itch that improves after avoiding the culprit allergen.

### Diagnosis

Patch tests can give a positive reaction but are usually eczematous in nature.

### Histopathology

Lymphomatoid CD shows more of spongiosis, and exocytosis predominantly of inflammatory lymphocytes, unlike atypical cells in MF and perivascular lymphocytic infiltrate, unlike band-like infiltrate of large lymphoid cells with cerebriform nuclei in MF. Features such as Pautrier's microabscesses are absent in lymphomatoid CD.

## Pigmented Contact Dermatitis

It is characterized by pigmentation which is present during the acute eczematous phase, and which persists even beyond the acute rash settles. Riehl's melanosis and poikiloderma of Civatte, are considered forms of pigmented ACD, both of which are associated with sensitizing fragrances **(Fig. 3)**.

### Causes

Azo-dyes, gums, and cinnamic alcohol derivatives are the allergens most commonly associated with this form.

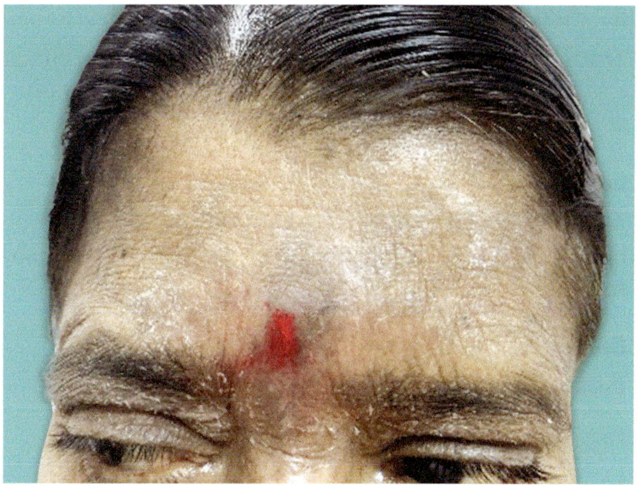

**FIG. 3:** Pigmented contact dermatitis due to *bindi* application.

### Dyes

Naphthol AS, Sudan I, Brilliant Lake Red, and Vacanceine Red.

### Cosmetics

Pigments and azoic solvents.

### Fragrances

Jasmine, hydroxycitronellal, and *Patchouli*.

### Antiseptics

Carbanilide.

### Miscellaneous

Formaldehyde, nickel, rubber, and musk ambrette.

### Clinical Features

It is characterized by intense pigmentation which usually occurs at the site of contact, after the acute eczematous phase subsides.

### Diagnosis

A positive patch test may induce a hyperpigmented area after the disappearance of an eczematous reaction.

### Histopathology

Atrophic epidermis, basal vacuolar degeneration, and pigment incontinence are the main histologic findings in pigmented contact dermatitis (PCD).[7]

## Pustular Contact Dermatitis

The characteristic lesions are sterile pustules on an erythematous base which can follow either an irritant or allergic reaction.

### Causes

Allergic pustular reactions are known from nitrofurazone, black rubber, and textile dyes, such as dispersed blue and red and minoxidil.[8]

### Diagnosis

Positive patch test usually as a pustular, reaction can occur.

### Histopathology

Histology showed perifollicular lymphocytes, histiocytes, and eosinophils. Pustules are sterile and transient and can displace subcorneally.

## Dyshidrosiform Contact Dermatitis

Dyshidrosiform allergic CD can be primitive or secondary.[9] Secondary form is contact sensitivity which complicates a preexisting primitive palmoplantar pompholyx.

Topical medicaments, paraphenylenediamine, chrome, cobalt, mercaptobenzothiazole, nickel, para-tert-butylphenol, and formaldehyde resin were the common causes. Primitive dyshidrosiform ACD is instead an expression of systemic contact allergy, of common observation in nickel-sensitized patients **(Fig. 4)**. Histologically, spongiosis and exocytosis are much more marked in ACD than in pompholyx.

## Granulomatous Allergic Contact Dermatitis

It clinically presents papulonodular infiltrative lesions after an initial eczematous eruption, 4–6 weeks after exposure to the culprit allergen. Zirconium-containing deodorants, chrome, cobalt, cadmium-containing tattoo dyes, aluminum hydroxide-containing vaccines, mercury, beryllium, gold, palladium, and titanium-containing pacemakers.[9] Histopathological examination shows sarcoid granulomas as seen in sarcoidosis. The patch test gives a positive result.

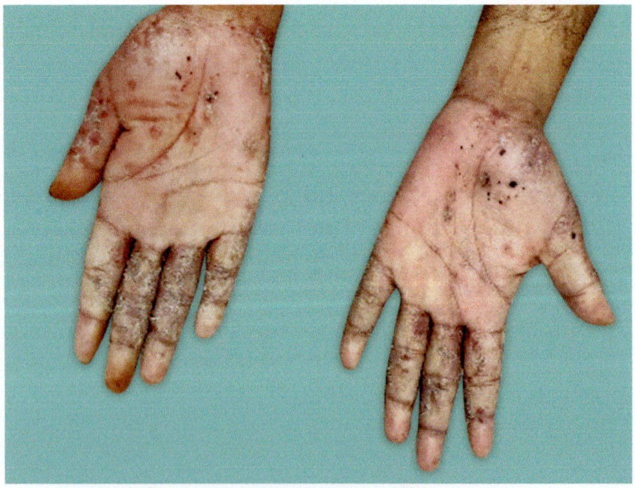

**FIG. 4:** Dyshidrosiform palmar rash in a farmer.

## Bullous Allergic Contact Dermatitis

This form is characterized by blisters localized at the contact site with the culprit allergen. Histopathologic examination with direct immunofluorescence may be performed to diagnose the same and exclude other autoimmune bullous disorders. This noneczematous form is often caused by sensitization with cinnamic aldehyde, potassium dichromate, thimerosal, and bufexamac and is usually associated with a positive patch test with the culprit agent characterized by a vesicular or bullous reaction **(Flowchart 1)**.

## Papular/Follicular Contact Dermatitis

Nickel, cosmetic products containing polyoxyethylene lauryl ether, textile products containing formaldehyde and, vitamin E, may be associated with follicular and papular type CD.

# NONECZEMATOUS IRRITANT CONTACT DERMATITIS

- *Bullous ICD*: Bullous phytophotodermatitis is a well-known form of noneczematous ICD and is characterized by erythema, blisters in a linear fashion, and postinflammatory pigmentation. It usually occurs after contact with a furanocoumarin-containing irritant plant and is activated by exposure to sunlight.

Noneczematous contact dermatitis

| Allergic | Irritant | Systemic |
|---|---|---|
| • Erythema multiforme-like<br>• Purpuric<br>• Lichenoid<br>• Lymphomatoid<br>• Pigmented<br>• Pustular<br>• Dyshydrosiform<br>• Granulomatous<br>• Bullous<br>• Papular/follicular | • Bullous<br>• Pustular<br>• Photoirritant pigment purpuric<br>• Granulomatous | • Dyshydrosiform<br>• Urticaria and anaphylaxis |

**FLOWCHART 1:** Types of noneczematous contact dermatitis.

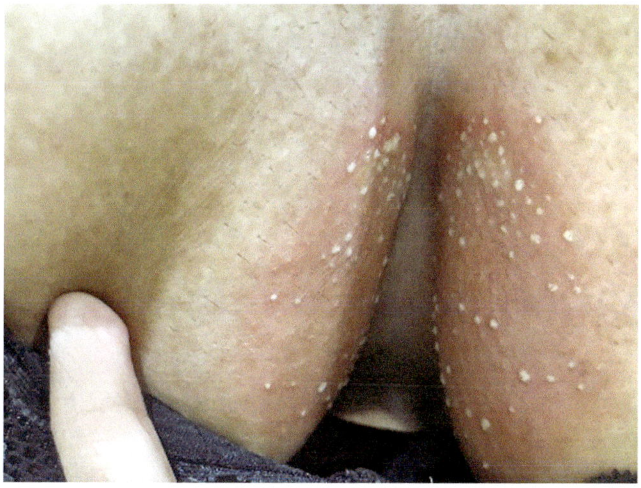

**FIG. 5:** Pustular rash on an erythematous base in paederus dermatitis.

- *Pustular ICD* is usually associated with croton oil. Paederus dermatitis, caused by contact exposure with the potent toxin of the pederin beetles, is also a form of pustular ICD **(Fig. 5)**. Metal salts, particularly nickel, copper, arsenic, and mercury represent the most common causes of these reactions.
- *Photoirritant-pigmented CD*, also known as Berloque dermatitis, is often caused by exposure to ultraviolet light after contact with perfumed cosmetic products.
- *Purpuric ICD*: Fiberglass particles in clothing may also cause purpuric ICD.
- *Granulomatous ICD*: Cases due to inoculation of talc, zinc, stearate, silicon, and magnesium have also been reported.

## NONECZEMATOUS SYSTEMIC CONTACT DERMATITIS

### Dyshidrosiform Rash

Recurring itchy eruptions of deep-seated vesicles on the fingers and palms can occur due to nickel, cobalt, or chromate ingestion. Atopic individuals are more prone. Oral provocation tests can help with diagnosis. Balsam of Peru, garlic, food colors, preservatives, and antioxidants are known causes.

### Urticaria and Anaphylaxis

It can rarely be seen in conjunction with typical eczematous lesions. Azo dyes, sulfonamides, and antihistamines have been reported to cause this.

## CONCLUSION

Clinical feature of ACD is generally polymorphic. Besides the classic eczematous form, different noneczematous clinical variants are possible. The causes for such variability in ACD clinical aspects are many. Noneczematous forms are slightly more common (52%) than the classic eczematous one (48%). Various clinical patterns of noneczematous of ACD have been described: some are linked to topical use of specific haptens and others more often dependent on allergens on systemic administration. Clinical suspicion followed by targeted patch test will help us to arrive at the correct diagnosis. Avoidance of the allergen, topical and in severe case a short course of oral steroid administration will help in the successful management of noneczematous contact dermatitis.

## REFERENCES

1. Goh CL. Urticarial papular and plaque eruptions. A noneczematous manifestation of allergic contact dermatitis. Int J Dermatol. 1989;28(3):172-6.
2. Raccagni AA, Bardazzi F, Baldari U, Righini MG. Erythema-multiforme-like contact dermatitis due to capsicum. Contact Dermatitis. 1995;33(5):353-4.
3. Garcia-Bravo B, Rodriguez-Pichardo A, de Pierola SF, Camacho F. Airborne erythema-multiforme-like eruption due to pyrethrum. Contact Dermatitis. 1995;33(6):433.
4. Schwartz RS, Downham TF 2nd. Erythema multiforme associated with Rhus contact dermatitis. Cutis. 1981;27(1):85-6.
5. Angelini G, Vena GA. Airborne contact dermatitis. Clin Dermatol. 1992;10(2):123-31.
6. Laine J, Kalimo K, Forssell H, Happonen RP. Resolution of oral lichenoid lesions after replacement of amalgam restorations in patients allergic to mercury compounds. Br J Dermatol. 1992; 126(1):10-5.
7. Elmas ÖF, Akdeniz N, Atasoy M, Karadag AS. Contact dermatitis: a great imitator. Clin Dermatol. 2020;38(2):176-92.
8. Sánchez-Motilla JM, Pont V, Nagore E, Rodríguez-Serna M, Sánchez JL, Aliaga A. Pustular allergic contact dermatitis from minoxidil. Contact Dermatitis. 1998;38(5):283-84.
9. Meneghini CL, Angelini G. Contact and microbial allergy in pompholyx. Contact Dermatitis. 1979;5(1):46-50.

3.9

CHAPTER

# Occupational Contact Dermatitis

*Lisa Jennifer Dsouza, Sathish Pai B*

## INTRODUCTION

Occupational diseases encompass any modifications in the skin, mucosa, and associated structures, stemming directly or indirectly from agents found in the workplace or occupational activities, contributing to their causation, conditioning, perpetuation, or exacerbation. Contact dermatitis, constituting the majority at 90%, dominates this category. The classifications include (1) irritant contact dermatitis (ICD) and (2) allergic contact dermatitis.

## IRRITANT CONTACT DERMATITIS

Irritant contact dermatitis constitutes 80% of occupational dermatitis cases,[1] resulting from the direct cytotoxic impact on skin cells. This process leads to skin alterations, causing barrier dysfunction and transepidermal water loss, ultimately leading to cell destruction. Additionally, nonimmunological release of proinflammatory cytokines further contributes to the pathology.

Irritants responsible for ICD include chemicals, minerals, or vegetable oils, and they can be categorized into immediate and cumulative types. The former, characterized by corrosive substances, manifests within minutes to hours, while the latter requires repeated exposure, as seen in the case of detergents.

Patients experiencing ICD typically report a burning sensation or pain rather than pruritus. The condition is marked by the development of vesicles, oozing, and crusting.

The common irritants are:

- Acids and alkali
- *Solvents*: Aliphatic—petroleum, kerosene, and gasoline
    - *Aromatic*: Benzene, toluene, and xylene.
    - *Halogenated*: Chloroform, trichloroethylene, methyl chloride.
    - *Miscellaneous*: Water, alcohols, ketones, glycols, and turpentine
- Soaps and detergents.
- *Plastics and resins*: Epoxy, phenolic, and acrylic monomers, amine catalysts, styrene, and benzoyl peroxide.
- *Plants*: Bristles, thorns, calcium oxalate—dieffenbachia, philodendron, daffodil, and agave.
- *Metal salts*: Nickel, chromium, cobalt, platinum, and arsenic.
- *Particles*: Sand, sawdust, fiberglass, and metal filings.
- *Phototoxic psoralens*: *Apiaceae* and *Rutaceae*.

## ALLERGIC CONTACT DERMATITIS

Allergic contact dermatitis (ACD), a less frequent occupational dermatosis, unfolds through two distinct phases: During the sensitization phase (lasting 10–15 days), easily absorbable, small, lipophilic particles infiltrate the stratum corneum. Antigen-presenting cells then take up these incomplete antigens (haptens), converting them into complete antigens by binding to proteins of the MHC complex. The transformed antigens migrate toward the lymph nodes, where naïve T cells differentiate into clusters of differentiation 4 (CD4) and CD8 suppressors, effectors, and memory cells.

In the subsequent elicitation phase (8–48 hours), individuals previously sensitized to the allergen experience reexposure, triggering the release of interleukin-1, interleukin-12, and interferon-gamma. This leads to the proliferation of cytotoxic T cells and the recruitment of macrophages, culminating in an inflammatory response in the skin.

The hallmark of ACD is intense pruritus, presenting as erythema, edematous plaques with lichenification, and excoriations. The skin may exhibit dryness, accompanied by a history of serous exudation.

The common allergens are:

- *Metals*: Nickel, chromium, cobalt, mercury, gold, and platinum
- *Biocides*: Formaldehyde and formaldehyde releasers, glutaraldehyde. Isothiazolinones, methyldibromo glutaronitrile, and iodopropynyl butylcarbamate
- *Plants*: Penta- and heptadecylcatechols, and sesquiterpene lactones
- *Cosmetics*: Paraphenylenediamine, glyceryl thioglycolate, cocamidopropyl betaine, and parabens
- *Plastics and resins*: Epoxy, phenolic and acrylic monomers, amine, anhydride, and peroxide, catalysts, colophony, turpentine, and catechols
- Fragrances and essential oils
- *Rubber additives*:
  - *Accelerators*: Mercaptobenzothiazole, carbamates, thiurams, and thioureas
  - *Antioxidants*: N-phenyl-N-isopropyl-paraphenylenediamine, etc.

## CLINICAL PRESENTATION OF OCCUPATIONAL CONTACT DERMATITIS

In the majority of cases, approximately 90%,[2] the presentation involves dermatitis-like lesions as detailed earlier. The remaining cases encompass various manifestations, including:[3]

- *Contact urticaria*: Characterized by the occurrence of transient wheals accompanied by pruritus.
- *Acne*: Specifically, chloracne.
- *Erythema multiforme type*: Linked to exposures to substances, such as rosewoods, balsam of Peru, formaldehyde, and paraphenyldiamine (PPD).
- *Lichen planus*: Noted for its distinctive violaceous, flat-topped, polygonal papules and plaques, often attributed to nickel, epoxy resin, acrylic, and PPD.
- *Purpuric contact dermatitis*: Resulting from the use of rubber (specifically mercaptobenzothiazole) and textile materials (azo dyes).

The sites predominantly affected are those exposed, with a notable occurrence over the hands, followed by the wrists and forearms. In instances involving transfer from the hands, the face, and distant sites may also become involved. Airborne allergens, such as sawdust and vapors, may accumulate over the eyelids and retroauricular area. Dermatitis can extend to involve less exposed areas such as the scalp and folds of the neck. Work uniforms, when saturated with allergens, have the potential to induce lesions on unexposed sites. Additionally, leather boots and improperly fitted footwear may contribute to the development of dermatitis.

Analyzing the pattern of dermatitis can provide crucial insights into identifying the causative agent. For instance, in cases of photocontact dermatitis, certain areas such as the upper eyelid, skin behind the ears, and the submental area may be spared. On the other hand, phytodermatitis might exhibit a distinct presentation with linear streaks of vesiculation and plaques. A comprehensive review of common occupations with the clinical features are summarized in **Table 1**.[3]

## APPROACH TO DIAGNOSIS AND MANAGEMENT

Gathering a comprehensive history is pivotal in understanding dermatological conditions. Key aspects include the timing of onset, the initial site of manifestation, and the subsequent evolution of the skin lesions. It is crucial to explore any temporal relationship between holidays and the appearance of skin issues, as well as the influence of work uniforms and safety equipment. A meticulous inquiry into the specific chemicals or substances encountered at work, along with details about soaps or detergents used, adds valuable insights. Documenting any prior history of dermatological diseases, atopy, or asthma is essential.

Furthermore, considering external factors such as chemical exposure and cosmetic use beyond the workplace is important. To capture a holistic picture, a detailed account of day-to-day activities is warranted. This comprehensive approach to history-taking aids in unraveling potential triggers and establishing a more accurate diagnosis.

The criteria set by Mathias[4] for determining the occupational causation of contact dermatitis encompass several key points:

- The clinical presentation should align with the typical features of contact dermatitis.
- There must be documented exposure to potential cutaneous irritants or allergens within the workplace.
- The anatomical distribution of the dermatitis should be coherent with cutaneous exposure associated with the job.
- The timing of exposure and the onset of symptoms should correlate, in accordance with the expected pattern of contact dermatitis.
- Other nonoccupational sources of exposure should be systematically ruled out as likely causes.
- Improvement of dermatitis upon removal from occupational exposure serves as a significant indicator.
- Positive results from patch or provocation tests specifically implicate workplace-related exposure as the cause of dermatitis.

Adhering to these criteria aids in establishing a robust foundation for linking contact dermatitis to occupational factors.

Four out of the seven are required to be positive to conclude occupational contact dermatitis.

**TABLE 1: Dermatitis associated with common occupations and its allergens.[3]**

| Occupation | Dermatitis | Allergen |
|---|---|---|
| Agricultural workers | • Parthenium dermatitis<br>• Pesticide handlers<br>• Cashew nut-related irritant contact dermatitis | • Parthenium hysterophorus (weed)—allergen is a sesquiterpene lactone called "Parthenin"<br>• Thiuram, organophosphorus compounds, synthetic pyrethroids, dithiocarbamates, propargite, and captan<br>• Anacardic acid in fruit shells of Anacardium occidentale |
| Automobile industry | Allergic contact dermatitis, irritant contact dermatitis, oil acne, skin infections, and callosities | Epoxy resins, cutting oil, and colophony |
| Construction industry | ICD, ACD, and callosities on palm | Cement, chromate, hydrochloric acids, epoxy resin, fiberglass, leather gloves, rubber, adhesives, wood preservatives, and cobalt |
| Plastic industry | ACD and ICD | Unsaturated polyester resin, stearic acid, waxes, alkylated phenols, benzoyl peroxide, methyl ethyl ketone peroxide, and formaldehyde |
| Rubber industry | ACD | Benzothiazole, paraphenylenediamine compounds, ethylene thiourea, and resorcinol |
| Paint industry/painters | | Epoxy resin, potassium dichromate, glue, and colophony |
| Food industry workers/ cooks | Irritant contact dermatitis, paronychia, contact urticaria, fingertip eczema, intertrigo, pitted keratolysis, and callosities | Soap, detergents, constant use of water, onion, garlic, spices, seafood, and continuous mechanical insult |
| Hairdressers | ACD/ICD | Paraphenylene diamine, nickel, ammonium persulfate (bleaching agent), glyceryl monothioglycolate (permanent wave agent), shampoos, preservatives, and fragrances |

During the examination, it is imperative for the physician to meticulously inspect the dermatitis lesions, assessing their severity and looking for additional signs indicative of atopic dermatitis or psoriasis. A comprehensive examination, encompassing a thorough evaluation of the entire body, including nails and the scalp, is essential for a comprehensive understanding. Diagnostic tests play a crucial role in confirming the diagnosis. The skin prick test is employed to assess immediate hypersensitivity. Nonirritating concentrations of substances, including the patient's own products or food, are applied to the skin for this purpose. For individuals with suspected allergic contact dermatitis, patch testing serves as a confirmatory diagnostic tool. This specialized testing aids in identifying specific allergens contributing to dermatitis, providing valuable insights for targeted management strategies.

The patient should receive written information detailing the identified allergen and materials that may potentially contain the allergen. Moving to the treatment phase, addressing acute, oozing lesions involves the use of wet dressings, which can be accomplished with either saline compresses or potassium permanganate soaks. Subsequent steps include the application of topical corticosteroid creams and the administration of sedative antihistamines for comprehensive management.

In cases where allergic contact dermatitis is extensive, a tailored approach to treatment is imperative.

Prevention strategies are pivotal in minimizing the risk of occupational dermatitis:

- Conducting health checks and screenings before employment serves to sensitize individuals about potential workplace hazards.
- Emphasizing the importance of personal protective wear and ensuring well-ventilated workspaces contributes to creating a safer environment.
- Promoting immediate removal of soaked clothing, practicing proper handwashing techniques, and incorporating the use of barrier creams are essential measures in reducing the likelihood of dermatitis in occupational settings.

Various occupational groups face distinct dermatitis challenges due to specific allergens:

Understanding these occupational dermatitis scenarios helps tailor preventive measures for specific workplace risks.

## CONCLUSION

The profession of an individual, with an emphasis on materials used and handled, is an important piece of information to a diagnostician to treat contact dermatitis.

## REFERENCES

1. Bains SN, Nash P, Fonacier L. Irritant contact dermatitis. Clin Rev Allergy Immunol. 2019;56:99-109.
2. Sasseville D. Occupational contact dermatitis. Allergy Asthma Clin Immunol. 2008;4(2):59-65.
3. Srinivas CR, Sethy M. Occupational dermatoses. Indian Dermatol Online J. 2022;14(1):21-31.
4. Mathias CGT. Contact dermatitis and workers' compensation: criteria for establishing occupational causation and aggravation. J Am Acad Dermatol. 1989;20(5 Pt 1):842-8.

CHAPTER 3.10

# Patch Testing

***Sathish Pai B, Lisa Jennifer Dsouza***

## INTRODUCTION

Patch testing was introduced as a simple diagnostic tool in the investigation of contact dermatitis. German physician Joseph Jadassohn played a pivotal role in introducing the technique and concepts of patch testing.[1] Since then, this method has undergone significant evolution and refinement, leading to standardization based on regional variations, testing devices, and protocols. In a notable development in 1967, the formation of the International Contact Dermatitis Research Group (ICDRG) marked a crucial milestone in the journey toward standardizing skin testing methodologies.

## DEFINITION

The patch test serves as a bioassay, a tool employed to confirm sensitization to a substance leading to allergic contact dermatitis (ACD). Despite being artificial and not duplicating real-world clinical exposure, it offers valuable insights. The application is for a fixed duration, utilizing a defined concentration of the allergen. In comparison to the clinical "trial and error" approach, the patch test is considered a superior method for determining sensitivities and identifying specific allergens responsible for dermatological reactions.

## PRINCIPLE OF PATCH TESTING

It is a diagnostic procedure employed to pinpoint specific allergens associated with ACD or, in certain instances, to establish the ACD diagnosis itself. The underlying principle of patch testing rests on the recognition that in sensitized individuals, circulating primed antigen-specific T lymphocytes of the Th1 phenotype possess the capability to reproduce a delayed-type hypersensitivity reaction. This occurs when nonirritating concentrations of the antigen are applied to unaffected skin. The antigen applied to the skin undergoes processing by local antigen-presenting cells. The TH1 effector cell recognizes the antigen, leading to the release of cytokines, which in turn affect the vascular endothelium. The recruitment of T cells and phagocytes, along with the accumulation of fluid and proteins at the site, results in visible lesions.

## WHAT IS THE ROLE OF PATCH TESTING?

The identification of triggering and/or aggravating allergens through patch testing plays a crucial role in providing accurate avoidance advice. This, in turn, contributes to reducing morbidity and enhancing the overall quality of life for individuals affected by ACD.

## WHAT IS AN IDEAL PATCH TEST?

An ideal patch test should possess the following characteristics:

- Indicate contact sensitization
- No false positive reactions
- Allergen-pure and right concentration
- Low risk of active sensitization
- Minimum irritant reaction
- Stable, easy to apply, easy to read

## WHAT ARE THE INDICATIONS?

- Eczematous disorders
- In cases where eczematous disorders show inadequate response to standard treatment, patch testing becomes valuable in uncovering potential contact allergens.
- For individuals experiencing chronic hand and foot eczema, patch testing is advisable to investigate and pinpoint the underlying causes.

- Patch testing is recommended when dealing with persistent or intermittent eczema affecting sensitive areas such as the face, eyelids, ears, and perineum.
- In cases of varicose eczema, patch testing is employed to explore potential contact allergens contributing to the condition.

## CONTRAINDICATIONS FOR PATCH TESTING

Patch testing is contraindicated under certain conditions:

- Presence of active dermatitis
- Dermatitis at the test site
- Immunodeficiency and autoimmune diseases
- Patients on immunosuppressive drugs
- Pregnancy and lactation

## TYPES OF PATCH TEST

- Closed test
- Open test
- Semiopen test
- Repeated open application test
- Usage test

The preferred site for patch testing is the upper back, although alternative locations include the upper arm and lower back. To ensure effective testing, hair removal from the chosen site is recommended. Hairy areas can be shaved 2–3 days before the test, or if preferred, avoided altogether. Prior to patch application, degreasing the site with mild solvents or ethanol is essential. It is crucial to allow sufficient time for the solvent to evaporate before applying the patch to ensure accurate and reliable results.

## PRETEST REQUISITES

Before undergoing patch testing, individuals should adhere to the following pretest requisites:

- Avoid bath or shower
- Avoid exercise
- Abstain from engaging in strenuous exercise
- Avoid activities likely to dislodge patches
- *Medication considerations*: Refrain from taking medications, particularly systemic steroids, for at least 4 weeks before the test. Additionally, discontinue the use of topical steroids for a minimum of 1 week. For topical immunomodulators like pimecrolimus, cessation for 1 week is recommended.

These precautions contribute to the accuracy and reliability of patch test results. Continuation of oral antihistamines during patch testing is permissible, as these medications exert minimal if any, impact on the mechanisms of delayed hypersensitivity.

Patients are advised to refrain from exposure to ultraviolet radiation prior to undergoing patch testing. In cases where patients exhibit a significant tan, it is recommended to defer patch testing. Furthermore, a waiting period of at least 2 weeks postsignificant sun exposure should be observed before initiating patch testing.

## PATCH TEST SERIES

- *Standard series*: Each country has its own standard series, e.g., Indian Standard series.
- Footwear series
- Dental series
- Cosmetic series
- Preservative series
- Corticosteroid series, etc.

### Indian Standard Series

Indian Standard series contains:

- Vaseline (100%)
- Wool alcohol (lanolin) 30%
- Balsam of Peru 10%
- Formaldehyde 2%
- Mercaptobenzothiazole 1%
- Potassium dichromate 0.1%
- Nickel sulfate 5%
- Cobalt sulfate 5%
- Colophony 10%
- Epoxy resin 1%
- Paraben mix 9%
- Paraphenylenediamine 1%
- Parthenium 15%
- Neomycin sulfate 20%
- Benzocaine 5%
- Chlorocresol 1%
- Fragrance mix 8%
- Thiuram mix 1%
- Nitrofurazone 1%
- Black rubber mix 0.60%

Nickel is the most frequent sensitizer surpassing Potassium dichromate in India[2] and worldwide[3].

## IDEAL VEHICLE FOR PATCH TESTING

The ideal vehicle for patch testing should allow occlusion, stabilize allergens, and be economical. Examples you mentioned include:

- Petrolatum
- Water
- Acetone
- Ethanol
- Hydrophilic gel

## PATCH TESTING CHAMBERS

- *Finn chamber* **(Figs. 1A to C)**:
  - Made with aluminum
  - Circular disc with 8 mm diameter and 0.5 mm depth
  - Mounted on micropore tape
  - Other chambers include Van der Bend and IQ chambers

Upper back is the preferred site for application of the patches **(Fig. 1D)**. There should not be active dermatitis at the site. For about 2–3 mm of the allergens are placed at the center of the chamber as shown above. Liquid allergens are placed over a filter paper inserted in the chamber **(Fig. 2)**.

The typical regimen involves the following steps:

**Day 1:** Apply Patches

**Day 3:** Remove Patches and Mark Areas **(Fig. 3)**

Wait for 30 minutes. After the 30-minute wait, take the initial reading, representing the 48-hour exposure.

**Day 4:** Second Reading (72 hours)
On the fourth day, take a second reading, representing the 72-hour exposure.

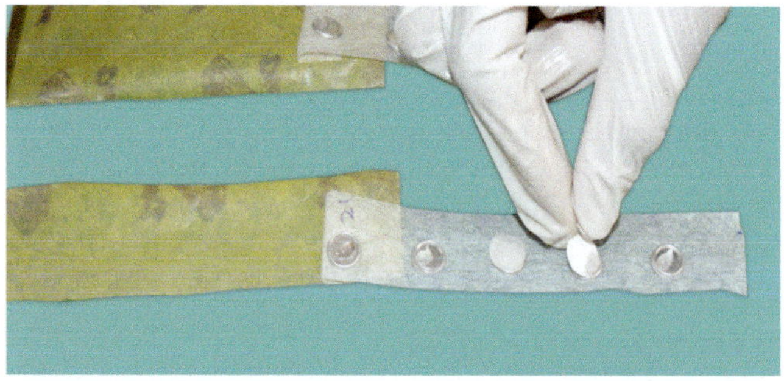

**FIG. 2:** Application of liquid allergen using the filter paper.

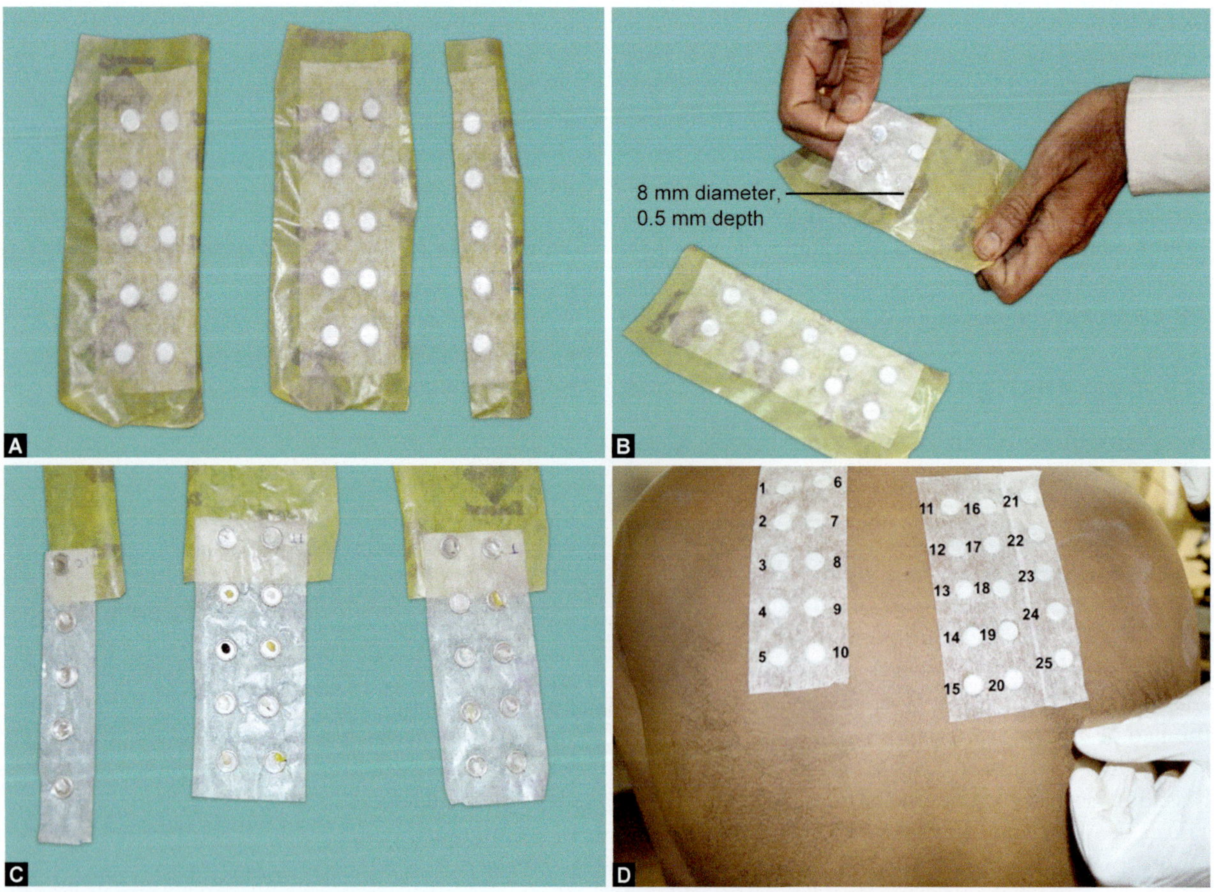


**FIGS. 1A TO D:** (A) Patch test material showing the aluminium chamber fixed to micropore tape and the plastic film; (B) Removal of the plastic film showing the diameter and depth of the aluminium chamber attached to the micropore tape; (C) Placing of 2–3 mm of allergen at the center of the chambers; and (D) Application of the patches over the back.

**Day 5 and 7:** Additional Readings Advisable

It is advisable to take additional readings on the 5th and 7th days.

Test results are measured using morphological criteria recommended by the International Contact Dermatitis Research Group (ICDRG).

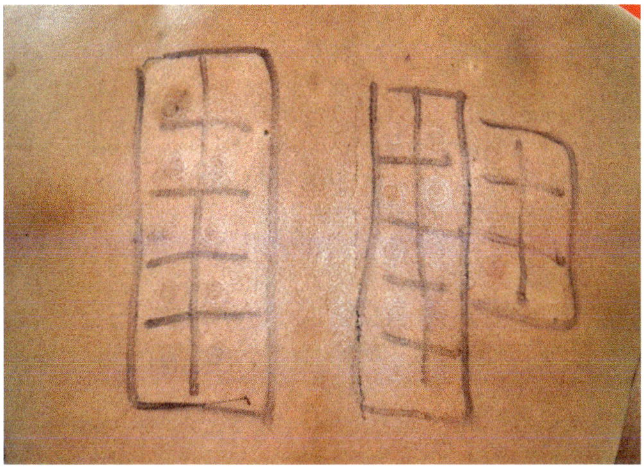

**FIG. 3:** Marking the test areas.

+? Doubtful

\+ Weak positive, palpable erythema, and infiltration **(Fig. 4A)**.

++ Strong positive, erythema, infiltration, papules and vesicles **(Fig. 4B)**.

+++ Very strong, intense erythema, infiltration, coalescing vesicles **(Fig. 4C)**.

IR irritant reaction, inflammation limited to the exposed area, petechiae, and pustules.

*False positive reactions*:
- Excessive concentration
- Presence of contaminants
- Excess allergen applied
- Current or recent dermatitis at the patch test site
- Current dermatitis at distant sites
- Adhesive tape reaction
- Angry back

*False negative reactions*:
- Insufficient concentration
- Insufficient amount applied
- Inappropriate vehicle
- Readings performed too early
- Poor adhesion of patches

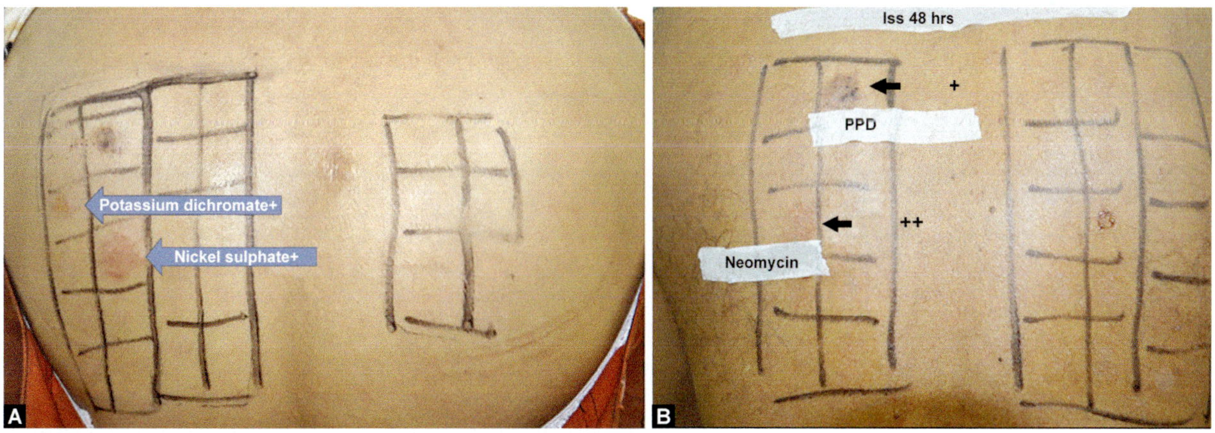


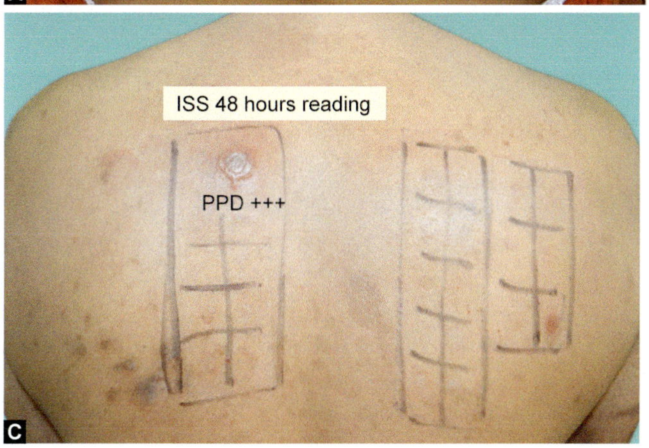


**FIGS. 4A TO C:** (A) Patch test showing + reaction to Potassium dichromate and nickel sulphate; (B) Patch test showing ++ reaction to neomycin and + reaction to PPD; (C) Patch test showing +++ reaction to PPD.

- Patches applied at the wrong site
- Systemic treatment with immunosuppressants

## RELEVANCE (COADEX)

- *C (current)*: The patient has been exposed to the allergen before the current episode of dermatitis, and there is improvement when the exposure is ceased.
- *O (old)*: Old or past relevance. This indicates past episodes of dermatitis resulting from exposure to the allergen.
- *A (active sensitization)*: The patient presents with a sensitization (late) reaction, suggesting an ongoing sensitivity to the allergen.
- *D (doubtful)*: Relevance is difficult to assess. There is no traceable relationship between the positive test and the disease.
- *E (exposed)*: History of previous exposures that did not cause dermatitis. This indicates a prior exposure that did not result in a skin reaction.
- *X (cross-reaction)*: The positive test is due to cross-reaction with another hapten that is clinically relevant. This suggests that the observed positive result is not directly related to the tested substance but is due to a reaction with a related compound.

## CONCLUSION

Patch testing is the only reliable test to identify the contact allergen. It is important to know the correct method of performing the test and also to do a proper reading and interpretation of the test. It is crucial to establish the relevance and advice the patients accordingly regarding avoidance of the allergens.

## REFERENCES

1. Fischer T, Maibach HI. Patch testing in allergic contact dermatitis: An update. Sem Dermatol. 1986;5:214-24.
2. Narendra G, Srinivas CR. Patch testing with Indian standard series. Indian J Dermatol Venereol Leprol. 2002;68:281-2.
3. Ahlström MG, Thyssen JP, Wennervaldt M, Menné T, Johansen JD. Nickel allergy and allergic contact dermatitis: A clinical review of immunology, epidemiology, exposure, and treatment. Contact Dermatitis. 2019;81:227-41.

SECTION

# 4

# Drug Allergy

***Section Editors:*** Kiran Godse and Anant Patil

4.1

CHAPTER

# Approach to Suspected Drug Reactions

*Maryam Khoshkhui, Rana Tafrishi*

## INTRODUCTION

Drug reactions present a significant challenge for clinicians, ranging from mild, self-limiting symptoms such as maculopapular rash to life-threatening conditions such as toxic epidermal necrolysis (TEN). A suspected adverse drug reaction (ADR) requires immediate and systematic evaluation to distinguish between harmless side effects, which are self-limited and serious adverse effects that need specific interventions. With the growing complexity of pharmacotherapy, including polypharmacy and new drug classes, the importance of understanding, diagnosing, and managing drug reactions has become paramount in patient care. ADRs not only affect patient outcomes but also lead to hospitalizations, longer treatment time, and increased healthcare costs. This chapter outlines a structured approach to diagnosing and managing common drug reactions, focusing on identifying onset, recognizing clinical manifestations, assessing causality, and applying management strategies based on evidence-based guidelines.[1]

## CLASSIFICATION OF DRUG REACTIONS

We can classify adverse drug reactions in different ways:

1. Adverse drug reactions are broadly organized into two subtypes: Type A reactions (predictable) and type B reactions (unpredictable). Predictable reactions are dose-dependent, related to the known pharmacologic actions, and although they may occur in otherwise normal individuals. Predictable reactions account for about 80% of ADRs including overdosage, side effects, and drug interactions.

   Unpredictable reactions are less related to dose, are unrelated to the pharmacologic action of the drug, and occur only in susceptible individuals. Unpredictable reactions are account for about 80% of ADRs including drug allergy (immunologically mediated responses), which are the main part of this chapter, and we will discuss more in detail later, drug intolerance (undesirable pharmacologic effect that occurs at low and sometimes subtherapeutic doses of the drug without underlying abnormalities of metabolism, excretion, or bioavailability of the drug), and nonallergic reactions with immunologic manifestations, which result from direct release of mediators from mast cells and basophils, rather than being triggered by specific immunoglobulin E (IgE) antibodies such as Redman syndrome due to vancomycin.[2]
2. Drug allergy can be classified based on their clinical manifestation (maculopapular rash, urticaria, TEN, fixed drug reaction, etc.).
3. They can also be classified based on basic immunologic mechanisms to type 1, type 2, type 3, and type 4 (Gell and Coombs Classification), which can help to understand the etiology, diagnostic tests, and treatment strategies.

   Type 1 or immediate reactions are IgE-mediated reactions that typically occur within 1 hour of drug dosing. IgE antibodies that bind to Fcε receptors on the surface of mast cells and basophils are formed. On reexposure to the same drug, cross-linking of cell-bound antibodies on mast cells and basophils occurs that leads to degranulation and the release of vasoactive mediators such as histamines and leukotrienes.

   Type 2 hypersensitivities are non-IgE antibody-mediated reactions that, like IgE-mediated reactions, typically occur within minutes to hours after drug dosing. These reactions occur in association with drugs that are able to rapidly haptenate host proteins such as beta-lactams. They result in antibody-mediated

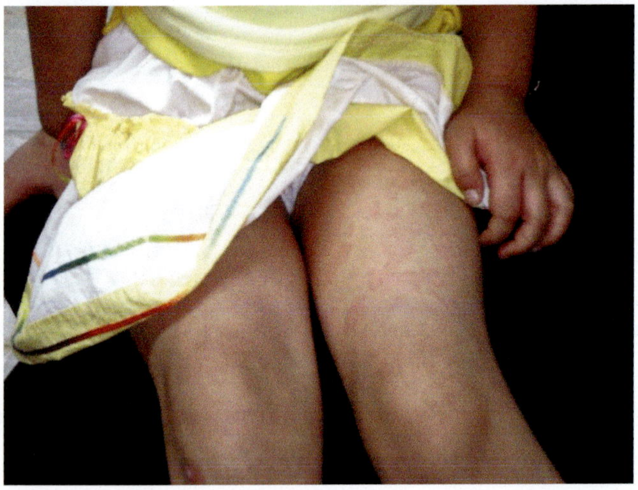

**FIG. 1:** Serum-sickness-like reaction with severe urticaria and arthralgia due to cefixime.

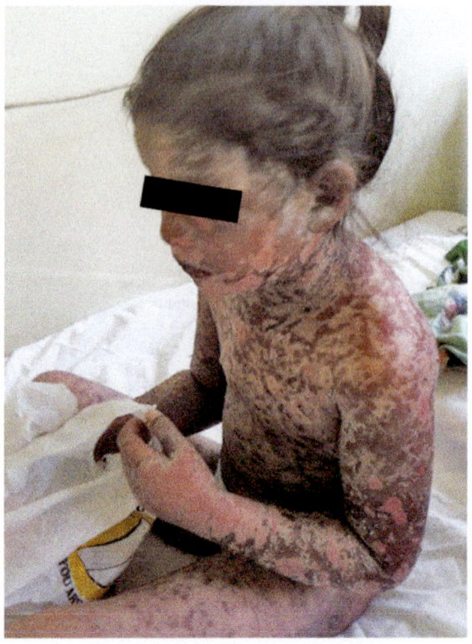

**FIG. 2:** Toxic epidermal necrolysis (TEN) due to phenobarbital with positive Nikolsky sign in a girl with epilepsy.

cytopenias, such as hemolytic anemia (penicillins and quinidine).

Type 3 reactions are immune complex reactions that result from high-dose prolonged therapy and may produce a serum-sickness-like reaction with severe urticarial rash and joint pain. They result when an antibody (IgG more than IgM) binds to a soluble antigen (a drug or metabolite), leading to circulating immune complexes that deposit in sites of disease such as skin, joints, and small vessels **(Fig. 1)**.

4. Type 4 reactions are the purely T cell–mediated type reactions that are delayed days to weeks after first exposure to a drug. Maculopapular rash, DRESS (drug reaction with eosinophilia and systemic symptom) syndrome, Stevens–Johnson syndrome (SJS), and TEN are the examples of type 4 reactions **(Figs. 2 and 3)**.

A useful practical classification is dividing reactions to immediate and delayed based on the time gap between drug usage and the onset of clinical manifestations. This later classification is critical for determining the urgency of the reaction and also for the appropriate management:

- *Immediate reactions*: These occur within minutes to hours of drug administration and typically involve IgE-mediated hypersensitivity (type 1 Gell and Coombs Classification) or non-IgE mechanisms, such as complement activation. Anaphylaxis, urticaria, and angioedema are the classic examples of immediate reactions.[3] These reactions are often life-threatening and need rapid intervention including epinephrine for treatment of anaphylaxis.
- *Delayed reactions*: Delayed reactions manifest hours, days, or even weeks after drug exposure. These reactions typically involve T-cell-mediated hypersensitivity (type 4 Gell and Coombs Classification) and include rashes, organ toxicity, and severe cutaneous adverse reactions (SCARs) such as DRESS syndrome, SJS, and TEN.[4] Delayed reactions often require more prolonged monitoring, and a more nuanced treatment approach compared to immediate reactions. As there is a long gap (1–8 weeks) between drug use and delayed adverse reactions, drugs as a cause may be neglected by the clinicians.

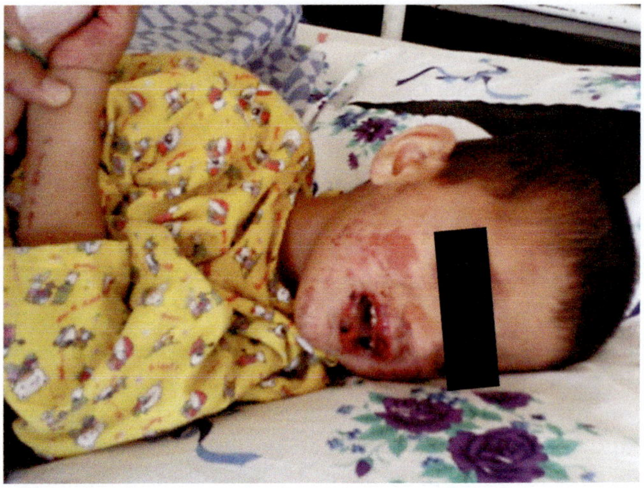

**FIG. 3:** Stevens–Johnson syndrome (SJS) due to carbamazepine in a boy with epilepsy.

## STEPWISE APPROACH TO DIAGNOSING DRUG REACTIONS

A systematic approach is necessary to accurately diagnose drug reactions. This involves a comprehensive clinical

**Clinical history and physical exam**
Gather details on onset, medication history, evaluation of all patient symptoms

↓

**Classify reaction type based on history and physical exam**
For example:
Type 1: Anaphylaxis,
Type 3: Serum sickness,
Type 4: Delayed reactions….

↓

**Management**
- *Immediate reactions*: Discontinue the drug, treat anaphylaxis with epinephrine
- *Delayed reactions*: Discontinue the drug, provide supportive care
- *Severe cutaneous reactions (e.g., SJS, TEN)*: Use corticosteroids, IVIG, and ICU care

To prevent drug allergies, it is crucial to accurately diagnose any suspected reactions

For IgE-mediated drug reactions, skin prick tests and intradermal tests can be used, but it is important to consider the positive and negative predictive values of these tests

For delayed type reactions, patch tests can be utilized. In cases of TEN and SJS, avoiding the suspected drug is of utmost importance

**FLOWCHART 1:** Practice flowchart for drug allergy diagnostic work-up and management

evaluation, identification of symptoms, causality assessment, and management **(Flowchart 1)**.

## History and Clinical Evaluation

The first step in evaluating a suspected drug reaction is obtaining a detailed clinical history. A careful history helps determine whether a drug could be the cause of the reaction and provides insight into the most likely diagnosis. It is important, especially when the patient takes several drugs simultaneously.

- *Onset and timing*: The timing of the reaction relative to drug administration is essential. Immediate reactions such as anaphylaxis occur within minutes to hours of exposure, while delayed reactions, such as TEN and Stevens-Johnson, may develop over days or weeks.[5] Serum sickness like reactions occur 1–3 weeks after exposure.
- *Medications history*: It is crucial to assess all medications the patient is currently taking, including over-the-counter drugs, herbal supplements, and biologics. Certain medications, such as antibiotics (e.g., penicillin), anticonvulsants, and nonsteroidal anti-inflammatory drugs (NSAIDs), are commonly associated with ADRs.[5]
- Understanding the patient's full medical history—including allergies and prior drug reactions—plays a significant role in predicting future reactions and avoiding harmful drug interactions.[2]

## Clinical Manifestations

Clinical manifestations of ADRs are diverse and can include a range of symptoms, from mild rashes to life-threatening conditions. Identifying these manifestations helps guide the diagnosis and management of the reaction.

- *Cutaneous reactions*: Maculopapular rashes are one of the most common ADRs. They range from benign maculopapular rashes to more severe reactions like SJS and TEN, which can involve mucosal surfaces and lead to systemic symptoms.[4] While mild rashes are benign and self-limited, severe cutaneous reactions require urgent intervention including corticosteroids, cyclosporine, or intravenous immunoglobulin (IVIG) due to their high morbidity and mortality rates.
- *Hypersensitivity reactions*: Immediate hypersensitivity reactions such as anaphylaxis involve symptoms like urticaria and angioedema, wheezing and dyspnea, vomiting and abdominal pain, and hypotension. These reactions are typically IgE-mediated and require immediate treatment with epinephrine.[3]
- *Organ toxicity*: Drug-induced liver injury (DILI) and nephrotoxicity are other common ADRs. Drugs like acetaminophen and NSAIDs are frequent culprits. Advancements in biomarkers to detect subclinical organ toxicity allow earlier intervention and prevention of severe outcomes.[6]

## Management

Management of ADRs varies depending on the type and severity of the reaction. Immediate cessation of the offending drug is the first and most important step in all cases. Symptomatic treatment and close monitoring are critical for minimizing harm and preventing further complications.

- *Immediate reactions*: For life-threatening reactions such as anaphylaxis, rapid administration of intramuscular epinephrine (0.3–0.5 mg in adults and 0.01 mg/kg in children) is essential, along with supplemental oxygen, intravenous fluids, and antihistamines for symptom control. Corticosteroids may also be used to reduce inflammation.[6]
- *Delayed reactions*: Discontinuation of the drug is the primary intervention. In cases such as drug-induced liver injury, the management may include supportive care, liver function monitoring.[4]
- *SCARs*: Supportive care, including fluid management, wound care, and possible corticosteroid, cyclosporine or IVIG use, is crucial for reactions such as DRESS, SJS, and TEN. ICU admission may be required for severe cases. TEN patients should be treated in burn wards.[4]

In life-threatening drug reactions and severe reactions (such as SJS and TEN), the patient must avoid the culprit drug. To determine the appropriate drug for future use, and if necessary, drug challenge tests, the patient should be referred to an allergy specialist.

## PREVENTION AND EDUCATION

Preventing ADRs involves both pre-emptive measures and patient education. Clinicians should carefully review a patient's medical history, including previous drug reactions and known allergies, to minimize the risk of ADRs. Avoidance of unnecessary drug prescription specially antibiotics are crucial.

- *Patient education*: Patients should be educated about recognizing early signs of ADRs and instructed to report any unusual symptoms to their healthcare provider. This is particularly important for high-risk drugs.[7]
- *Alternative therapies*: For patients with known drug allergies or a history of ADRs, alternative medications should be considered. Rechallenging a patient with a suspected drug reaction should only be done cautiously, under supervision, and when protocols like desensitization are available.[8]

## CONCLUSION

The optimal approach to a patient suspected of having a drug allergy begins with a thorough history-taking and physical examination. This is followed by the classification of lesions, selection of appropriate diagnostic tests as needed, and initiation of appropriate treatment modalities.

## REFERENCES

1. Uetrecht J, Naisbitt DJ. Idiosyncratic drug reactions: Current concepts. Pharmacol Rev. 2013;65(2):779-808.
2. Burks AW, O'Hehir RE, Broide DH, Holgate ST, Bac LB (Eds). Middleton's Allergy: Principles and Practice, 9th edition. Elsevier; 2020.
3. Jeimy S, Wong T, Ben-Shoshan M et al. Drug allergy. Allergy Asthma Clin Immunol. 2024;20 (Suppl 3):78.
4. Warrington, R., Silviu-Dan, F. & Wong, T. Drug allergy. Allergy Asthma Clin Immunol 14 (Suppl 2), 60 (2018). https://doi.org/10.1186/s13223-018-0289-y
5. Sullivan TJ, Leeder JS. Drug-induced liver injury: Mechanisms and management. Ann Intern Med. 2017;166(11):783-92.
6. Nelson JC. Comprehensive Drug Allergy and Reactions. 2024.
7. World Health Organization. International drug monitoring: The role of the WHO. [online] Available from https://www.who.int [Last accessed January, 2025].
8. Ho SS, Lee SL. Managing allergic drug reactions: A guide for clinicians. Am J Clin Dermatol. 2019;20(6):859-68.

4.2

CHAPTER

# Approach to Exanthematous Drug Reactions

***Muhammed Burak Yücel, Özlem Su Küçük***

## INTRODUCTION

Exanthematous drug reactions, also known as morbiliform or maculopapular drug rashes, are the most common type of adverse cutaneous drug reaction. These reactions are usually benign and self-limiting, but sometimes they may be the first signs of more serious systemic reactions such as drug reaction with eosinophilia and systemic symptoms (DRESS) or Stevens–Johnson syndrome (SJS)/toxic epidermal necrolysis (TEN), which carry a potential risk of morbidity and mortality. Therefore, rapid identification and accurate diagnosis of an adverse drug reaction is essential for optimal patient's management to prevent potentially significant complications. Exanthematous drug reactions occur in 1–5% of first-time users of the drugs responsible, particularly antibiotics, nonsteroidal anti-inflammatory drugs (NSAIDs), and antiepileptic drugs (carbamazepine, phenytoin, and lamotrigine).

The underlying mechanism is likely to be immunological via cell-mediated hypersensitivity. A drug antigen or hapten may be presented directly to T lymphocytes via Langerhans cells, or it may bind covalently (e.g., β-lactam antibiotics) or noncovalently (e.g., sulfamethoxazole and lidocaine) to major histocompatibility complex class II (MHC II) peptide complexes, activating both CD4- and CD8-positive T cells and leading to a cytotoxic effect.[1]

Recent studies have highlighted the role of genetic predisposition in exanthematous drug reactions **(Table 1)**. While the main genetic predisposition to hypersensitivity reactions has been attributed to variations in the regulation and expression of the cytochrome P-450 enzyme system, these genetic associations may be both drug and phenotype specific. In this context, specific human leucocyte antigen (HLA) alleles, such as HLA-B*1502 in carbamazepine-induced reactions, HLA-B*5701 in abacavir-induced reactions, or HLA-B*3101 in Europeans, provide insights into the pathogenesis of hypersensitivity and preventive opportunities. Future pharmacogenomic studies will pave the way for personalized therapeutic approaches.[2,3]

**TABLE 1: Common drugs linked to exanthematous drug reactions.[6]**

| Reaction patterns | Causative drugs |
|---|---|
| Exanthematous (maculopapular) reaction | Allopurinol, barbiturates, benzodiazepines, captopril, carbamazepine, cephalosporins, gentamicin, gold, lithium, NSAIDs, penicillin, phenytoin, sulfonamides, and thiazides |
| Urticaria | ACE inhibitors, aspirin, cephalosporins, contrast media, monoclonal antibodies, NSAIDs, opiates, penicillin, phenytoin, quinine, tetracycline, and sulfonamides |
| Acute generalized exanthematous pustulosis (AGEP) | β-lactams, carbamazepine, diltiazem, doxycycline, isoniazid, macrolides, nystatin, penicillin, quinolones, sulfonamides, and terbinafine |
| DRESS/DIHS | Anticonvulsants (many), allopurinol, cotrimoxazole, dapsone, minocycline, sulfonamides, and terbinafine (lamotrigine combined with valproate = high risk) |
| SJS/TEN | Allopurinol, barbiturates, carbamazepine, cephalosporins, lamotrigine, nevirapine, NSAIDs (oxicams), penicillin, pentamidine, phenytoin, and sulfonamides |

(ACE: angiotensin-converting enzyme; DIHS: drug-induced hypersensitivity syndrome; DRESS: drug reaction with eosinophilia and systemic symptoms; NSAIDs: nonsteroidal anti-inflammatory drugs; SJS: Stevens–Johnson syndrome; TEN: toxic epidermal necrolysis)

## CLINICAL FEATURES

*Onset:* Symptoms usually begin 4–14 days after starting the culprit drug. However, in cases of re-exposure, the reaction may occur within 24–48 hours.

*Associated symptoms:* Mild signs of systemic involvement such as pruritus, low-grade fever (<38.5°C), fatigue, and lymphadenopathy may be seen. Mucosal involvement is usually absent.

The rash is usually self-limiting and subsides rapidly after discontinuation of the culprit drug, and systemic symptoms are rare in pure exanthematous reactions. However, the presence of facial edema, mucosal involvement, blistering, palpable purpura, or ulcerations should be considered red flags and a warning of serious systemic reactions.

*Laboratory findings* such as leukocytosis, eosinophilia, or elevated liver enzymes may be present, but special care should be taken in the differential diagnosis because of overlapping clinical features, especially in severe reactions such as DRESS, SJS/TEN, and viral exanthemas.[4]

## DIAGNOSTIC APPROACH

### History Taking

- Identification of new medications, especially those started within the last 2 weeks.
- Assessment of dosage, duration, and previous drug reactions.
- Consideration of concomitant factors such as infections or concomitant diseases and examination of the patient's immune status.

### Physical Examination

- The distribution and morphology of the rash, preservation of mucosal membranes and absence of vesicles or pustules, and resolution after discontinuation of the culprit drug support the diagnosis.
- Evaluation of fever, lymphadenopathy, and systemic involvement is important to exclude differential diagnoses.

### Laboratory Investigations

- Routine blood tests may reveal eosinophilia in some cases, but it is not always present and often there is no specific laboratory marker.
- Skin biopsy, although rarely needed and nonspesific, shows perivascular lymphocytic infiltrates with eosinophils and spongiform changes.[5]
- Genetic screening is becoming increasingly important in high-risk populations. In this context, pharmacogenetic testing for HLA-B alleles in patients before starting high-risk drugs such as carbamazepine has been shown to be significantly effective in preventing hypersensitivity reactions.[2]

## GENERAL FEATURES OF DIFFERENTIAL DIAGNOSES

*Viral exanthems:* The common clinical manifestations of drug-induced morbiliform rashes, i.e., maculopapular exanthema and urticaria, are similar to those of viral-induced rashes and are difficult to distinguish in the acute phase. Viral infections can also cause or aggravate drug-associated rashes [e.g., Epstein–Barr virus (EBV)-ampicillin, DRESS-human herpes virus (HHV)-6 associations]. Differential diagnosis is therefore important. The most common clinical presentations of the six classical viral exanthems [measles, scarlet fever, rubella, Filatow–Dukes disease (fourth disease), erythema infectiosum (fifth disease) and exanthema subitum (sixth disease)] and other atypical viral exanthems (enteroviruses, herpesviruses, etc.) are maculopapular, purpuric, and vesicular exanthems.

Some clinical features are important in the differential diagnosis. In measles, mild fever and prodrome with cough, catarrh, conjunctivitis, and bright Koplik spots on the buccal mucosa and centrifugal maculopapular rashes on the body; in scarlet fever, sore throat, peripheral pallor, pastia line, strawberry tongue and scarlatiniform rashes on the body; in rubella, subfebrile fever with mild constitutional symptoms, small red spots on the soft palate (Forchheimer spots) and maculopapular rash on the body with posterior auricular lymphadenopathy; in the fifth disease (erythema infectiosum) caused by parvovirus B19, there is a slapped cheek-red rash on the face and a lace-like retiform rash on the body; and in exanthema subitum (the sixth disease), after several days of high fever, there is an itchless, pink maculopapular rash on the body, followed by a drop in temperature. For most viral exanthema, the clinical features should be well known, a detailed drug history should be taken and symptomatic treatment is usually sufficient **(Figs. 1A and B)**.[7]

*Urticaria/Angioedema:* Drug-induced urticaria is the second most common type of drug reaction and presents as a transient acute eruption of erythematous itchy wheals.

The erythematous itchy wheals usually disappear within 24 hours and do not leave scarring, but may develop if the culprit drug is continued. The clinical picture may present as isolated urticaria, angioedema or a combination of the two. In severe cases, particularly those associated with penicillin and latex, the reaction may progress to anaphylaxis. This is typically a type I hypersensitivity

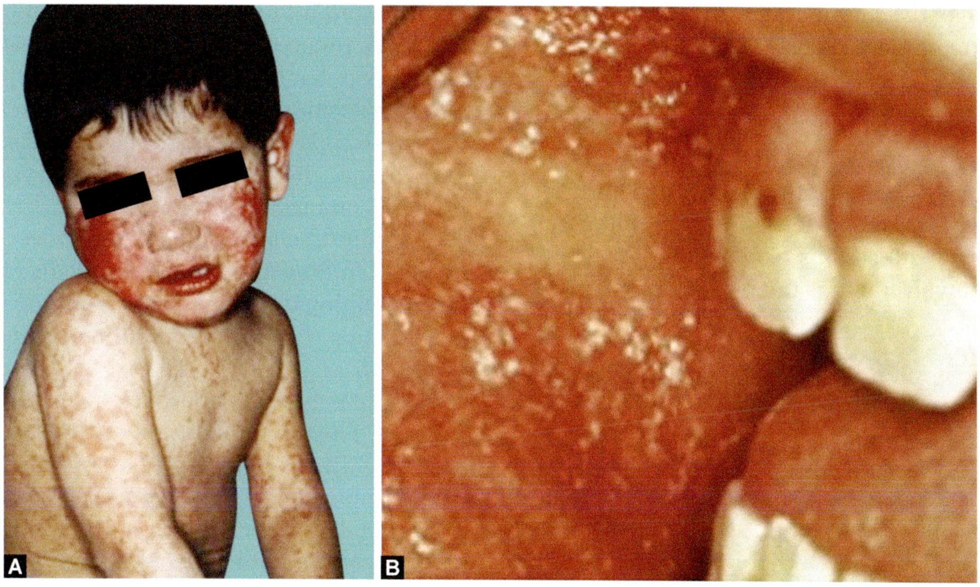

**FIGS. 1A AND B:** Diffuse morbilliform rash and white papules on the buccal mucosa seen in measles.[7]

reaction. The reaction is mediated by immunoglobulin E (IgE) antibodies, which cause activation and degranulation of mast cells. In the absence of IgE antibodies, similar clinical features are associated with the use of opiates and radiocontrast agents, resulting in the direct release of histamine and other inflammatory mediators and is coined an "anaphylactoid" reaction.

Urticaria usually develops within 24–36 hours of exposure to the culprit drug, but can sometimes develop within a few hours or minutes. In general, urticarial lesions develop with repeated exposure to the culprit drug, which is related to the production of IgE antibodies to the drug from previous exposure and immune sensitization. On the other hand, isolated drug-induced angioedema is usually related to the bradykinin-mediated pathway and may develop after the use of ACE inhibitors and may occur at any time. Treatment involves the use of nonsedating second-generation oral antihistamines and discontinuation of the culprit drug. In cases of severe angioedema or anaphylaxis, corticosteroids and intramuscular epinephrine are used **(Fig. 2)**.[8]

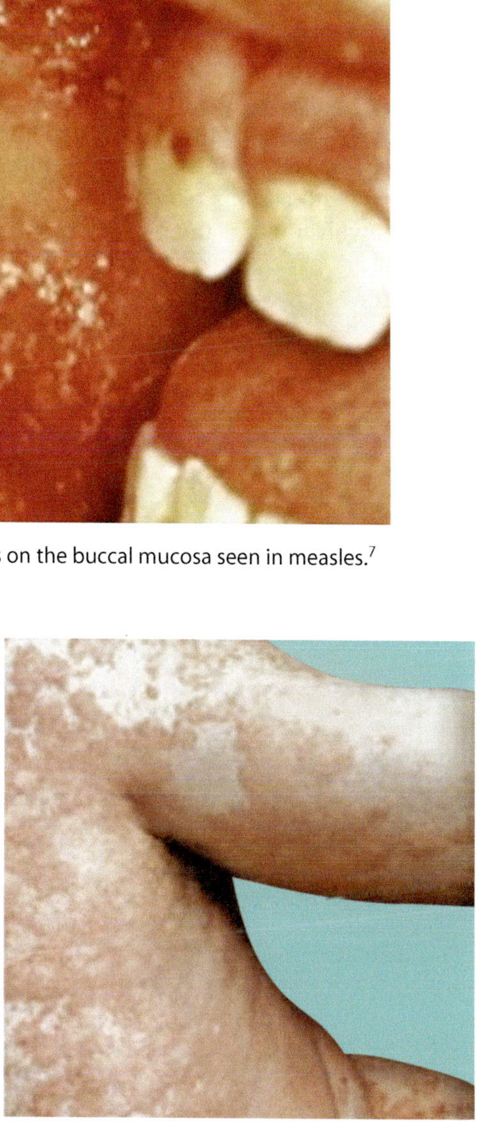

**FIG. 2:** Typical urticarial rash characterized by itchy wheals.[8]

*Acute generalized exanthematous pustulosis (AGEP):* This relatively rare acute pustular eruption may clinically resemble pustular psoriasis. It is characterized by multiple nonfollicular pustules on a background of fever and widespread erythema.

It mainly affects the major body folds and the upper trunk. The association with drugs is acute, with most cases occurring within 24 hours of exposure. The pathophysiology is uncertain, but neutrophil-activating cytokines such as interleukin (IL)-3 and IL-8 induced by drug-specific T lymphocytes are likely to play a role. The rash lasts 1–2 weeks and is followed by superficial desquamation without scarring. The main differential diagnosis is pustular psoriasis, and biopsy is required for definitive diagnosis. On histopathological examination, dermal edema, eosinophilic exocytosis, and necrotic keratinocytes support the diagnosis of AGEP, whereas the presence of acanthosis, papillomatosis, and hypogranulosis suggests pustular psoriasis. In addition, other factors such as a personal or family history of psoriasis and the possibility of a particular drug causing AGEP should be carefully considered in the medical history. Drug history in the anamnesis and resolution of the rash after discontinuation of the culprit drug is an important finding and should support the diagnosis of AGEP **(Fig. 3)**.[9]

*DRESS syndrome:* DRESS/DIHS is a severe drug hypersensitivity reaction associated with systemic and constitutional symptoms such as fever, malaise, lymphadenopathy, hepatitis, myocarditis, interstitial nephritis, and pneumonitis. Anticonvulsants are the most common cause of the syndrome, with serious reactions occurring in 1% of cases. Liver involvement is the most common visceral involvement and the most serious complication, with a few cases progressing to fulminant hepatitis. The rash is maculopapular, may be accompanied by purpuric lesions, and the reaction may sometimes progress to exfoliative dermatitis. It is usually associated with facial involvement and edema. The diagnosis of DRESS syndrome is based primarily on regiSCAR criteria.

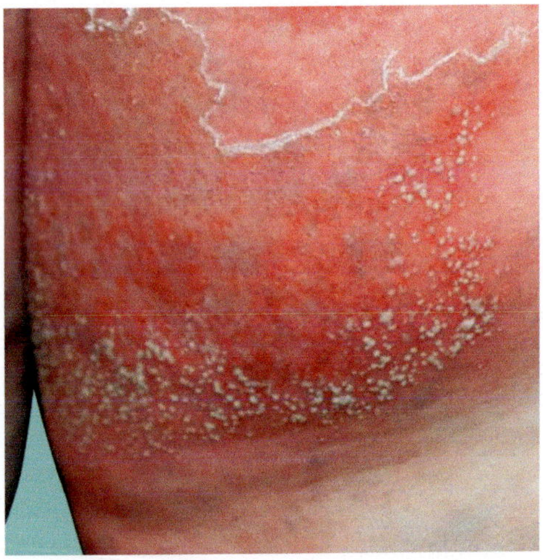

**FIG. 3:** Typical acute generalized exanthematous pustulosis with widespread nonfollicular pustules on an erythematous base.

Peripheral eosinophilia is the most common hematological finding and may be markedly elevated in some cases, helping to distinguish it from the mildly elevated eosinophilia seen in other exanthematous drug eruptions **(Table 2)**.

Atypical lymphocytes are seen in almost half of patients. Fever is subfebrile (<38.5°C) and may be seen in about three quarters of patients. It is important to discontinue the culprit drug as soon as it is suspected. Activated drug-specific T lymphocytes and their release of IL-5 are thought to play an important role in the pathophysiology through their attraction to eosinophils. Some evidence suggests a possible role for HHV-6 and HHV-7 and reactivation of EBV. Recent studies suggest a pharmacogenetic association between HLA-B*5801 and allopurinol, although the role of genetic predisposition remains to be established. DRESS/DIHS typically has a long latency period after drug administration. Oral steroids and supportive care are required, but relapses are common after dose reduction or withdrawal, often leading to prolonged systemic therapy **(Figs. 4A and B)**.[10]

**TABLE 2: General characteristics of drug eruption of differential diagnosis.**[6]

| Diagnosis | Latency period | Clinical features | Histological features | Laboratory abnormalities | Differential diagnoses | Treatment |
|---|---|---|---|---|---|---|
| SJS/TEN | 1–4 weeks | Fever, dusky purpuric macules, atypical target lesions, flaccid blisters, and mucosal involvement | Full-thickness epidermal necrosis, subepidermal blistering, and sparse dermal inflammation | Fever and poor prognosis factors: advanced age, renal impairment, metabolic acidosis, and tachycardia | Staphylococcal scalded skin syndrome, pemphigus vulgaris, and erythema multiforme | Withdrawal of culprit drug, intensive care, and IV immunoglobulins |
| DRESS/ DIHS | 2–8 weeks | Maculopapular eruption, vesicles, bullae, facial edema, exfoliative rash, and fever | Superficial lymphocytic infiltrate and dyskeratotic keratinocytes | Fever, eosinophilia, atypical lymphocytes, and HHV-6/EBV reactivation | Early SJS/TEN, viral infections, and pseudolymphoma | Withdrawal of culprit drug and systemic corticosteroids |
| AGEP | 1–7 days | Nonfollicular pustules on erythematous background, fever, and facial involvement | Subcorneal pustules, dermal edema, and mixed infiltrate with eosinophils | Fever and neutrophilia | Pustular psoriasis | Withdrawal of culprit drug and symptomatic treatment |

*Continued*

*Continued*

| Diagnosis | Latency period | Clinical features | Histological features | Laboratory abnormalities | Differential diagnoses | Treatment |
|---|---|---|---|---|---|---|
| Drug exanthem | 1–2 weeks | Symmetrical erythematous macules and papules, and mild fever | Perivascular lymphocytic infiltrate and occasional eosinophils | Low-grade fever and eosinophilia (in some cases) | Viral exanthema and lymphocyte recovery syndrome | Withdrawal of drug, topical corticosteroids, and antihista-mines |
| Urticaria | Minutes–48 hours | Transient wheals and flares lasting <24 hours | Dermal edema, neutrophils, and absence of leukocytoclasia | RAST and skin prick tests (selected cases) | Physical urticaria and serum sickness | Withdrawal of drug, antihistamines, and systemic corticosteroids |
| Fixed drug eruption | 24–48 hours (re-exposure) | Sharply demarcated erythematous plaques, blistering, and recurrence at same site | Lymphocytic infiltrate, interface dermatitis, and few apoptotic keratinocytes | Recurrence within 48 hours upon re-exposure | Generalized variant may mimic SJS/TEN | Withdrawal of drug and symptomatic treatment |

(AGEP: acute generalized exanthematous pustulosis; DIHS: drug-induced hypersensitivity syndrome; DRESS: drug reaction with eosinophilia and systemic symptoms; EBV: Epstein–Barr virus; HHV: human herpes virus; RAST: radioallergosorbent test; SJS: Stevens–Johnson syndrome; TEN: toxic epidermal necrolysis)

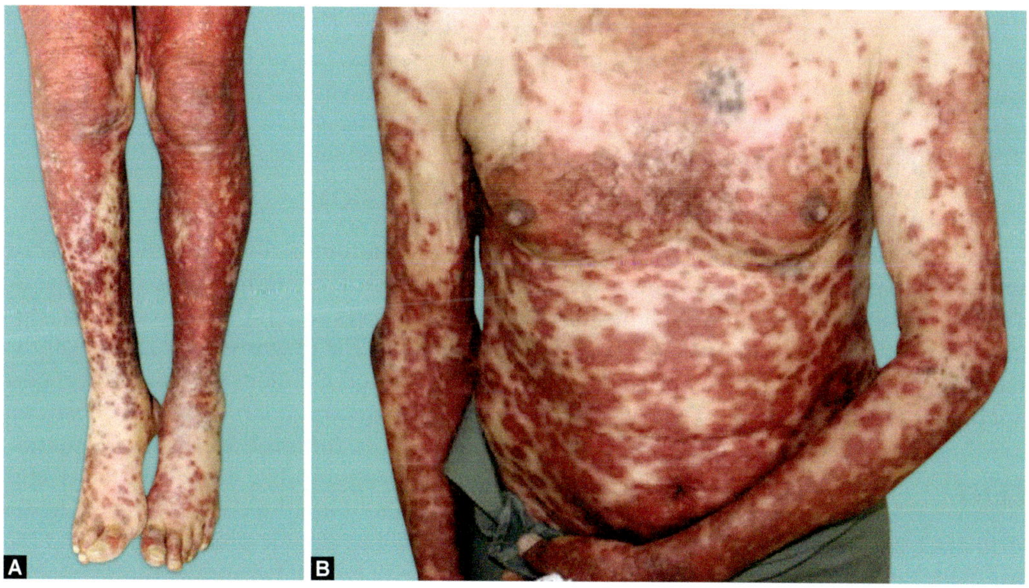


**FIGS. 4A AND B:** Erythematous widespread maculopapular and occasionally purpuric skin rash seen in DRESS syndrome.[11]

*Stevens-Johnson syndrome/Toxic epidermal necrolysis:* These two cutaneous hypersensitivity reactions are rare but serious drug reactions and are considered to be variants of the same disease with different severity. CD8(+) T-cell-mediated cytotoxic reactions against epidermal cells are the main immunopathological etiology.

Although it is emphasized that cytokines such as interferon (IFN)-α and tumor necrosis factor (TNF), granule-mediated exocytosis (perforin and granzyme B) and Fas–Fas ligand interactions and granulysin may lead to apoptosis of epidermal cells in the pathogenesis, this is still not fully understood. In addition, the role of genetics has been emphasized and, in particular, the relationship between HLA-B*1502 and carbamazepine and SJS/TEN has been investigated.

Clinically, SJS/TEN begins within 4 weeks of the first-drug exposure. Initial skin lesions are erythematous purpuric macules that tend to coalesce. As the reaction progresses, necrotic lesions coalesce, widespread erythema develops, and this erythema thickens and sloughs off, leaving eroded areas. Loss of skin integrity and full thickness epidermal necrosis may lead to sepsis

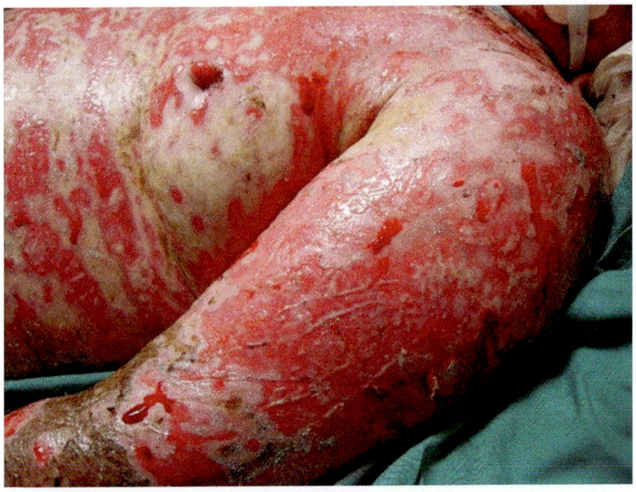

**FIG. 5:** Full-thickness necrosis and separation of the epidermis toxic epidermal necrolysis (TEN).[13]

and fluid loss. Fever, malaise, arthralgia, and headache may accompany the rash and mucosal involvement is common.

The mortality rate is approximately 5–10% in SJS and 30% in TEN. Early withdrawal of all suspected drugs is essential. The classification of SJS/TEN is based on the body surface area (BSA) affected by epidermal necrosis. SJS indicates that <10% of the BSA is affected, TEN involves >30% of the BSA, and the SJS/TEN overlap is used when the affected area is between 10 and 30%.

Intensive treatment is required to maintain fluid and electrolyte balance, nutritional support, and to prevent infection. Active interventions remain controversial; intravenous immunoglobulins are commonly used but evidence is conflicting, systemic corticosteroids are used variably (but may also predispose to infection) and cyclosporine is sometimes helpful **(Fig. 5)**.[12]

## MANAGEMENT

Management focuses on identifying and discontinuing the culprit drug, which usually results in resolution within 1–2 weeks.

### First-line Treatment

- *Discontinuation of the drug:* Prompt discontinuation of the causative agent is essential.
- *Symptomatic relief:* Topical emollients, antihistamines for pruritus (e.g., cetirizine or loratadine), and low- to moderate-potency topical corticosteroids (e.g., hydrocortisone or mometasone).

### Severe Cases

Systemic corticosteroids (e.g., prednisone 0.5–1 mg/kg/day) may be considered in extensive or refractory cases. However, this approach remains controversial in uncomplicated reactions because it is prudent to avoid systemic steroids, which may obscure the picture if there is any differential diagnosis or underlying infection.

Hospitalization for monitoring may be required if systemic symptoms develop.

### Supportive Care

Maintenance of hydration, avoidance of secondary infections, and provision of patient's education are vital components. New treatments that target specific inflammation pathways, such as biologics, may offer alternatives in severe or refractory cases, but their applications are still being investigated.[14]

## CONCLUSION

Exanthematous drug reactions can result in clinical presentations ranging from typically mild and self-limiting to severe and life-threatening. Up to now, there are no specific diagnostic tools for exanthematous drug reactions and a patient's history of reaction patterns and drugs is essential. A structured diagnostic and therapeutic approach is required to ensure patient's safety. Early diagnosis, appropriate drug withdrawal, and symptomatic management are the cornerstones of treatment. Further research into genetic predisposition and biomarkers may improve diagnostic accuracy and preventive strategies in the future.

## REFERENCES

1. Pichler WJ, Yawalkar N. Allergic reactions to drugs: involvement of T cells. Thorax. 2000;55(suppl 2):S61-5.
2. Stern RS. Exanthematous drug eruptions. N Engl J Med. 2012; 366(26):2492-501.
3. Wilke RA, Lin DW, Roden DM, Watkins PB, Flockhart D, Zineh I, et al. Identifying genetic risk factors for serious adverse drug reactions: current progress and challenges. Nat Rev Drug Discov. 2007;6(11):904-16.
4. Pichler WJ, Adkinson NF, Feldweg AM. An approach to the patient with drug allergy. UpToDate. 2016;24(3):151-72.
5. Naim M, Weyers W, Metze D. Histopathologic features of exanthematous drug eruptions of the macular and papular type. Am J Dermatopathol. 2011;33(7):695-704.
6. Al-Niaimi F. Drug eruptions in dermatology. Expert Rev Dermatol. 2011;6(3):273-86.

7. Keighley CL, Saunderson RB, Kok J, Dwyer DE. Viral exanthems. Curr Opin Infect Dis. 2015;28(2):139-50.
8. Sabroe RA. Acute urticaria. Immunol Allergy Clin. 2014;34(1):11-21.
9. Szatkowski J, Schwartz RA. Acute generalized exanthematous pustulosis (AGEP): a review and update. J Am Acad Dermatol. 2015;73(5):843-8.
10. Husain Z, Reddy BY, Schwartz RA. DRESS syndrome: Part I. Clinical perspectives. J Am Acad Dermatol. 2013;68(5):693-e1.
11. Bahloul E, Trimeche K, Sellami K, Hammami F, Hayder F, Chaabouni R, et al. Characteristics of DRESS Syndrome in the Elderly: A Comparative Study of 55 Patients. Dermatitis. 2024;35(1):55-60.
12. Marks ME, Botta RK, Abe R, Beachkofsky TM, Boothman I, Carleton BC, et al. Updates in SJS/TEN: collaboration, innovation, and community. Front Med (Lausanne). 2023;10:1213889.
13. Harris V, Jackson C, Cooper A. Review of toxic epidermal necrolysis. Int J Mol Sci. 2016;17(12):2135.
14. Bottlaender L, Amini-Adle M, Maucort-Boulch D, Robinson P, Thomas L, Dalle S. Cutaneous adverse events: a predictor of tumour response under anti-PD-1 therapy for metastatic melanoma, a cohort analysis of 189 patients. J Eur Acad Dermatol Venereol. 2020;34(9):2096-105.

# Anaphylaxis

***Jie Shen (Jason) Fok***

## INTRODUCTION

Anaphylaxis is a serious and life-threatening systemic hypersensitivity reaction.[1] It has a rapid onset, usually ranging from a few minutes to hour following exposure to an allergen, which triggers a cascade of mediator release. This results in symptoms, typically multisystemic, involving the mucocutaneous, respiratory, cardiovascular, gastrointestinal, and central nervous system **(Fig. 1)**. Though mucocutaneous features are common, such as flushing, urticaria and angioedema, they may not occur in all cases. On the most severe spectrum, loss of consciousness and confusion may occur. Anaphylaxis is a medical emergency and a clinical diagnosis. Untreated and significant morbidity or mortality may ensue. It is therefore of paramount importance to recognize features of acute allergic reaction and diagnose anaphylaxis accordingly in a prompt manner to commence the appropriate management plans.

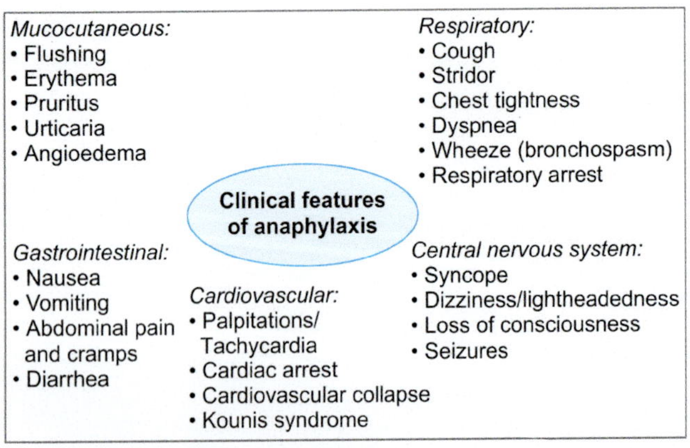


**FIG. 1:** Clinical features of anaphylaxis.

There are published criteria to help clinicians to diagnose anaphylaxis.[1-3] In essence, anaphylaxis is highly likely when there is an acute onset of an illness with simultaneous skin involvement after exposure to an allergen, coupled with either respiratory compromise, reduced blood pressure or severe gastrointestinal symptoms. In other criteria where cutaneous features are absent, anaphylaxis is considered highly likely if there is an acute onset of hypotension, bronchospasm or laryngeal involvement after being exposed to a known or highly likely allergen.

The estimated lifetime prevalence of anaphylaxis ranges from 0.3 to 5.1%.[1,4,5] An increasing trend has been observed in the Asia Pacific region.[6-8] It is estimated that 0.1% of emergency presentation of anaphylaxis cases have a fatal outcome.[9]

Food is a common trigger for anaphylaxis, especially in the pediatric population, where peanut and cashew are implicated.[10] Shellfish and fish allergy follow tree nut and peanuts as the next most common offending agents in food-induced anaphylactic reaction.[11] Previous studies have identified several risk factors in anaphylaxis fatality, including lack of access to epinephrine, presence of asthma, peanut and tree nut allergy, as well as standing position when anaphylaxis occurs.[12] The empty ventricle syndrome is caused by hypoperfusion in an upright position, potentially resulting in death within seconds.[13] In the assessment of anaphylaxis, a cause may not be apparent in preliminary history taking. Further evaluation of food packaging label is therefore crucial to unravel a hidden allergen, such as buckwheat allergy.[14] Food allergy acquired through cutaneous sensitization is not uncommon. A classic example is goat's milk or goat's cheese anaphylaxis with a background history of cutaneous application of goat's milk-based skin care products.[15]

Rarely, delayed onset of anaphylaxis may occur. This has been observed in red meat allergy primed by tick bite seen in the α-Gal syndrome, involving the carbohydrate galactose-α-1,3-galactose.[16]

Once history of food allergy is established, investigations with skin prick testing and specific immunoglobulin E (IgE) testing usually follow. Oral food challenges are performed when there is a strong suspicion for food anaphylaxis and preliminary investigations are negative. Oral food challenges remain the gold standard to confirm or exclude a food allergy in doubtful circumstances. The potential risk of inducing a systemic allergic reaction must always be explained to patients. An informed consent is needed.

Anaphylaxis caused by drugs is a common referral to allergy/immunology clinic. Drug-induced anaphylaxis accounts for 35% of cases in the adult population.[5] Commonly implicated drugs include penicillins, cephalosporins, nonsteroidal anti-inflammatory drugs (NSAIDs), and anesthetic drugs. It is common to observe mucocutaneous features in drug allergy, such as urticaria, morbilliform rashes and angioedema. Cutaneous features may be easily missed in perioperative anaphylaxis as skin changes may not be apparent when a patient is covered in surgical drape, further masking the diagnosis, especially a drop in blood pressure is the only observed or documented feature, which may also be a pharmacological effect of a patient's existing medications, such as β-blockers. Recognized risk factors for severity or fatality in drug anaphylaxis include cardiovascular comorbidity, older age, β-lactam antibiotics, and general anesthetic agents.[4]

Like assessment of all anaphylaxis cases, careful history taking, with special focus to prior exposure, timing of exposure, and presenting characteristics are all important aspects to be explored. Drug skin test that consists of skin prick and intradermal testing with standard, recommended diluents are important steps in investigating penicillin and cephalosporin anaphylaxis. Ultimately, oral challenge is required to prove tolerance to a drug, such as amoxicillin oral challenge. In some circumstances, intravenous challenge may be required, depending on assessment and at the clinician's discretion. With penicillin or cephalosporin allergy assessment, consideration should be given to explore potential cross-reactivity between specific group of penicillin and cephalosporin based on their side chain structures, such as the R1-side chain. A blanket rule of labeling a patient with "cephalosporin allergy" is indeed misleading.[17]

Once a drug allergy is confirmed and established, a Medic Alert device is highly recommended. In the setting of perioperative anaphylaxis, a review of anesthetic record, including timing of changes of vital signs following administration of certain medications and lists of medications received, must be undertaken meticulously. Chlorhexidine should always be included in the testing panel as it is a hidden allergen commonly missed. In the uncommon scenario in which obvious culprit is not readily identified or recognized following an initial comprehensive testing, excipient allergy must always be considered. This is especially true when there have been repeated anaphylactic reactions in the context of at least two structurally different drugs or products.[18] For drug allergy investigations, specific IgE testing is available for certain drugs, such as penicillins, cefaclor, chlorhexidine, and suxamethonium. Availability of or accessibility to assay may vary in different geographical regions. It should be noted that specific IgE to drugs decline over time, therefore optimal sampling time is essential for optimal interpretation.[19]

Worldwide, insect venom is an important cause of anaphylaxis. This is common in both the northern and southern hemispheres. Important species accounting for this phenomenon are those from the order Hymenoptera, including honeybee (*Apis mellifera*), European wasp/yellow jacket (*Vespula sp.*) and paper wasp (*Polistes sp.*). The Jack jumper ant (*Myrmecia pilosula*) is a venomous species native to Australia, found mostly in Tasmania, Victoria, and South Australia. There are four primary categories of clinical reactions to insect stings, i.e., normal response, large local swellings, minor immediate generalized reactions (IGR), and major IGR/anaphylaxis.[20] A burning or painful swelling or wheal seen in normal response usually self-resolves in hours, though it may take days. A large local swelling occurs when the sting site progresses to involve swelling of the adjacent structure. The most common presentation of a minor IGR is a cutaneous reaction with generalized urticaria and facial angioedema in the absence of cardiovascular or respiratory features. Specific alarming features such as hypotension, a sense of impending doom, and collapse and abdominal cramps may be seen in anaphylaxis (i.e., major IGR). Estimated deaths from sting anaphylaxis are in the range of 1–10/10 million/annum based on data from Australia and the States.[21] Venom immunotherapy or desensitization has a strong role in anaphylaxis to reduce likelihood of severe reaction upon future stings. There are established protocols for venom immunotherapy. Prior to commencing venom immunotherapy, identification of culprit organism responsible for the episode must be undertaken. Patient's recollection of the species involved may not be reliable in some cases. To further evaluate, specific IgE testing to honey, yellow jacket, paper wasp, and Jack jumper ant may be utilized. If required, venom skin test may be performed to provide more clarity. Insect venom anaphylaxis may be the first presentation of systemic mastocytosis, therefore the role of establishing baseline serum tryptase cannot be emphasized enough in the complete evaluation of anaphylaxis. Important risk factors for fatality include mastocytosis, cardiovascular comorbidities, older age, and use of antihypertensive medication.[22]

The role of cofactors in anaphylaxis must not be neglected. Eliciting the presence of potential risk-multiplier in history taking is useful as these factors may cause severe anaphylaxis. Examples of cofactors are alcohol consumption, nonsteroidal anti-inflammatory drugs (NSAIDs), intercurrent infection, physical exercise, and menstruation.[23] Epidemiological studies had previously demonstrated that cofactors contributed to 30% of anaphylactic reactions in adults.[24] Cofactors may augment the severity of or lower the threshold of anaphylactic reaction through specific mechanisms.

Tryptase is a serine protease released from mast cells which are activated and degranulated during an anaphylactic reaction. A rise in serum tryptase level following an allergic reaction might provide clinicians a clue regarding activation of mast cells. This is a useful test when interpreted in the right context or when the samples are collected at the right time for comparison of values. Persistently elevated baseline tryptase levels following recovery from anaphylaxis should prompt clinicians to further investigate for mastocytosis, a systemic clonal disease that has both immunological and nonimmunological implications on the affected patients.

There are pitfalls in diagnosing anaphylaxis. It is important to consider an array of conditions that give rise to symptoms that resemble anaphylaxis. In clinical practice, laryngeal involvement or respiratory distress may be seen in vocal cord dysfunction (inducible laryngeal obstruction) and severe bronchial asthma. Acute or chronic urticaria, with or without angioedema, may be misdiagnosed as anaphylaxis. Carcinoid syndrome and pheochromocytoma may present with gastrointestinal features. Vasovagal syncope and panic attack should be considered as a differential diagnosis too.

The key principle of future anaphylaxis prevention involves avoidance of the offending allergen. Prescribing an epinephrine autoinjector is essential as it is lifesaving when a misadventure happens. This is especially true when dining out as cross-contamination of food allergen could potentially occur, or in the setting of insect sting anaphylaxis in a remote area. Providing an action plan and travel plan for patients are recommended. Details on the anaphylaxis action plan may vary in different countries; however, the contents generally include recognition of features of allergic reaction, and the dos and don'ts during anaphylaxis.[25] The current standard of care in managing anaphylaxis is intramuscular epinephrine. Use of intranasal epinephrine is on the horizon.[26]

## CONCLUSION

Anaphylaxis is a potentially fatal condition. Recognition is important. Investigations must be carried out to identify the offending agent causing the allergic reaction. Referral to a centre specialising in allergy assessment is strongly recommended.

## REFERENCES

1. Cardova V, Ansotegui IJ, Ebisawa M, El-Gamal Y, Rivas MF, Fineman S, et al. World Allergy Organisation anaphylaxis Guidance 2000. World Allergy Organ J. 2020;13(10):100472.
2. Muraro A, Worm M, Alviani C, Cardona V, DunnGalvin A, Garvey LH, et al. EAACI guidelines: Anaphylaxis (2021 update). Allergy. 2022; 77(2):357-77.
3. ASCIA. (2024). ASCIA Guidelines - Acute Management of Anaphylaxis. [online] Available from https://www.allergy.org.au/hp/papers/acute-management-of-anaphylaxis-guidelines [Last accessed Jan., 2025].
4. Turner PJ, Jerschow E, Umasunthar T, Lin R, Campbell DE, Boyle RJ. Fatal anaphylaxis: mortality rate and risk factors. J Allergy Clin Immunol Pract. 2017;5(5):1169-78.
5. Wood RA, Camargo CA, Lieberman P, Sampson HA, Schwartz LB, Zitt M, et al. Anaphylaxis in America: the prevalence and characteristics of anaphylaxis in the United States. J Allergy Clin Immunol. 2014;133:461-7.
6. Liew WK, Williamson E, Tang ML. Anaphylaxis fatalities and admissions in Australia. J Allergy Clin Immunol. 2009;123:434-42.
7. Yang MS, Kim JY, Kim BK, Park HW, Cho SH, Min KU, et al. True rise in anaphylaxis incidence: Epidemiologic study based on a national health insurance database. Medicine (Baltimore). 2017; 96(5):e5750.
8. Li L, Huang N, Li W, Yang Y, Ma D, Chen H, et al. Incidence and trends of anaphylaxis among inpatients from 2003 to 2023 in Wuhan, China: A multicenter retrospective study. W Allergy Orgen J. 2024;17(11):100980.
9. Ma L, Danoff TM, Borish L. Case fatality and population mortality associated with anaphylaxis in the United States. J Allergy Clin Immunol. 2014;133:1075-83.
10. de Silva IL, Meh SS, Tey D, Tang ML. Paediatric anaphylaxis: a 5 year retrospective review. Allergy. 2008;63:1071-6.
11. Hompes S, Kohli A, Nemat K, Scherer K, Lange L, Rueff F, et al. Provoking allergens and treatment of anaphylaxis in children and adolescents—data from the anaphylaxis registry of German-speaking countries. Pediatr Allergy Immunol. 2011;22:568-74.
12. Fishbein A. Anaphylaxis to food. Immunol Allergy Clin North Am. 2015;35(2):231-45.

13. Pumphrey RS. Lessons for management of anaphylaxis from a study of fatal reactions. Clin Exp Allergy. 2000;30(8):1144-50.
14. Fok JS, Kette F, Smith WB, Smith A, Ahmadie A, Heddle RJ, et al. Buckwheat allergy in Australia. Intern Med J. 2019;49(12):1552-3.
15. Volkamp AL, Zubrinich CN, Abramovitch JB, Rolland JM, O'Hehir RE. Goat's cheese anaphylaxis after cutaneous sensitisation by moisturiser that contained goat's milk. J Allergy Clin Immunol Pract. 2014;2(5):629-30.
16. Platts-Mills TAE, Li RC, Keshavarz B, Smith AR, Wilson JM. Diagnosis and management of patients with the alpha-gal syndrome. J Allergy Clin Immunol Pract. 2020;8(1):15-23e1.
17. Yuson C, Katelaris CH, Smith W. Cephalosporin allergy label is misleading. Aust Prescr. 2018;41(2):37-41.
18. Khan DA, Banerji A, Blumenthal KG, Phillips EJ, Solensky R, White AA, et al. Deug allergy: a 2022 practice parameter update. J Allergy Clin Immunol. 2022;150(6):1333-93.
19. Opstrup MS, Poulsen LK, Malling HJ, Jensen BM, Garvey LH. Dynamics of plasma levels of specific IgE in chlorhexidine allergic patients with and without accidental re-exposure. Clin Exp Allergy. 2016;46(8):1090-8.
20. Heddle RJ, Le TA. Beware of allergic reactions to stings and bites. Medicine Today. 2022;23(7 Suppl):24-33.
21. Heddle RJ, David BK. Allergy to insect stings and bites. World Allergy Organ J. 2008.
22. Stoevesandt J, Sturm GJ, Bonadonna P, Oude Elberink JNG, Traumann A. Risk factors and indicators of severe systematic insect sting reactions. Allergy. 2019;75(3):535-45.
23. Smith PK, Hourihane JO'B, Lieberman P. Risk multipliers for severe food anaphylaxis. World Allergy Organ J. 2015;8(1):30.
24. Wölbing F, Fischer J, Koberle M, Kaesler S, Biedermann T. About the role and underlying mechanisms of cofactors in anaphylaxis. Allergy. 2013;68:1085-92.
25. ASCIA. (2025). ASCIA Action Plans and First Aid Plans for Anaphylaxis. [online] Available from https://www.allergy.org.au/hp/anaphylaxis/ascia-action-plan-for-anaphylaxis [Last accessed Jan., 2025].
26. Tal Y, Ribak Y, Rubin L, Talmon A, Shamriz O, Hershko AY, et al. Fast acting, dry powder, needle-free, intranasal epinephrine spray: a promising future treatment for anaphylaxis. J Allergy Clin Immunol Pract. 2023;11(10):3047-54.

CHAPTER 4.4

# Management of Stevens–Johnson Syndrome and Toxic Epidermal Necrolysis

*Vesna Trajkova, Natasa Teovska Mitrevska, Hristina Breshkovska*

## INTRODUCTION

Stevens-Johnson syndrome (SJS) and toxic epidermal necrolysis (TEN) are severe, mucocutaneous, adverse reactions in most cases induced by medications.[1] Clinical features include fever, prodromal symptoms, mucositis, and extensive epidermal detachment. SJS and TEN are considered a disease continuum and are collectively known as epidermal necrolysis.[1]

The classification of the disease is based on the total body surface area (BSA) involved with skin detachment:[1,2]

- SJS is defined as skin detachment affecting <10 percent of the BSA
- TEN is defined as skin detachment affecting >30 percent of the BSA
- SJS/TEN overlap is defined as skin detachment involving 10 to 30 percent of the BSA.

## CLASSIFICATION

The management of Stevens–Johnson syndrome (SJS)/ toxic epidermal necrolysis (TEN can be broadly classified into two phases:[1,2]

1. *Acute phase*: Lasting 5–7 days with worsening cutaneous detachment and mucositis, this phase is critical with risks including fluid imbalance, sepsis, organ failure, and potentially death (10–50% mortality). Focus is on supportive care and preventing complications.
2. *Chronic phase*:Occurring during recovery, this phase involves managing physical and psychological sequelae to maintain life quality **(Flowchart 1)**.

## INITIAL IN-HOSPITAL EVALUATION

Patients suspected of having SJS/TEN require *immediate in-hospital evaluation.* An initial assessment includes evaluation of airway, breathing, and circulation, urinary output, and clinical evidence of septicemia. *Prompt withdrawal of the offending drug* may improve the prognosis. *Assessment of the extent of skin detachment* is used for estimation of the percentage of the total body surface area (BSA), and *assessment of severity and prognosis* is determined by using the score of toxic epidermal necrolysis (SCORTEN) within the first 24 hours. Patients with ≥10% BSA detachment or rapidly worsening conditions should *be transferred to specialized* dermatology units, burn centers, or intensive care units and monitoring of vital signs.[2,3]

## ACUTE MANAGEMENT

The management of SJS/TEN is multidisciplinary. *Supportive care* is the cornerstone of management, additionally variety of *systemic agents* have been utilized for the treatment **(Figs. 1 and 2)**.[2,3]

### Supportive Care

Supportive care includes wound care, fluid and electrolyte management, nutritional support, temperature management, pain control, infection prevention and management, ocular care, and organ support, if needed. Mucosal surfaces of the eyes, mouth, and urogenital tract are frequently affected, and multidisciplinary care is recommended.[3]

- *Wound care*: It varies among centers and can be broadly divided into surgical and conservative approaches.
  - *Surgical approach* (the devitalized epidermis is removed via debridement, manual scrubbing, or applied whirlpools biologic membranes following debridement).[3]
  - *Conservative approach* ("antishear" approach): The detached/detachable epidermis is left in situ with additional care including gentle cleansing

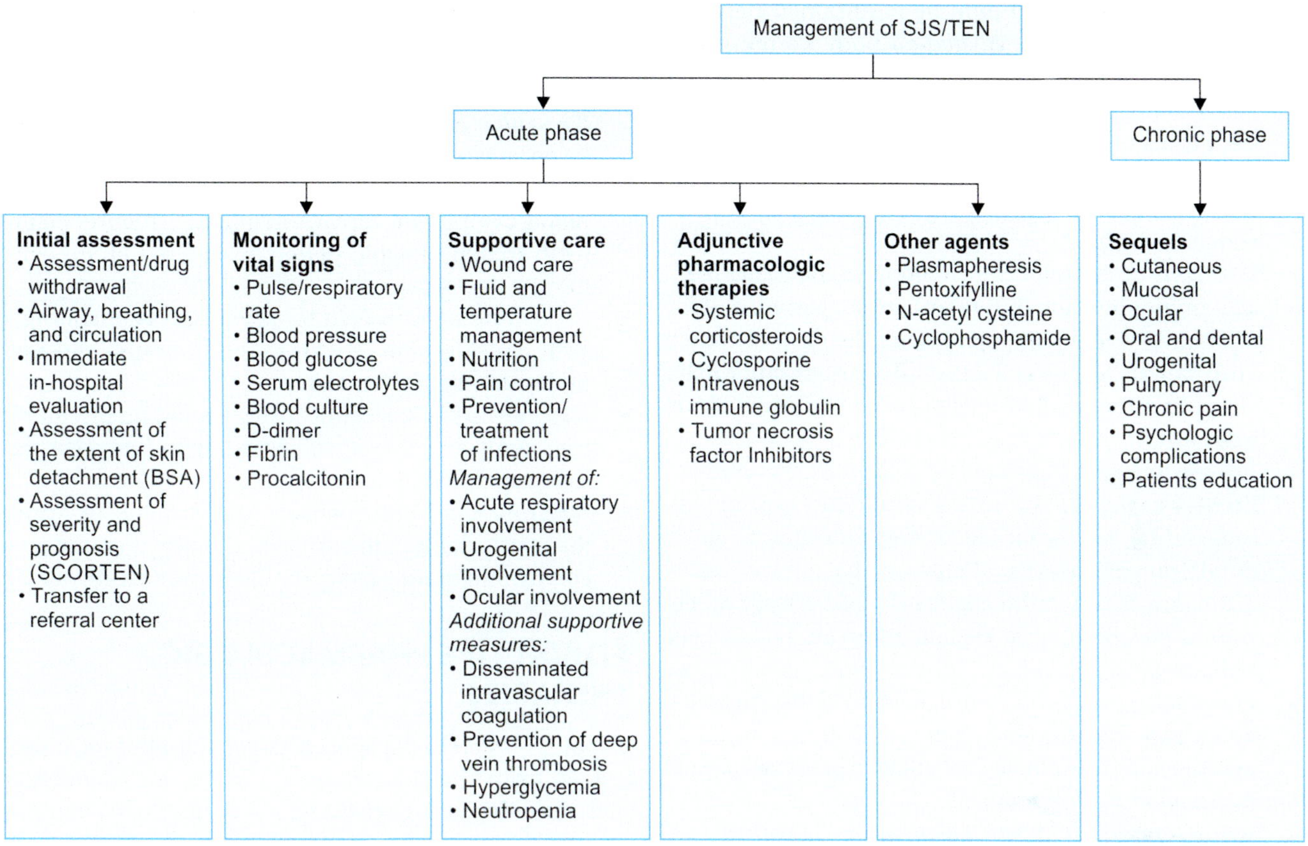


**FLOWCHART 1:** Management of Stevens–Johnson syndrome (SJS) and toxic epidermal necrolysis (TEN).
(BSA: body surface area; SCORTEN: score of toxic epidermal necrolysis)

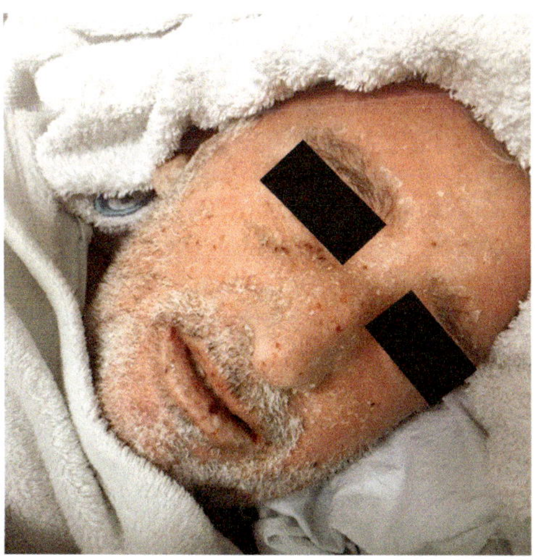

**FIG. 1:** Patient with toxic epidermal necrolysis (TEN) (erythema, blisters, and erosions on the face including lips and eyes).[8]

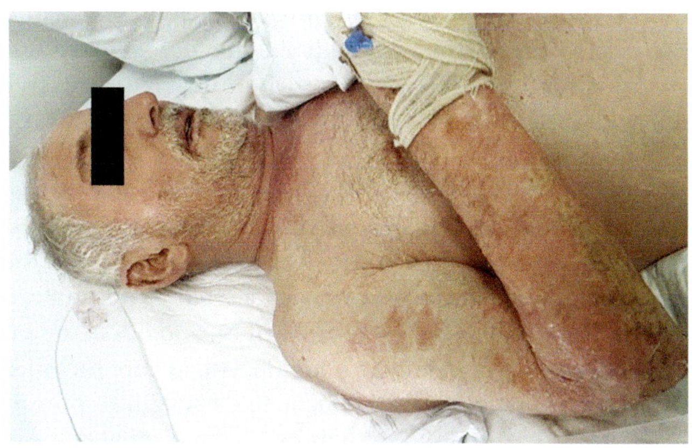

**FIG. 2:** Patient with toxic epidermal necrolysis (TEN) (erythematous rush, blisters, and erosions on the body and face).[8]

with sterile water or diluted chlorhexidine, large bullae may be ruptured, petrolatum-impregnated gauze is used daily or modern dressings (e.g., nonadherent nanocrystalline silver gauze materials and biosynthetic dressings) left up to 7 days, and air-fluidized beds are also useful.[3]

- *Fluid and temperature management*: In the first 24 hours, essential fluid requirements are estimated to be 2 mL/kg/BSA percent affected and should be titrated according to the patient's response and urine output, aiming for urine volume of 0.5–1 mL/kg/h.

Room temperature should be maintained between 82.4° to 89.6°F (28–32°C). Heated-air body warmers may also be used.

- *Nutrition*: Caloric requirement is 20–25 kcal/kg per day during the early catabolic phase and 25–30 kcal/kg per day during the anabolic phase of the disease. If required, nasogastric feeding should be initiated as soon as possible.[3]
- *Pain control*: For mild pain, nonopioid analgesics (e.g., acetaminophen and ibuprofen) are suggested, and for moderate/severe pain, opioids are the drug of choice and can be delivered enterally, subcutaneously, via patient-controlled analgesia, or via intravenous infusions.[3,4]
- *Prevention and treatment of infections*: Prevention involves: Sterile handling and skin antisepsis (octenidine, polyhexanide, or chlorhexidine or silver nitrate preparations), and repeated bacterial cultures of the skin, blood, catheters, gastric, and urinary tubes, should be obtained at regular intervals (e.g., every 48 hours).[3,4]
- *Treatment*: Antibiotic choice should be directed by culture results whenever possible. Commonly isolated pathogens include *Staphylococcus aureus* and *Pseudomonas aeruginosa.*
- *Management of acute respiratory involvement*: Evaluation includes chest radiographs and arterial blood gases. Bronchoscopy may be warranted for bronchial involvement, evaluate the presence of pulmonary infection, prevent atelectasis, and airway obstruction through the mechanical removal of sloughed bronchial epithelium. Noninvasive ventilation is contraindicated, oral intubation may be challenging.[3,4]
- *Management of urogenital involvement*: Nonadhesive dressings should be applied to urogenital erosions; moderate-potency topical corticosteroids can be applied daily, estrogen and barrier creams (petrolatum and zinc oxide) for re-epithelization, and lidocaine for mucosal pain. In female patients, vulvar care includes water washes or sitz baths, intravaginal potent corticosteroid ointment, and silicone vaginal dilators and urinary catheter. In uncircumcised male patients, daily retraction of the foreskin can prevent preputial adhesions.
- *Management of ocular involvement*: Saline rinses, lubricants (artificial tears) or ointments, topical corticosteroids, and/or broad spectrum antibiotics—preparations (e.g., moxifloxacin hydrochloride 0.5%) 4–6 times per day, adhesion separation daily with forceps, squint hooks, or scissors. Amniotic membrane transplantation (AMT) can be performed.

*Additional supportive measures*:

- *Stress ulcer prophylaxis* with proton pump inhibitor may be necessary in those who are unable to feed enterally.
- *Disseminated intravascular coagulation*: In these cases, blood component replacement (e.g., cryoprecipitate, fresh frozen plasma, platelets, and red blood cells) may be necessary.
- *Prevention of deep vein thrombosis:* It is encouraged with compression stockings, calf pumps, and low-molecular-weight heparin.
- *Hyperglycemia*: Glycemic levels should be monitored frequently and managed according to intensive care unit principles.
- *Neutropenia*: Neutropenia is known to occur during the acute phase of the disease. The use of granulocyte colony-stimulating factor (G-CSF) has been advocated.

## ADJUNCTIVE PHARMACOLOGIC THERAPIES

The progression in the acute phase is self-limiting, lasting 8 days from the onset, and there are no established pharmacologic treatments. A variety of systemic agents, such as systemic corticosteroids, intravenous immunoglobulin (IVIG), cyclosporine, plasmapheresis, and anti-tumor necrosis factor (TNF) agents, have been utilized for the treatment.[5]

- *Systemic corticosteroids*: Varying regimens have been including—prednisolone 60–250 mg/day for 2–12 days, intravenous dexamethasone 1.5 mg/kg/day for 3 days, and intravenous methylprednisolone 250–1,000 mg/day for 3 days. In pregnancy, it should be avoided in the first trimester, and early and short IV course is recommended. The efficacy of systemic corticosteroids has not been proven.
- *Cyclosporine:* Recommended usage of cyclosporine is 3–5 mg/kg/day as adjunctive therapy within 24–48 hours of symptom onset. In pregnancy, it is considered as second-line treatment.[5]
- *Intravenous immunoglobulin*: It is given at a dose of 2–4 g/kg over 2–5 days, which is initially proposed as a treatment. In pregnancy, it is safe and effective, in children and in HIV patients, it is recommended in low doses 0.2–0.5 mg/kg. Systemic corticosteroids and IVIG have been administered in combination to patients, but the data remain limited.[5,6]
- *Tumor necrosis factor inhibitors*: Limited data exist that a single infusion of 5 mg/kg of TNF-alpha

inhibitor infliximab halted the progression of skin detachment and induced a rapid re-epithelization of the denuded skin. If cyclosporine is contraindicated, a single dose of TNF inhibitor etanercept given in a single 50 mg subcutaneous injection twice weekly is an alternative option. There are initial studies evaluating combinations of etanercept and systemic corticosteroids.

- *Other agents*: These include plasmapheresis, pentoxifylline, N-acetyl cysteine, cyclophosphamide.
- *Harmful agents*: Thalidomide, a potent inhibitor of TNF-alpha, should *not* be used for the treatment of SJS/TEN because of excess mortality.
- *Prognosis*: The overall mortality rate is approximately 25%, ranging from approximately 10% for SJS to >30% for TEN. Sepsis, acute respiratory distress syndrome, and multiple organ failure are the most common causes of in-hospital death.

## LONG-TERM SEQUELAE

These include cutaneous, mucosal, ocular, visceral, and psychologic complications, which are increasingly reported as survival improves.[5,7]

- *Cutaneous sequelae* include postinflammatory hypo- or hyperpigmentation, scarring, eruptive nevi, telogen effluvium, and chronic pruritus and nail changes.
- *Ocular sequelae* include dry eye, photophobia, trichiasis, corneal neovascularization or scaring, lid margin changes, keratitis, and symblepharon. Management involves the use of artificial tears and scleral lenses. Surgical interventions include limbal stem cell transplantation, amniotic membrane transplantation (AMT), cultivated oral mucosal epithelial transplantation, and corneal transplant.[7]
- *Oral and dental sequelae* include mouth discomfort, xerostomia, gingival inflammation and synechiae, caries, and periodontal disease. Severe dental growth abnormalities (e.g., dental agenesia, root dysmorphia, root-building abortion, microdontia) may occur.[7]
- *Urogenital sequelae*: These include adhesion formation, scarring, urethral stenosis, and strictures. In females, introital stenosis, vaginal dryness, dyspareunia, urinary retention, hematocolpos, and vaginal adenosis can be seen, and in males phimosis is observed.[7]
- *Pulmonary sequelae:* These include chronic bronchitis/bronchiolitis with obstructive changes (including bronchiolitis obliterans and organizing), bronchiectasis, and obstructive disorders.[7]
- *Chronic pain:* It has been reported in approximately one-third of patients at mucocutaneous sites of involvement.[6,7]
- *Psychiatric sequelae*: Long-term psychosocial complications and psychiatric disorders (e.g., anxiety and depression), post-traumatic stress disorder, and decreased health-related quality of life have been reported.[5,7]

## FUTURE DRUG AVOIDANCE

- *Patient education*: Educating patients on avoiding the culprit drug is vital. Wearing medical alert jewelry and updating medical records are recommended. Further alergotesting on suspected drug is not recommended.[7]
- *Future use of related medications*: The risk of recurrent SJS/TEN with structurally distinct agents (within the same therapeutic class of drugs) is unknown but probably very low.[8]

## CONCLUSION

Stevens-Johnson syndrome (SJS) and toxic epidermal necrolysis (TEN) require prompt recognition and multidisciplinary management to improve patient outcomes.[1] Supportive care, particularly in burn units, is crucial to maintaining fluid balance, preventing infections, and ensuring proper wound care.[2] Early withdrawal of the offending drug is essential to halt disease progression.[3] Systemic therapies, such as IV immunoglobulin (IVIG) or cyclosporine, may help modulate the immune response, though their efficacy remains debated.[5] Close monitoring for complications, including sepsis and multi-organ failure, is necessary for timely interventions.[6] A standardized approach to TEN management can enhance survival rates and reduce long-term morbidity.[7,8]

## REFERENCES

1. Ingen-Housz-Oro S, Duong TA, Bensaid B, Bellon N, de Prost N, Lu D, et al. Epidermal necrolysis French national diagnosis and care protocol (PNDS; protocole national de diagnostic et de soins). Orphanet J Rare Dis. 2018;13:56.
2. McPherson T, Exton LS, Biswas S, Creamer D, Dziewulski P, Newell L, et al. British Association of Dermatologists' guidelines for the management of Stevens-Johnson syndrome/toxic epidermal necrolysis in children and young people, 2018. Br J Dermatol. 2019;181:37.
3. Brüggen MC, Le ST, Walsh S, Toussi A, de Prost N, Ranki A, et al. Supportive care in the acute phase of Stevens-Johnson syndrome and toxic epidermal necrolysis: an international, multidisciplinary Delphi-based consensus. Br J Dermatol. 2021;185:616.

4. Lee HY. Wound management strategies in Stevens-Johnson syndrome/toxic epidermal necrolysis: An unmet need. J Am Acad Dermatol. 2018;79:e87.
5. Torres-Navarro I, Briz-Redón Á, Botella-Estrada R. Systemic therapies for Stevens-Johnson Syndrome and Toxic Epidermal Necrolysis: a SCORTEN-based systematic review and meta-analysis. J Eur Acad Dermatol Venereol. 2021;35:159.
6. Finkelstein Y, Macdonald EM, Li P, Hutson JR, Juurlink DN. Recurrence and mortality following severe cutaneous adverse reactions. JAMA. 2014;311(21):2231.
7. Gupta LK, Martin AM, Agarwal N, DSouza P, Das S, Kumar R, et al. Guidelines for the management of Stevens–Johnson syndrome/ toxic epidermal necrolysis: An Indian perspective. Indian J Dermatol Venereol Leprol. 2016;82:603-25.
8. Breshkovska H, Duma S, Nikolovska S, Dohceva-Karajovanov I, Telenta-Mitrova J, Duma H, et al. Toxic Epidermal Necrolysis: Case Report and Review. SEE J Immunol. 2024;7:56-60.

4.5

CHAPTER

# Management of Drug Reaction with Eosinophilia and Systemic Symptoms

***Hüseyin Bahadır Şenol, Emine Aylin Yılmaz, Öner Özdemir***

## INTRODUCTION

"*Drug rash with eosinophilia and systemic symptoms (DRESS)*" is a rare but serious adverse drug reaction characterized by fever and skin involvement as initial manifestations. The condition can progress systemically, potentially affecting any organ system.[1] Systemic involvement frequently includes renal and hepatic manifestations; however, lungs, heart, and nervous system may also be affected.[2] Laboratory parameters include leukocytosis, atypical lymphocytes, eosinophilia, as well as impairment of renal or hepatic functions.[1] The incidence of DRESS syndrome is estimated at 0.01%.[3] Genetic predisposition, metabolic pathway disturbances of drugs, and the reactivation of viruses like human herpes virus-6 (HHV-6) are known factors involved in its pathogenesis.[4]

## DIAGNOSIS

The RegiSCAR scoring system is used for diagnosis.[5] Diagnosis of DRESS is established with three mandatory criteria (the first three) and the fulfillment of at least six out of seven criteria in total **(Box 1)**.

## MANAGEMENT

The clinical variability inherent in such a severe and multisystemic disease makes the diversity of treatment protocols inevitable. In this chapter, the management of DRESS has been presented based on the latest evidence from the current literature. Three well-established algorithms guide the management approach to DRESS syndrome.

**BOX 1 Diagnostic criteria for drug reaction with eosinophilia and systemic syndrome (DRESS) by the RegiSCAR Group.[5]**

1. Acute rash
2. Reaction suspected drug-related
3. Hospitalization
4. Fever (>38°C)
5. Laboratory abnormalities (at least one present)
    i. Lymphocyte above or below normal
    ii. Low platelet
    iii. Eosinophilia
6. Involvement of ≥1 internal organ
7. Enlarged lymph nodes ≥2 sites

The first of these was developed in Japan by Mizukawa et al. They suggested a severity scoring system for DRESS patients to assess complication risks and improve management strategies. In this scoring system, early detection, particularly when the score is 4 or higher, is emphasized as essential in preventing severe complications, especially those related to cytomegalovirus (CMV) reactivation. For high-risk patients, prompt initiation of anti-CMV therapy was strongly recommended. Additionally, they highlighted the importance of carefully managing corticosteroid treatments, advocating for gradual dose reductions to prevent relapses. The authors underscored that CMV reactivation is a major contributor to complications, including late-onset issues such as myocarditis and gastrointestinal bleeding, which could be mitigated with appropriate interventions. Their recommendations suggest that utilizing the scoring system can help to identify high-risk patients early and guide timely therapeutic measures.[2]

An another group from France, led by Descamps et al., provides a comprehensive overview of DRESS syndrome, emphasizing its association with viral reactivation and immune response dysregulation. They discuss the importance of early diagnosis through standardized criteria and highlight the need for a comprehensive algorithm to management. This involves immediate cessation of the responsible drug, monitoring of organ involvement and specific therapeutic interventions based on the severity of the disease, similar to other algorithms. For severe cases, systemic glucocorticoids and, when necessary, intravenous immunoglobulins (IVIGs) are recommended. They also explores the potential role of antiviral agents in managing herpesvirus reactivation, though their routine use remains limited by toxicity concerns.[6]

Cabañas et al. established a recognized protocol in Spain, structuring similar findings into a systematic algorithm for the management.[7] The primary step of this protocol is the cessation of the responsible drug, followed by symptomatic management. The severity of the disease is assessed based on the degree of organ involvement, with special attention to vital systems such as the liver, kidneys, and lungs **(Box 2)**. Therefore, the treatment plan is customized to the severity score. For nonsevere cases, close monitoring is sufficient, with clinical and laboratory evaluations conducted every 48 hours. In severe cases, systemic corticosteroids are preferred as the main treatment, while IVIG is recommended for cases that do not respond to standard treatment **(Box 3)**. The protocol also acknowledges the role of antiviral treatments in managing cases with viral reactivation, particularly herpesviruses like HHV-6. Treatment plans are designed to be flexible, adapting to the patient's evolving clinical status, with regular follow-up to monitor for potential relapses or long-term complications. This structured approach ensures comprehensive care, addressing both acute management and future health risks.

The most widely accepted treatment for DRESS is the early initiation of systemic corticosteroids.[8] To prevent relapses, the dose should be gradually tapered over 3–6 months.[9] In particularly severe cases, a dose of 30 mg/kg can be administered for 3 days.[10]

Although the mechanism of IVIG in treatment is not clearly known, it has been reported to be effective in cases.[11] Yet, IVIG is associated with serious potential side effects, and in cases where no clinical response is achieved, oral steroid regimens are preferred. Therefore, its use as monotherapy is not recommended.[12]

Case reports highlight cyclosporine as another second-line treatment option.[13,14] Although the number of patients receiving this treatment is limited, its rapid response rate is noteworthy.[15]

**BOX 2 Severity criteria for drug reaction with eosinophilia and systemic symptoms (DRESS) syndrome.[7]**

- ALT > 5 × URL or ALP ≥ 2 × URL and TB ≥ 2 × URL
- sCr > 2–2.9 times baseline or UO < 0.5 mL/kg/h for >12 hours
- The other organ involvements:
  - Hemophagocytosis
  - Pulmonary system
  - Cardiac system

*Note*: The presence of at least one of the three criteria listed in Box 2 defines a severe case. The remaining cases are classified as nonsevere.

(ALP: alkaline phosphatase; ALT: alanine aminotransferase; sCR: serum creatinine; TB: total bilirubin; UO: urine output; URL: upper reference limit)

**BOX 3 Treatment approach for severe cases.[7]**

*First-line treatment*:
- *Prednisolone*: Administered at a dose of 0.8–1 mg/kg/day for an initial period of 2–3 weeks, followed by a gradual reduction over the course of 4–6 weeks.

*Second-line treatment*: In cases where corticosteroids are contraindicated or ineffective—
- Cyclosporine: 4–5 mg/kg/day for 5–7 days, followed by tapering
- IVIG: 2 g/kg over 5 days
- Plasmapheresis

*In cases of viral reactivation*:
- *Intravenous ganciclovir*: 5 mg/kg administered twice daily for 7 days.
- *Subsequent valganciclovir therapy*: 900 mg orally every 12 hours.

(IVIg: intravenous immunoglobulin)

In addition, interleukin (IL)-5 plays a significant role in eosinophilic pathophysiology and is proposed as a novel therapeutic target for hypereosinophilic conditions.[16] The use of biological agents targeting the IL-5 or IL-5R axis in the treatment of DRESS syndrome is considered a novel option for corticosteroid-dependent or resistant cases.[17] Reslizumab, mepolizumab, and benralizumab are case-based treatment options that have been used and deemed successful.[18-20]

Follow-up of DRESS patients should focus on identifying and managing long-term complications, particularly autoimmune diseases, which can emerge months or even years after the acute phase. Factors like severe liver involvement or atypical lymphocytosis are associated with prolonged recovery times and increased relapse risks. Regular monitoring for these complications is essential, along with patient's education on recognizing late-onset symptoms to facilitate early intervention.[1]

## CONCLUSION

DRESS syndrome is a rare but severe adverse drug reaction with significant systemic effects. Early identification and diagnosis using well-defined criteria, such as the RegiSCAR scoring system, are crucial for prompt intervention. Various management protocols emphasize the importance of drug discontinuation, corticosteroid therapy, and careful monitoring of organ involvement. While systemic corticosteroids remain the cornerstone of treatment, alternative therapeutic options, including IVIG, cyclosporine, and IL-5 inhibitors, may be utilized in refractory cases. Given the risk of relapse and long-term complications, including autoimmune sequelae, extended follow-up is necessary to ensure comprehensive patient management. Ongoing research into the pathogenesis and treatment of DRESS will contribute to the development of optimized management strategies and improved patient outcomes.

## REFERENCES

1. Husain Z, Reddy BY, Schwartz RA. DRESS syndrome: Part I. Clinical perspectives. J Am Acad Dermatol. 2013;68:693.e1-693.e14.
2. Mizukawa Y, Hirahara K, Kano Y, Shiohara T. Drug-induced hypersensitivity syndrome/drug reaction with eosinophilia and systemic symptoms severity score: A useful tool for assessing disease severity and predicting fatal cytomegalovirus disease. J Am Acad Dermatol. 2019;80(3):670-8.e2.
3. Shiohara T, Mizukawa Y. Drug-induced hypersensitivity syndrome (DiHS)/drug reaction with eosinophilia and systemic symptoms (DRESS): An update in 2019. Allergol Int. 2019;68:301-8.
4. Calle AM, Aguirre N, Ardila JC, Cardona Villa R. DRESS syndrome: A literature review and treatment algorithm. World Allergy Organ J. 2023;16(3):100673.
5. Eshki M, Allanore L, Musette P, Milpied B, Grange A, Guillaume JC, et al. Twelve-Year Analysis of Severe Cases of Drug Reaction With Eosinophilia and Systemic Symptoms A Cause of Unpredictable Multiorgan Failure [Internet]. Arch Dermatol. 2009;145(1):67-72.
6. Descamps V, Ranger-Rogez S. DRESS syndrome. Joint Bone Spine. 2014;81(1):15-21.
7. Cabañas R, Ramírez E, Sendagorta E, Alamar R, Barranco R, Blanca-López N, et al. Spanish guidelines for diagnosis, management, treatment, and prevention of dress syndrome. J Investig Allergol Clin Immunol. 2020;30(4):229-53.
8. Rubin L, Talmon A, Ribak Y, Kessler A, Martin Y, Haran TK, et al. Novel targeted inhibition of the IL-5 axis for drug reaction with eosinophilia and systemic symptoms syndrome. Front Immunol. 2023;14:1134178.
9. Barbaud A, Collet E, Milpied B, Assier H, Staumont D, Avenel-Audran M, et al. A multicentre study to determine the value and safety of drug patch tests for the three main classes of severe cutaneous adverse drug reactions. Br J Dermatol. 2013;168(3):555-62.
10. Husain Z, Reddy BY, Schwartz RA. DRESS syndrome: Part II. Management and therapeutics. J Am Acad Dermatol. 2013;68(5):709.e1-9.
11. Galvão VR, Aun MV, Kalil J, Castells M, Giavina-Bianchi P. Clinical and laboratory improvement after intravenous immunoglobulin in drug reaction with eosinophilia and systemic symptoms. J Allergy Clin Immunol: In Practice. 2014;2(1):107-10.
12. Joly P, Janela B, Tetart F, Rogez S, Picard D, D'Incan M, et al. Poor Benefit/Risk Balance of Intravenous Immunoglobulins in DRESS. Arch Dermatol. 2012;148(4):543-4.
13. Joo HL, Park HK, Heo J, Tae OK, Gwang HK, Dae HK, et al. Drug Rash with Eosinophilia and Systemic Symptoms (DRESS) syndrome induced by celecoxib and anti-tuberculosis drugs. J Korean Med Sci. 2008;23(3):521-5.
14. Shaughnessy KK, Bouchard SM, Mohr MR, Herre JM, Salkey KS. Minocycline-induced drug reaction with eosinophilia and systemic symptoms (DRESS) syndrome with persistent myocarditis. J Am Acad Dermatol. 2010;62:315-8.
15. Kirchhof MG, Wong A, Dutz JP. Cyclosporine treatment of drug-induced hypersensitivity syndrome. JAMA Dermatol. 2016;152(11):1254-7.
16. Shamriz O, Hershko AY, Talmon A, Ribak Y, Elazary AS, Horev L, et al. The efficacy of off-label IL-5-modulating treatment in rare eosinophil-mediated diseases. Allergol Int. 2021;70(2):266-8.
17. Gschwend A, Helbling A, Feldmeyer L, Mani-Weber U, Meincke C, Heidemeyer K, et al. Treatment with IL5-/IL-5 receptor antagonists in drug reaction with eosinophilia and systemic symptoms (DRESS). Allergo J Int. 2023;32(4):104-11.
18. Mesli F, Dumont M, Soria A, Groh M, Turpin M, Voiriot G, et al. Benralizumab: A potential tailored treatment for life-threatening DRESS in the COVID-19 era. J Allergy Clin Immunol Pract. 2021;9(9):3529-31.e1.
19. Thein OS, Sutton B, Thickett DR, Parekh D. Mepolizumab rescue therapy for acute pneumonitis secondary to DRESS. BMJ Case Rep. 2019;12(10):e231355.
20. Park H, Choi GS, Lee EM. Successful Treatment of Imatinib-Induced DRESS Syndrome Using Reslizumab without Cessation of Imatinib: A Case Report. Case Rep Oncol. 2021;14(3):1548-54.

CHAPTER 4.6

# Penicillin Desensitization

***Busra Kocali, Umit Murat Sahiner***

## INTRODUCTION

The penicillin allergy label is a common clinical entity, associated with many potential adverse outcomes. Alternative drugs used instead of penicillin may lead to treatment failure and more adverse drug reactions. The use of alternative overly broad-spectrum antibiotics increases the risk of antimicrobial resistance. Patients with penicillin allergy labels more frequently detect multi-drug-resistant organisms such as *Clostridioides difficile*, methicillin-resistant *Staphylococcus aureus*, and vancomycin-resistant *Enterococcus* species. Decreased efficacy and unintended adverse effects of second-line treatments lead to increased healthcare costs **(Flowchart 1)**.[1]

The process of desensitization involves administering a drug at predetermined intervals, starting with doses below the threshold dose to trigger a reaction and gradually increasing the dose until it reaches a therapeutic dose. This alters the response of the immune system and creates a temporary tolerance to the allergic drug. When there is no acceptable alternative treatment, patients with a penicillin allergy label should undergo desensitization to safely take the drug.[2]

In this text, we will first discuss what to consider when deciding to use desensitization, then how to prepare the protocol, and what to do during and after the procedure.

The first step in deciding whether to desensitize a patient is to assess the risk. The classification is made according to the data obtained from the patient's detailed history and allergy evaluation. This is particularly important for penicillin desensitization because most

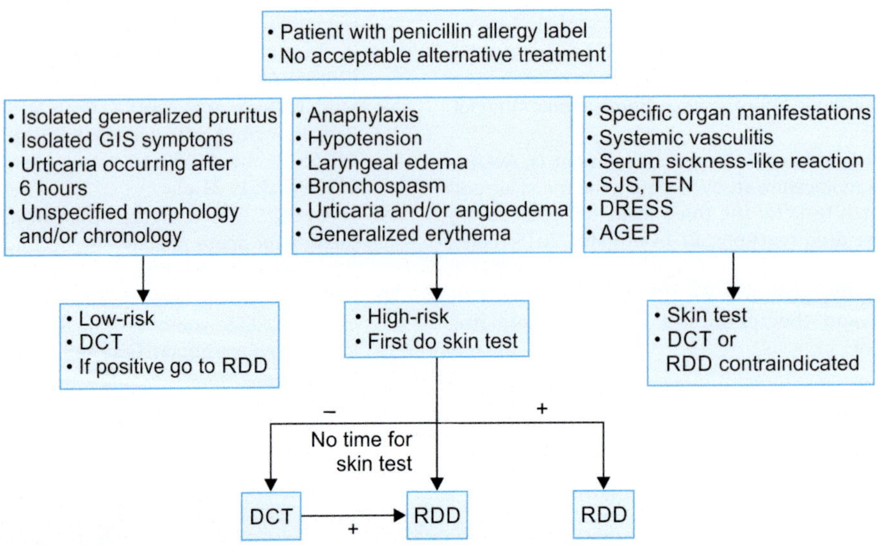


**FLOWCHART 1:** Risk stratification for desensitization in patients with a penicillin allergy label.

(AGEP: acute generalized exanthematous pustulosis; DCT: drug challenge test; DRESS: drug reaction with eosinophilia and systemic symptoms; GIS: gastrointestinal; RDD: rapid drug desensitization; SJS: Stevens–Johnson syndrome; TEN: toxic epidermal necrolysis)

patients with a penicillin allergy label are found not to be genuinely allergic to penicillin. Conditions classified as low risk include isolated generalized pruritus that did not require treatment, isolated gastrointestinal symptoms such as nausea, vomiting, and diarrhea, urticaria that manifested after 6 hours, and mild-to-moderate maculopapular erythema, a condition more common in children. We may classify patients with unclear morphology and/or chronology as low risk once we rule out danger indications. We can conduct drug challenge testing in these patients without the need for skin testing. If there is a history of anaphylaxis, hypotension, laryngeal edema, bronchospasm, urticaria and/or angioedema, and generalized erythema, these patients are considered at high risk of having an immunoglobulin E (IgE)-mediated reaction. We recommend performing skin testing first in these cases. Should the skin test yield a negative result, we can proceed with drug challenge tests. However, if medical urgency prevents testing or there is a history of positive skin and drug challenge tests, we may perform desensitization. Patients with a history of specific organ manifestations (e.g., drug-induced anemia, granulocytopenia, thrombocytopenia, hepatitis, and nephritis), systemic vasculitis, serum sickness-like reaction, Stevens–Johnson syndrome, toxic epidermal necrolysis, drug reaction (or rash) with eosinophilia and systemic symptoms, acute generalized exanthematous pustulosis are considered at high risk. Desensitization is not recommended in these patients as it may induce potentially life-threatening reactions.

## DESENSITIZATION DECISION

Desensitization is indicated when alternative treatments are less effective or adverse reactions are more severe. Syphilis infection during pregnancy or resistant to alternative therapies, listeriosis, the treatment of susceptible and deep-seated staphylococcal or enterococcal infections are examples of indications for penicillin desensitization.[1,3]

The first step is to take a careful history (underlying disease and comorbidities, characteristics of the drug involved, age of the patient), physical examination, and to obtain details of the index reaction. This information, together with an appropriate allergy assessment, may allow the underlying mechanism to be identified and the desensitization strategy to be determined accordingly. A risk assessment should be carried out for each patient. This is particularly important for penicillin desensitization because most patients with a penicillin allergy label are found not to be genuinely allergic to penicillin after appropriate evaluation. This is either due to improper diagnosis or resolution of the previous allergy over time.[2,4,5]

Conditions classified as low-risk include isolated generalized pruritus that did not require treatment, isolated gastrointestinal symptoms such as nausea, vomiting, and diarrhea, urticaria that manifested after 6 hours, and mild-to-moderate maculopapular erythema, a condition more common in children. We may classify patients with unclear morphology and/or chronology as low risk once we rule out danger indications. We can conduct drug challenge testing in these patients without the need for skin testing. Desensitization may be necessary if the drug challenge test results are positive, but this is typically not the case.[6,7]

If there is a history of anaphylaxis, hypotension, laryngeal edema, bronchospasm, urticaria, and/or angioedema, generalized erythema, these patients are considered at high risk of having an IgE-mediated reaction. We recommend performing skin testing first in these cases. Should the skin test yield a negative result, we can proceed with drug challenge tests; however, if medical urgency prevents testing or there is a history of positive skin and drug challenge tests, we may perform desensitization.[6,7]

Patients with a history of specific organ manifestations (e.g., drug-induced anemia, granulocytopenia, thrombocytopenia, hepatitis, and nephritis), systemic vasculitis, serum sickness-like reaction, Stevens–Johnson syndrome, toxic epidermal necrolysis, drug reaction (or rash) with eosinophilia and systemic symptoms, acute generalized exanthematous pustulosis are considered at high risk. Desensitization is not recommended in these patients as it may induce potentially life-threatening reactions.[6-9]

Furthermore, patient characteristics are essential for risk assessment. Subjects with severe cardiovascular, renal, and/or respiratory compromise or those on beta-blocker therapy should be regarded as at high risk regardless of index reactions. Pregnant women and those with systemic mastocytosis are also considered at high risk.[6]

There is always a risk of developing a hypersensitivity reaction during desensitization. The decision to desensitize should be made by an experienced allergist in agreement with the patient's primary care physician, following a risk-benefit assessment. The risks and benefits of the procedure must be discussed in detail with the patient and/or caregivers, and a joint decision must be made.[8]

## DESENSITIZATION PROTOCOL PREPARATION

Desensitization is not a one-size-fits-all method. It must be tailored to the needs of the individual patient. Drug characteristics are also important, including route of administration, total intended dose, maximum infusion rate, drug concentration, and half-life.[4]

Premedication before desensitization should also be individualized. Medications are chosen according to each patient's history of hypersensitivity. For example, if the patient has a history of hives/angioedema, an H1 blocker might be given; if bronchospasm has occurred, montelukast and/or inhaled albuterol might be given.[4,10]

Desensitization is usually carried out as a 12-step protocol using three preparations with progressive concentrations, usually named bags A to C. Bag A containing a 1/1,000 to 1/100 dilution of the drug is used to administer the starting dose (step 1), which may range from 1/1,000,000 to 1/100 of the target dose. The starting dose should be determined according to the severity of the index reaction. Progressively doubling doses of the drug are administered over 15-minute periods, until the full cumulative therapeutic dose has been delivered.[4,8,10] **Tables 1 and 2** show examples of oral and intravenous desensitization protocols, respectively.[7]

**TABLE 1: Oral penicillin desensitization protocol.**

| Step | Penicillin dilution (mg/mL) | Time (minutes) | Volume administered (mL) | Penicillin dose (mg) | Penicillin dose units | Cumulative dose (mg) | Cumulative dose units |
|---|---|---|---|---|---|---|---|
| 1 | 0.5 | 15 | 0.1 | 0.05 | 80 | 0.05 | 80 |
| 2 | 0.5 | 15 | 0.2 | 0.1 | 160 | 0.15 | 240 |
| 3 | 0.5 | 15 | 0.4 | 0.2 | 320 | 0.35 | 560 |
| 4 | 0.5 | 15 | 0.8 | 0.4 | 640 | 0.75 | 1,200 |
| 5 | 0.5 | 15 | 1.6 | 0.8 | 1,280 | 1.55 | 2,480 |
| 6 | 0.5 | 15 | 3.2 | 1.6 | 2,560 | 3.15 | 5,040 |
| 7 | 0.5 | 15 | 6.4 | 3.2 | 5,120 | 6.35 | 10,160 |
| 8 | 5 | 15 | 1.2 | 6.0 | 9,600 | 12.35 | 19,760 |
| 9 | 5 | 15 | 2.4 | 12.0 | 19,200 | 24.35 | 38,960 |
| 10 | 5 | 15 | 4.8 | 24.0 | 38,400 | 48.35 | 77,360 |
| 11 | 50 | 15 | 1.0 | 50.0 | 80,000 | 98.35 | 157,360 |
| 12 | 50 | 15 | 2.0 | 100.0 | 160,000 | 198.35 | 317,360 |
| 13 | 50 | 15 | 4.0 | 200.0 | 320,000 | 398.35 | 637,360 |
| 14 | 50 | 15 | 8.0 | 400.0 | 640,000 | 798.35 | 1,277,360 |

*Source*: Castells M, Khan DA, Phillips EJ. Penicillin Allergy. N Engl J Med. 2019;381(24):2338-51.

**TABLE 2: 12-step intravenous penicillin desensitization protocol.**

| Three-bag, 12-step Intravenous Penicillin Desensitization Protocol | | | | | | |
|---|---|---|---|---|---|---|
| **Step** | **Bag** | **Rate (mL/h)** | **Time (minutes)** | **Volume infused (mL)** | **Dose administered units** | **Cumulative dose units** |
| 1 | 1 | 2.0 | 15 | 0.50 | 200 | 200 |
| 2 | 1 | 5.0 | 15 | 1.25 | 500 | 700 |
| 3 | 1 | 10.0 | 15 | 2.50 | 1,000 | 1,700 |
| 4 | 1 | 20.0 | 15 | 5.00 | 2,000 | 3,700 |
| 5 | 2 | 5.0 | 15 | 1.25 | 5,000 | 8,700 |
| 6 | 2 | 10.0 | 15 | 2.50 | 10,000 | 18,700 |
| 7 | 2 | 20.0 | 15 | 5.00 | 20,000 | 38,700 |
| 8 | 2 | 40.0 | 15 | 10.00 | 40,000 | 78,700 |
| 9 | 3 | 10.0 | 15 | 2.50 | 98,032.5 | 176,732.5 |
| 10 | 3 | 20.0 | 15 | 5.00 | 196,065 | 372,797.5 |
| 11 | 3 | 40.0 | 15 | 10.00 | 392,130 | 764,927.5 |
| 12 | 3 | 80.0 | 15 | 82.50 | 3,235,072.5 | 4,000,000 |

*Source*: Castells M, Khan DA, Phillips EJ. Penicillin Allergy. N Engl J Med. 2019;381(24):2338-351.

This protocol can be used with all oral penicillins. Up to 20% of patients may experience mild breakthrough reactions. About > 99% of patients receive the target dose. This includes those with initial anaphylactic reactions. Furthermore, anaphylaxis occurs in <1% of patients.

The frequency of breakthrough reactions is similar to the oral penicillin desensitization protocol. Up to 20% of patients may experience mild breakthrough reactions. About > 99% of patients receive the target dose. This includes those with initial anaphylactic reactions. Furthermore, anaphylaxis occurs in <1% of patients.

In patients with severe reactions, it is advisable to modify the protocol by decreasing the initial dose, decreasing the infusion rate, increasing the interval between doses, and/or increasing the number of steps up to 16. The number of steps, the dose at each step, and the time to complete the entire procedure should be determined according to a mandatory risk assessment.[4,10]

## PERFORMING DESENSITIZATION

Before starting the desensitization procedure, it is important to obtain signed informed consent from the patient and/or caregivers. An allergist must be involved in all steps of the process, including monitoring the drug preparations, checking the stability of the solutions, and confirming the total therapeutic dose. It is important to ensure that emergency medicines (e.g., antihistamines, corticosteroids, adrenaline, bronchodilators, with calculated doses) and resuscitation equipment are readily accessible.[4,8]

Most drug desensitization protocols can be performed outside the intensive care unit (ICU). The most critical aspects of the procedure are the administration of drugs according to the desensitization protocol, continuous telemetry monitoring, and 1:1 nursing care. The nurse should be trained and experienced in desensitization and be able to recognize hypersensitivity reactions if they occur. If the patient has a history of a severe reaction, the initial desensitization can be administered in the ICU, but if this is uneventful, subsequent courses do not need to be administered in the ICU. Vital signs should be recorded at the beginning of desensitization and reassessed every 15 minutes during the procedure before proceeding to the next step.[8,10]

At any stage of desensitization, or even at multiple stages, a breakthrough reaction can occur. The most common time for a breakthrough reaction to occur is during the final step. If a reaction is observed, healthcare professionals should stop the infusion immediately and then check vital signs and assess the patient for signs and symptoms of anaphylaxis. If the patient is not in anaphylaxis and vital signs are normal, treatment will be given as appropriate for the developing symptom. If the patient's symptoms resolve, the infusion is continued. If the patient is having anaphylaxis, anaphylaxis treatment will be given according to current guidelines. After the targeted cumulative dose is administered, the patient continues to be observed for 1–2 hours.[4,8,10]

Desensitization provides a temporary tolerance, and its effect is over after approximately three to four half-lives of the medication. If the drug is to be given again at a longer interval than this, desensitization should be repeated.[7,9,10]

## CONCLUSION

Drug desensitization is a clinical procedure that allows the safe administration of a drug to patients who have had a hypersensitivity reaction to the drug in the past. It is an individually tailored procedure to make use of first-line treatments. The use of first-line therapy results in higher efficacy, fewer side effects, and improved quality of life. In addition, desensitization is cost-effective when compared with second-line treatment.[8]

## REFERENCES

1. Stone CA Jr, Trubiano J, Coleman DT, Rukasin CRF, Phillips EJ. The challenge of de-labeling penicillin allergy. Allergy. 2020;75(2):273-88.
2. Solensky R, Phillips EJ. Drug allergy. In: Burks AW, Holgate ST, O'Hehir R, Broide DH, Bacharier LB, Hershey GKK (Eds). Allergy: Principles and Practice, 9th edition. Amsterdam: Elsevier; 2020. pp. 1261-82.
3. Pham MN, Ho HE, Desai M. Penicillin desensitization: Treatment of syphilis in pregnancy in penicillin-allergic patients. Ann Allergy Asthma Immunol. 2017;118(5):537-41.
4. Cernadas J, Vasconcelos MJ, Carneiro-Leão L. Desensitization in children allergic to drugs: Indications, protocols, and limits. Pediatr Allergy Immunol. 2023;34(6):e13965.
5. Shenoy ES, Macy E, Rowe T, Blumenthal KG. Evaluation and Management of Penicillin Allergy: A Review. JAMA. 2019;321(2):188-99.
6. Romano A, Atanaskovic-Markovic M, Barbaud A, Bircher AJ, Brockow K, Caubet JC, et al. Towards a more precise diagnosis of hypersensitivity to beta-lactams—an EAACI position paper. Allergy. 2020;75(6):1300-15.
7. Castells M, Khan DA, Phillips EJ. Penicillin allergy. N Engl J Med. 2019;381(24):2338-51.
8. Alvarez-Cuesta E, Madrigal-Burgaleta R, Broyles AD, Cuesta-Herranz J, Guzman-Melendez MA, Maciag MC, et al. Standards for practical intravenous rapid drug desensitization & delabeling: A WAO committee statement. World Allergy Organ J. 2022;15(6):100640.
9. Minaldi E, Phillips EJ, Norton A. Immediate and Delayed Hypersensitivity Reactions to Beta-Lactam Antibiotics. Clin Rev Allergy Immunol. 2022;62(3):449-62.
10. Yang BC, Castells MC. The Who, What, Where, When, Why, and How of Drug Desensitization. Immunol Allergy Clin North Am. 2022;42(2):403-20.

# 4.7

CHAPTER

# Intradermal Tests and Skin Prick Tests in Drug Allergy

*Aleksandra Wardzyńska, Anna Zalewska-Janowska*

## INTRODUCTION

Skin tests are a simple, inexpensive, and relatively safe method used in allergy diagnosis. Skin prick tests (SPTs) and intradermal tests (IDTs) are frequently used in the diagnosis of immediate drug hypersensitivity reactions. It should be mentioned that IDTs with delayed reading can be useful in such drug reactions as maculopapular exanthema (MPE), acute generalized exanthematous pustulosis (AGEP) or drug rash with eosinophilia and systemic symptoms (DRESS).[1] Skin tests are a valuable step in the diagnosis of drug hypersensitivity, and in many cases allow avoidance of high-risk procedures such as drug provocation or desensitization. Their educational value is significant, as when they are performed, the patient has a direct opportunity to see whether a particular drug/substance causes a reaction, which facilitates subsequent compliance with medical recommendations.

## UTILITY OF SKIN PRICK TESTS AND INTRADERMAL TESTS WITH IMMEDIATE READING

The use of SPTs and IDTs with immediate reading is only justified in situations where the clinical picture of the reaction indicates an immunoglobulin E (IgE)-dependent mechanism. This includes reactions occurring up to 6 hours after exposure to the drug/substance, which can consist of skin symptoms such as pruritus, urticaria, angioedema, or symptoms from other organs most often from the respiratory, circulatory or gastrointestinal systems, sometimes in the form of a systemic reaction or anaphylaxis.[2] In practice, most reactions of this type occur after exposure to β-lactam antibiotics. Less frequently other drugs and chemicals among them nonsteroid anti-inflammatory drugs (NSAIDs) including metamizole and propionic acid derivatives, iodine contrast agents, general anesthetics, drugs used in cancer therapy, such as platinum derivatives are involved.

The specificity and sensitivity of SPTs/IDTs for most drugs is unknown, one of the few exceptions being β-lactam antibiotics. In the latter case, the tests have low specificity but high sensitivity.[3] The lack of knowledge about the predictive value of skin tests in the diagnosis of hypersensitivity to other drugs may be related to various factors (the use of ready-made drug than metabolites, different methodologies for performing tests, or, finally, the lack of research on the subject). Taking into consideration the above, it should be emphasized that skin tests are only a step in the diagnosis of drug hypersensitivity. Drug provocation has remained the gold standard for either hypersensitivity definitive confirmation or exclusion.[4] The diagnostic regimen for immediate drug hypersensitivity is presented in **Flowchart 1**. In general, SPTs are the first step of this diagnostic algorithm. In case SPTs give negative

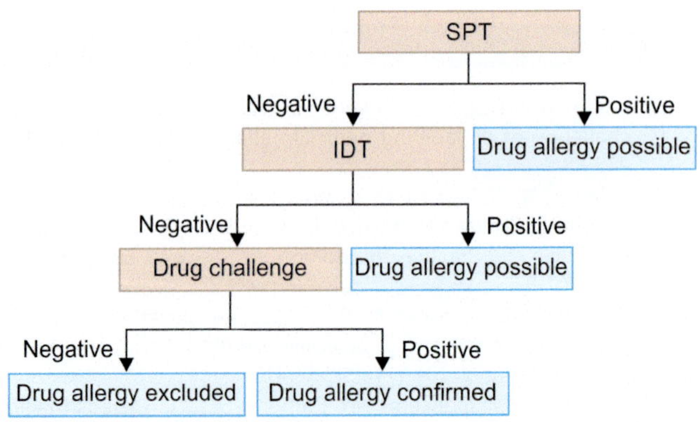


**FLOWCHART 1:** Skin prick tests and intradermal tests in the diagnosis of immediate drug-induced hypersensitivity reactions.

(IDT: intradermal tests; SPT: skin prick tests)

results, IDTs (usually with successive dilutions of the drug) are followed. Then, if IDTs results are also negative, drug provocation should be considered in order to obtain a definitive diagnosis. Of importance, in clinical practice, due to risk of occurrence of symptoms of similar or even greater severity to primary reaction, drug provocations are very rarely performed after a positive skin test result.

## INDICATIONS AND CONTRAINDICATIONS FOR SKIN PRICK TESTS AND INTRADERMAL TESTS IN THE DIAGNOSIS OF IMMEDIATE DRUG HYPERSENSITIVITY

Indications for performing SPTs and IDTs include confirmation or exclusion of drug/substance involvement in the initiation of the hypersensitivity reaction. Another indication for skin testing is the search for an alternative drug.

Increasingly, attention is being paid to the need for risk assessment before proceeding with drug hypersensitivity diagnosis.[5] This concept is complex, translating into the probability of reaction during the in vivo diagnostic procedure and determining the choice of strategy (de-labeling based on history, direct provocation test, provocation test preceded by skin tests, or desensitization when urgent drug administration is required). The risk depends primarily on the likelihood of whether the drug was the primary culprit of the reaction, in addition to the mechanism and phenotype of hypersensitivity, and may also be due to individual patient's characteristics (presence and severity of comorbidities, pregnancy, etc.). It should be noted that in the case of immediate reactions, anaphylaxis is not an absolute contraindication to SPTs/IDTs with the drug/substance, it only qualifies a patient to a high-risk group.[6] The relative contraindications to skin testing include unstable condition of the patient, active inflammation, skin lesions at the site of potential test application, treatment with β-blockers, pregnancy, current use of medications that prevent interpretation of the test. It should be noted that there is no clear-cut regimen for the list of drugs and the timing of their discontinuation. Among the drugs that reduce skin reactivity are antihistamines, topical glucocorticosteroids (GCSs), immunosuppressants and some psychotropic drugs, as well as ultraviolet (UV) radiation **(Table 1)**.

## TIMING OF SKIN TESTS PERFORMANCE IN DIAGNOSIS OF IMMEDIATE DRUG HYPERSENSITIVITY REACTIONS

It is generally believed that SPTs and IDTs should be performed optimally 4 weeks after hypersensitivity symptoms resolution but before 1 year after reaction to a given drug,[1,6] This is due to the well-documented phenomenon of sIgE disappearance with the time elapsed after the reaction, which has been best described for β-lactam antibiotics.[7]

**TABLE 1: Timing of drug withdrawal before skin and intradermal tests in the diagnosis of drug hypersensitivity.**

| Drug | Drug withdrawal |
|---|---|
| Antihistamines | 4 days (7 days for loratadine or desloratadine) |
| Topical corticosteroids (on the skin test site) | 7 days |
| Systemic corticosteroids | 1 month |
| Immunosuppressive drugs | 1 month |
| Phenothiazines | Up to 10 days |
| Imipramine | Up to 21 days |
| Ultraviolet (UV) exposure | Up to 4 weeks |

*Source*: Based on Barbaud A et al. (2022).[1]

## TECHNIQUE FOR PERFORMING SKIN TESTS IN DIAGNOSIS OF IMMEDIATE DRUG HYPERSENSITIVITY REACTIONS

Skin prick tests can be performed with any form of drug/substance. This includes intravenous drug, powdered tablet, ointment, and other drug forms. Usually tests are performed with undiluted drug, however, in justified cases, like in high-risk patients, it is recommended to perform the test with a diluted one, such as 1:10. In some cases, the highest nonirritating concentrations of a substance are known.[6]

Intradermal tests are performed only with parenteral forms of drugs, with successive dilutions, usually 1:100 and, in β-lactams, 1:1,000. In high-risk patients, these tests can be started with even lower concentrations. If there is no response, IDTs are stopped at the highest nonirritating concentration of the drug **(Table 2)**.

The technique for performing SPTs is generally known. In brief, SPTs are performed on the volar surface of the forearm, a drop/small amount of the substance is applied and then the skin is punctured with a 1-mm thick lancet to introduce the test substance into the deeper regions of the epidermis. The positive control is histamine at the concentration of 10 mg/mL, and the negative control can be saline. The technique of performing IDTs varies, and attention is drawn to the considerable variability in their performance between different centers. The recently recommended scheme

**TABLE 2: Maximum and nonirritant concentrations for drug prick tests and intradermal tests.**

| Drug type | Maximum SPT concentration | Maximum IDT concentration |
|---|---|---|
| *Antibiotics* | | |
| Amoxicillin, ampicillin, and other semisynthetic penicillins | – | 20 mg/mL |
| Benzylpenicillin | – | 10,000 IU/mL |
| Cephalosporins except cefepime | – | 20 mg/mL |
| Ciprofloxacin | – | 0.006 mg/mL |
| Levofloxacin | – | 0.025 mg/mL |
| Azithromycin | – | 0.01 mg/mL |
| Clarithromycin | – | 0.05 mg/mL |
| Clindamycin | – | 15 mg/mL |
| Cotrimoxazole | – | 0.8 mg/mL |
| *Drugs used in general anesthesia* | | |
| Atracurium | 1 mg/mL | 0.01 mg/mL |
| Rocuronium | 10 mg/mL | 0.05 mg/mL |
| Suxamethonium | 10 mg/mL | 0.1 mg/mL |
| Etomidate | 2 mg/mL | 0.2 mg/mL |
| Ketamine | 100 mg/mL | 0.1 mg/mL |
| Midazolam | 5 mg/mL | 0.05 mg/mL |
| Propofol | 10 mg/mL | 1 mg/mL |
| Thiopental | 25 mg/mL | 2.5 mg/mL |
| Sugammadex | – | 10 mg/mL |
| *Local anesthetics* | | |
| Articaine | – | 2 mg/mL |
| Lidocaine | – | 1 mg/mL |
| Mepivacaine | – | 2 mg/mL |
| *Other drugs* | | |
| Platinum salts | – | 1 mg/mL |
| Heparins | – | 1:10 of the usage concentration |
| Insulins | – | 1:10 of the usage concentration |
| Diclofenac | – | 2.5 mg/mL |
| Ketoprofen | – | 2 mg/mL |
| Pyrazolones | – | 0.1 mg/mL |
| Iodinated contrast media | – | 1/10th of the usage concentration |
| Gadolinium derivatives | – | 1/10th of the usage concentration |
| Proton pump inhibitors | – | 0.4 or 4 mg/mL |

(IDT: intradermal tests; SPT: skin prick tests)

*Source*: Based on Barbaud A et al. (2022).[1]

involves performing IDTs using a tuberculin syringe with a very thin needle. The test substance is drawn into the syringe, and the excess is removed to obtain only 0.02 mL of the solution. The needle is then inserted intradermally, and the injected volume allows for a 3- to 5-mm diameter wheal, which should be measured immediately after the test substance is introduced (called initial wheal, Wi). When IDTs are preceded by SPTs (and this is usually the case), the histamine test can be waived (positive control), however, test with solvent should be performed (negative control).[1]

## INTERPRETATION OF SKIN PRICK TESTS AND INTRADERMAL TESTS WITH IMMEDIATE READING

The SPTs and IDTs are read after 20 minutes. In the case of SPTs, a positive result is evidenced by a wheal ≥ 3 mm in diameter from the negative control's wheal. The wheal must be surrounded by erythema. For intradermal testing, a positive result is evidenced by a wheal diameter measured after 20 minutes (W20), which must be ≥3 mm than the initial wheal (Wi). The wheal must be surrounded by erythema, which should be also measured.[1]

## SAFETY OF PERFORMING SKIN PRICK TESTS AND INTRADERMAL TESTS WITH DRUGS

Skin tests are believed to be a relatively safe procedure, although there are few studies on the subject. In a prospective study involving more than 30,000 SPTs with inhaled allergens, foods, venoms, and drugs, the rate of systemic reactions was 0.08%, most of which were related to food allergens, but one severe case of anaphylaxis was related to the SPT with a drug (piperacillin/tazobactam).[8] A study that included 1,073 children with suspected drug hypersensitivity found only four reactions with suspected immune mechanism occurring after SPTs or IDTs with drugs.[9] Skin tests in low-risk patients can be performed in an outpatient allergy clinic equipped with the necessary tools to treat immediate reactions including anaphylaxis. In patients whose risks have been assessed as high, it is recommended to perform the procedure in an allergology department with access to an intensive care unit. It is recommended to obtain informed consent from the patient before performing drug skin tests. After testing, the patient should be observed, although the length of observation time varies among authors (20-60 min).[6,10] In any case, procedure should be done by properly trained medical team with the knowledge and experience to assist not only in the technical performance of the tests, but also in assessing symptoms indicative of hypersensitivity and being able to respond to them appropriately.[10]

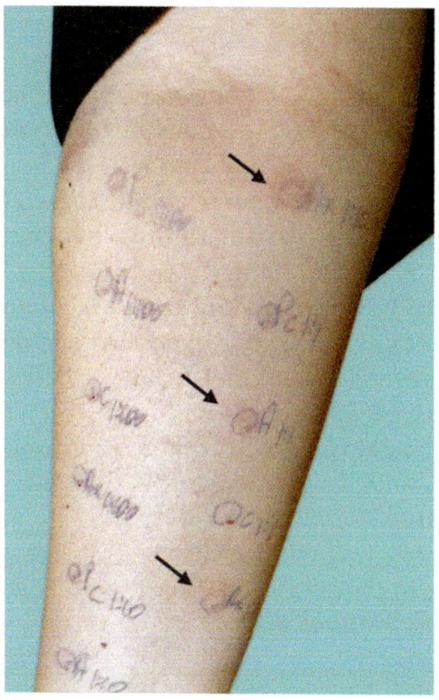

**FIG. 1:** Results of intradermal tests with a delayed reading in a 24-year-old female patient with a history of maculopapular exanthema to amoxicillin. The photo shows redness and swelling at the site of application of amoxicillin (1:10 and 1:1) and ampicillin (1:1) at 12 hours after application of the tests.

## UTILITY OF SKIN PRICK TESTS AND INTRADERMAL TESTS IN THE DIAGNOSIS OF DELAYED HYPERSENSITIVITY

In recent years, the phenomenon of reactions occurring after several hours at the site of drug insertion when performing SPTs/IDTs in patients with delayed forms of drug hypersensitivity has begun to attract attention.[1] While the diagnostic significance of SPTs for delayed reactions is undetermined, delayed-read IDTs are being used more widely. The technique for performing these tests is the same as immediate-read IDTs, however, they are evaluated at least after approximately 24 hours. A positive result is indicated by any infiltration/swelling at the site of allergen introduction **(Fig. 1)**. As already mentioned in the introductory paragraph, IDTs with delayed reading have applications in the diagnosis of such drug reactions as MPE, DRESS, and AGEP.

## CONCLUSION

Skin prick tests and intradermal tests are useful tools in the diagnosis of drug hypersensitivity. They allow determination of drug tolerance status in a relatively simple, inexpensive and safe manner. However, there is a need for further research in this area to standardize the methods of performing and interpreting these tests.

## REFERENCES

1. Barbaud A, Castagna J, Soria A. Skin tests in the work-up of cutaneous adverse drug reactions: A review and update. Contact Dermatitis. 2022;86(5):344-56.
2. Mayorga C, Ariza A, Muñoz-Cano R, Sabato V, Doña I, Torres MJ. Biomarkers of immediate drug hypersensitivity. Allergy. 2024;79(3):601-12.
3. Sousa-Pinto B, Tarrio I, Blumenthal KG, Araújo L, Azevedo LF, Delgado L, et al. Accuracy of penicillin allergy diagnostic tests: A systematic review and meta-analysis. J Allergy Clin Immunol. 2021;147(1):296-308.
4. Demoly P, Adkinson NF, Brockow K, Castells M, Chiriac AM, Greenberger PA, et al. International Consensus on drug allergy. Allergy. 2014;69(4):420-37.
5. Copaescu AM, Li L, Blumenthal KG, Trubiano JA. How to Define and Manage Low-risk Drug Allergy Labels. J Allergy Clin Immunol Pract. 2024;12(5):1095-106.
6. Barbaud A, Garvey LH, Torres M, Laguna JJ, Arcolaci A, Bonadonna P, et al. EAACI/ENDA position paper on drug provocation testing. Allergy. 2024;79(3):565-79.
7. Shenoy ES, Macy E, Rowe T, Blumenthal KG. Evaluation and Management of Penicillin Allergy: A Review. JAMA. 2019;321(2):188-99.
8. Sellaturay P, Nasser S, Ewan P. The incidence and features of systemic reactions to skin prick tests. Ann Allergy Asthma Immunol. 2015;115(3):229-33.
9. Karavaizoglu C, Suleyman A, Yavuz Alic R, Dolu KO, Yucel E, Demirkale ZH, et al. Drug Allergy in Children: Adverse Reactions after Skin Testing. Int Arch Allergy Immunol. 2024;185(1):56-62.
10. Kowalski ML, Ansotegui I, Aberer W, Al-Ahmad M, Akdis M, Ballmer-Weber BK, et al. Risk and safety requirements for diagnostic and therapeutic procedures in allergology: World Allergy Organization Statement. World Allergy Organ J. 2016;9(1):33.

# INDEX

Page numbers followed by *b* refer to box, *f* refer to figure, *fc* refer to flowchart, and *t* refer to table.

## A

## B



## C

## F



## G



## H



## I

## J



## K



## L



## M

## Q



## R



## S